Physics in
Nuclear Medicine

Second Edition

Physics in
Nuclear Medicine
Second Edition

James A. Sorenson, Ph.D.
Director, Medical Physics
Professor of Radiology
Department of Radiology
University of Utah Medical Center
Salt Lake City, Utah

Michael E. Phelps, Ph.D.
Jennifer Jones Simon Professor
Chief, Division of Nuclear Medicine
and Biophysics
Department of Radiological Sciences
UCLA School of Medicine
Chief, Laboratory of Nuclear Medicine
Laboratory of Biomedical and
Environmental Sciences, UCLA
Los Angeles, California

W.B. SAUNDERS COMPANY
A Division of Harcourt Brace & Company
Philadelphia   London   Toronto   Montreal   Sydney   Tokyo

W. B. SAUNDERS COMPANY
A Division of
Harcourt Brace & Company

The Curtis Center
Independence Square West
Philadelphia, PA 19106

Library of Congress Cataloging-in-Publication Data

Sorenson, James A., 1938-
  Physics in nuclear medicine.

  Includes bibliographies and index.
  1. Nuclear medicine. 2. Radioisotopes in medical
diagnosis. 3. Nuclear medicine—Instruments.
4. Medical physics. I. Phelps, Michael E. II. Title.
[DNLM: 1. Nuclear Medicine. 2. Physics. WN110 S713p]
R895.S58 1987   616.07′57   86-19597
ISBN 0-8089-1804-4

Library of Congress Catalog Number 86-19597
International Standard Book Number 0-8089-1804-4
Printed in the United States of America
              10 9 8 7 6

Contents

Chapter 3   DECAY OF RADIOACTIVITY   38

Chapter 4   RADIATION DETECTORS

**Chapter 7   PRODUCTION OF
                   RADIONUCLIDES   143**

**Chapter 8   PASSAGE OF CHARGED PARTICLES
                   THROUGH MATTER   161**

Preface

Physics and instrumentation impact all of the subspecialty areas of nuclear medicine. Because of their fundamental importance, they usually are taught as a separate course in nuclear medicine training programs. The authors have taught such courses to physicians, technologists, and scientists for a number of years. In our experience there is a need for an introductory text covering the physics and instrumentation of nuclear medicine in sufficient depth to be of permanent value to the trainee or student, but not at such depth as to be of interest only to the physics or instrumentation specialists.

This textbook was prepared with the hope of meeting this need. The goals of the second edition remain the same as they were for the first edition, with a number of important additions to keep pace with the evolving technology and applications of nuclear medicine. The book is designed to be used in training programs for physicians, technologists, and other scientists who desire to become specialists in nuclear medicine. We have assumed that the student or trainee will have had introductory courses in basic physics and mathematics, including an introduction to basic algebra. Knowledge of calculus is not required, although a few examples employing the methods of calculus are presented for the interest of those having a knowledge of this subject.

Nuclear medicine physics and instrumentation are complex subjects, especially when presented to students or trainees who are not specialists in these areas. Therefore, we have at all times tried to make our presentations as clear and understandable as possible. On the other hand, we also have attempted to be thorough and accurate in our discussions of important basic principles, believing this approach to be of more permanent value than a superficial or oversimplified one designed to make these complex topics more "palatable" to the student or trainee.

The organization of this text proceeds from basic principles to more practical aspects. We begin with a review of atomic and nuclear physics (Chapter 1) and basic principles of radioactivity and radioactive decay (Chapters 2 and 3). Basic principles of radiation detectors (Chapter 4), radiation counting electronics (Chapter 5), and statistics (Chapter 6) are treated next. The treatment of statistics has been expanded in the second edition to include basic statistical tests as well as nuclear counting statistics. The topics of the first six chapters appear early in the text to permit the introduction of laboratory exercises involving simple nuclear counting experiments in those training programs incorporating laboratory sections.

Radionuclide production methods are discussed in Chapter 7, followed by radiation interactions in Chapters 8 and 9. Radiation dosimetry, which is closely related to radiation interactions, is treated in Chapter 10.

Pulse-height spectrometry, which plays an important role in many nuclear medicine procedures is described in Chapter 11, followed by general problems in nuclear radiation counting in Chapter 12. The next two chapters are devoted to specific types of nuclear radiation counting instruments, for both in vivo and in vitro measurements. Chapter 13 deals exclusively with systems incorporating NaI(Tl) detectors, and Chapter 14 with systems employing other types of detectors: chiefly, semiconductor, liquid scintillation, and gas filled.

Chapters 15 through 21 discuss topics in radionuclide imaging, beginning with a description of the principles and performance characteristics of the Anger camera (Chapters 15 and 16), then other imaging instruments and techniques (rectilinear scanners, and multicrystal scanners and cameras) (Chapter 17), and general problems in radionuclide imaging (Chapter 18). The purpose of this last chapter is to tie together and relate the many interacting factors affecting the quality of radionuclide images obtained with virtually any radionuclide imaging instrument. There follow two new chapters for the second edition, covering the principles of nuclear medicine tomography (Chapter 19), and tomographic instruments (Chapter 20). An introduction to digital image processing (Chapter 21) completes the section on imaging. Our discussion of imaging instruments is limited to those which now enjoy or appear to have the potential for achieving clinical acceptance. Instruments that seem to be of research interest only are not described.

We then include a chapter introducing the concepts and some applications of tracer kinetic modeling (Chapter 22). Tracer kinetic modeling and its applications embody two of the most important strengths of nuclear medicine techniques: the ability to perform studies with minute (tracer) quantities of labeled substances, and the ability to extract quantitative physiologic data from these studies. We feel that tracer kinetic modeling will become an increasingly important topic in the future of nuclear medicine and include this chapter for that reason.

The text concludes with an introduction to the problems of radiation safety and health physics (Chapter 23). We did not deal with more general problems in radiation biology, believing this topic of sufficient importance to warrant its own special treatment, as has been done already in several excellent books on the subject.

Additional reading for more detailed information is suggested at the end of each chapter. We also have included sample problems with solutions to illustrate certain quantitative relationships and to demonstrate standard calculations that are required in the practice of nuclear medicine. Metric units are used throughout the text. SI units (Systeme Internationale) are introduced and also are employed along with conventional units in some of the sample problems to familiarize the student with them. Because they do not yet enjoy widespread popularity, however, they are not used as the standard for this text.

As is usually the case, the authors received much valuable assistance in preparing this textbook. We continue to be indebted to Drs. Gerry Hine and Bill Hendee, who reviewed several of the chapters and offered many constructive criticisms and suggestions in the preparation of the first edition. Drs. Dev Chakraborty and Wes Wooten provided helpful suggestions that have been included in the second edition. Dr. Randy Hawkins provided valuable assistance in the preparation of several new chapters (19–22) for the second edition. Artwork and photographic materials were skillfully prepared by Mr. Julian Maack, director of the University of Utah Medical Illustrations Service, and by Mrs. Lee Griswold at UCLA. We are indebted to Mrs. Lucy Sorenson, Mrs. Vicky Allen, Mrs. Maureen Kinney, and Ms. Magdalena Marquez for their secretarial assistance in preparation of the manuscript for the second edition. Finally, we express our gratitude to the staff of Grune & Stratton, Inc., who encouraged us to prepare this textbook and its second edition, and then patiently waited through the usual delays and extended deadlines until the project was finally completed.

1

Basic Atomic and Nuclear Physics

Radioactivity is a process involving events in individual atoms and nuclei. Before discussing radioactivity, therefore, it is worthwhile to review some of the basic concepts of atomic and nuclear physics.

A. QUANTITIES AND UNITS

1. Types of Quantities and Units

Physical properties and processes are described in terms of *quantities* such as time and energy. These quantities are measured in *units* such as seconds and joules. Thus, a quantity describes *what* is measured whereas a unit describes *how much*.

Physical quantities are characterized as fundamental or derived. A *fundamental* quantity is one that "stands alone", i.e., no reference is made to other quantities for its definition. Usually, fundamental quantities and their units are defined with reference to standards kept at national or international laboratories. Time, distance and mass are examples of fundamental quantities. *Derived* quantities are defined in terms of combinations of fundamental quantities. Energy (kg m^2/sec^2) is an example of a derived quantity.

The international scientific community has agreed to adopt so-called SI (Systeme International) units as the standard for scientific communication. This system is based on the use of fundamental quantities of mass, length, time, and electrical current in metric units, with all other quantities and units derived by appropriate definition from them. The use of specially defined quantities (e.g., "atmospheres" of barometric pressure) is specifically discouraged. It is hoped that this will improve scientific communication, as well as eliminate some of the more irrational units (e.g., feet and pounds). Table 1-1 lists some fundamental and derived SI quantities and units.

In most cases in this text we use SI units or their metric subunits (e.g., centimeters, grams, etc.); however, in some cases we use traditional or other non-SI units. In some instances this is done because the traditional units continue to be the more commonly used in the day-to-day practice of nuclear medicine, e.g., units of activity and absorbed dose. Because the nuclear medicine community currently is in a "transition period" between traditional and SI units for these quantities, we will indicate SI units in parentheses in selected examples. We also provide nomograms in Appendix F for conversions between these traditional and SI units. In other instances, SI units are unreasonably large (or small) for describing the processes of interest and specially defined units are more convenient. This is particularly true for units of mass and energy, as discussed below.

2. Mass and Energy Units

Events occurring at the atomic level, such as radioactive decay, involve amounts of mass and energy that are very small when described in SI or other conventional units. Therefore, they often are described in terms of specially defined units that are more convenient for the atomic scale.

The basic unit of mass is the *universal mass unit,* abbreviated u. One u is defined as being equal to exactly $1/12$ the mass of a ^{12}C atom.† A slightly different unit, commonly used in chemistry, is the *atomic mass unit* (amu), based on the average weight of oxygen isotopes in their natural abundance. In this text, except where indicated, masses will be expressed in universal mass units, u.

The basic unit of energy is the *electron volt,* abbreviated eV. One eV is defined as the amount of energy acquired by an electron when it is accelerated through an electrical potential of one volt. Basic multiples are the keV (*k*ilo *e*lectron *v*olt; 1 keV = 1000 eV) and the MeV (*M*ega *e*lectron *v*olt; 1 MeV = 1000 keV = 1,000,000 eV).

Mass m and energy E are related to each other by Einstein's equation $E = mc^2$, where c is the velocity of light. According to this equation, 1 u of mass is equivalent to 931.5 MeV of energy.

---

† Atomic notation is discussed in Section D.2 of this chapter.

Relationships between various units of mass and energy are summarized in Table 1-2. Universal mass units and electron volts are very small, yet, as we shall see, they are quite appropriate to the atomic scale.

B. RADIATION

The term *radiation* refers to "energy in transit." In nuclear medicine, we are interested principally in two specific forms of radiation:

1. *Particulate radiation,* consisting of atomic or subatomic particles (electrons, protons, etc.) which carry energy in the form of kinetic energy of mass in motion, and
2. *Electromagnetic radiation,* in which energy is carried by oscillating electrical and magnetic fields traveling through space at the speed of light.

Radioactive decay processes, discussed in Chapter 2, result in the emission of radiation in both of these forms.

The wavelength, λ, and frequency, ν, of the oscillating fields of electromagnetic radiation are related by

$$\lambda\nu = c \qquad (1\text{-}1)$$

where c is the velocity of light (approximately 3×10^8 meters/sec in vacuum). Table 1-3 list various types of electromagnetic radiation and their wavelengths.

Most of the more familiar types of electromagnetic radiation (visible light, radio waves, etc.) exhibit "wave-like" behavior in their interactions with matter (e.g., diffraction patterns, transmission and detection of radio signals, etc.). In some cases, however, electromagnetic radiation behaves as discrete "packets" of energy, called *photons* (also called *quanta*). This is particularly true for interactions involving individual atoms. Photons have no mass or electrical charge and also travel at the velocity of light. These characteristics distinguish them from the forms of particulate radiation mentioned above. The energy of the photon E and the wavelength λ of its associated electromagnetic field are related by

$$E(\text{keV}) = 12.4/\lambda(\text{Å}) \qquad (1\text{-}2)$$

$$\lambda(\text{Å}) = 12.4/E(\text{keV}) \qquad (1\text{-}3)$$

Table 1-3 also lists photon energies for different regions of the electromagnetic spectrum. Note that x and γ rays occupy the highest-

Table 1-1
Fundamental Quantities and Units

Quantity	Usual Symbol	Definition	SI Units	Relationships and Special Units
		Fundamental Units		
mass	m	*	kilogram (kg)	
length	l	*	meter (m)	
time	t	*	second (s, or sec)	
current	I	*	ampere (A)	
		Derived Units		
velocity	v	$\Delta l/\Delta t$	m/s	
acceleration	a	$\Delta l/\Delta t$	m/s^2	
force	F	$m \cdot a$	newton (N)**	$1N = 1kg \cdot m/s^2$
work or energy	E	$F \cdot l$, $1/2\ mv^2$	joule (J)	$1J = 1kg \cdot m^2/s^2$
power	P	E/t	watt (W)	$1W = 1J/S$
frequency	f	number per second	hertz (Hz)	$1Hz = 1s^{-1}$

Electrical Units

charge	Q	$I \cdot t$	coulomb (C)	$1C = 1A \cdot S$
potential	V	E/Q	volt (V)	$1V = 1J/C$
capacity	C	Q/V	farad (F)	$1F = 1C/V$
resistance	R	V/I	ohm (Ω)	$1\Omega = 1V/A$

Radiation Units

absorbed dose	D	energy absorbed from ionizing radiation per unit mass	gray (Gy)	$1Gy = 1J/kg$, rad (r)***, $1r = 10^{-2}$ Gy
exposure	X	charge liberated by ionizing radiation per unit mass of air	C/kg	roentgen (R)***, $1R = 2.58 \times 10^{-4}$ C/kg
activity	A	disintegrations of radioactive material per second	bequerel (Bq)	$1Bq = 1s^{-1}$, curie (Ci)***, $1Ci = 3.7 \times 10^{10}$ Bq

This table is adapted from Johns HE and Cunningham JR, The Physics of Radiology (4th Ed.). Springfield, Ill., Charles C. Thomas, 1983, p. 5. With permission.

*Basic physical units, defined arbitrarily and maintained in standardization laboratories.

**It is customary to capitalize abbreviations for units named after persons (N) but not when spelled out (newtons).

***These are special radiation units, defined here for convenience. It is recommended that usage of these units be gradually abandoned.

Table 1-2
Mass and Energy Units

Multiply → To Obtain	By	To Obtain ← Divide
u	1.66043×10^{-27}	kg
u	1.00083	amu
eV	1.6021×10^{-19}	joules
u	931.478	MeV

energy, shortest-wavelength end of the spectrum; x- and γ-ray photons have energies in the keV-Mev range, whereas visible light photons, for example, have energies of only a few eV. As a consequence of their high energies and short wavelengths, x and γ rays interact with matter quite differently from other, more familiar types of electromagnetic radiation. These interactions are discussed in detail in Chapter 9.

C. ATOMS

1. Composition and Structure

All matter is comprised of atoms. An atom is the smallest unit into which a chemical element can be broken down without losing its chemical identity. Atoms combine to form molecules and chemical compounds, which in turn combine to form larger, macroscopic structures.

The existence of atoms was first postulated on philosophical grounds by Ionian scholars in the 5th century B.C. The concept was formalized into scientific theory early in the 19th century, owing largely to the work of the chemist Dalton and his contemporaries. The exact structure of

Table 1-3
Approximate Photon Energy and Wavelength Ranges
for Different Types of Electromagnetic Radiation

Type	Energy (eV)	Wavelength
Radio, TV, radar	10^{-9}–10^{-3}	10^{-1}–10^5 cm
Infrared	10^{-3}–2	10^{-4}–10^{-1} cm
Visible	2–3	4000–7000 Å†
Ultraviolet	3–25	50–4000 Å
x rays	25–10^5	10^{-1}–50 Å
γ rays	10^4–10^6	10^{-2}–1 Å

† 1 Å = 10^{-8} cm.

atoms was not known, but at that time they were believed to be indivisible. Later in the century (1869), Mendeleev produced the first *periodic table,* and ordering of the chemical elements according to the weights of their atoms and arrangement in a grid according to their chemical properties. For a time it was believed that completion of the periodic table would represent the final step in understanding the structure of matter.

Events of the late 19th and early 20th centuries, beginning with the discovery of x rays by Roentgen (1895) and radioactivity by Bequerel (1896), revealed that atoms had a substructure of their own. In 1910, Rutherford presented experimental evidence indicating that atoms consisted of a massive, compact, positively charged core, or *nucleus,* surrounded by a diffuse cloud of relatively light, negatively charged *electrons.* This model came to be known as the *nuclear atom.* The number of positive charges in the nucleus is called the *atomic number* of the nucleus (Z). In the electrically neutral atom, the number of orbital electrons is sufficient to balance exactly the number of positive charges, Z, in the nucleus. The chemical properties of an atom are determined by orbital electrons; therefore the atomic number Z determines the *chemical element* to which the atom belongs. A listing of chemical elements and their atomic numbers is given in Appendix A.

According to classical theory, orbiting electrons should slowly lose energy and spiral into the nucleus, resulting in atomic "collapse." This obviously is not what happens. The simple nuclear model therefore needed further refinement. This was provided by Niels Bohr in 1913, who presented a model that has come to be known as the *Bohr atom.* In the Bohr atom there is a set of stable electron orbits or "shells" in which electrons can exist indefinitely without loss of energy. The diameters of these shells are determined by *quantum numbers,* which can have only integer values ($n = 1, 2, 3, \ldots$). The innermost shell ($n = 1$) is called the K shell, the next the L shell ($n = 2$), followed by the M shell ($n = 3$), N shell ($n = 4$), and so forth.

Each shell is actually comprised of a set of orbits, called substates, which differ slightly from one another. Each shell has $2n - 1$ substates, where n is the quantum number of the shell. Thus the K shell has only one substate; the L shell has three substates, labeled L_I, L_{II}, L_{III}; and so forth. Figure 1-1 is a schematic representation of the K and L shells of an atom. The M shell and other higher shells have larger diameters.

The Bohr model of the atom was further refined with the statement of the *Pauli Exclusion Principle* in 1925. According to this principle, no two orbital electrons in an atom can move with exactly the same motion. Because of different possible electron "spin" orientations, more than one electron can exist in each substate (Figure 1-1); however, the number of

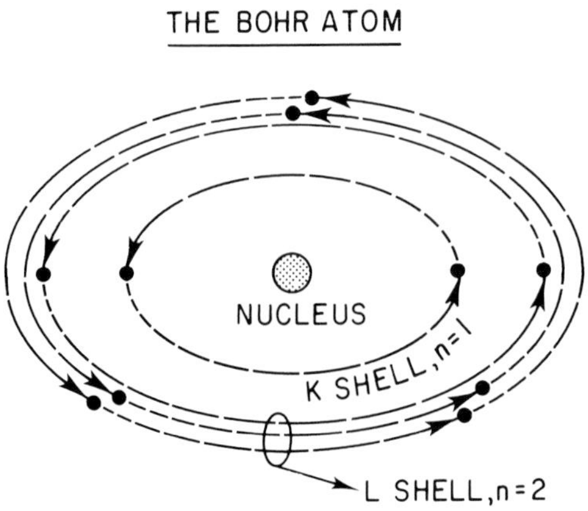

THE BOHR ATOM

Fig. 1-1. Schematic representation of the Bohr model of the atom; *n* is the quantum number of the shell. The K shell has one substate and the L shell has three substates. Each substate has two electrons.

electrons that can exist in any one shell or its substates is limited. For a shell with quantum number *n,* the maximum number of electrons allowed is $2n^2$. Thus the K shell ($n = 1$) is limited to two electrons, the L shell ($n = 2$) to eight electrons, and so forth.

The Bohr model is actually an oversimplification. According to modern theories the orbital electrons do not move in precise circular orbits, but rather in imprecisely defined "regions of space" around the nucleus, sometimes actually passing through the nucleus; however, the Bohr model is quite adequate for the purposes of this text.

2. Electron Binding Energies and Energy Levels

In the most stable configuration, orbital electrons occupy the innermost shells of an atom, where they are most "tightly bound" to the nucleus. For example, in carbon, which has six electrons, two electrons (the maximum number allowed) occupy the K shell, and the four remaining electrons are found in the L shell. Electrons can be moved to higher shells or completely removed from the atom, but doing so requires an energy input to overcome the forces of attraction that "bind" the electron to the nucleus. The energy may be provided, for example, by a particle or a photon striking the atom.

The amount of energy required to completely remove an electron from a given shell in an atom is called the *binding energy* of that shell. It

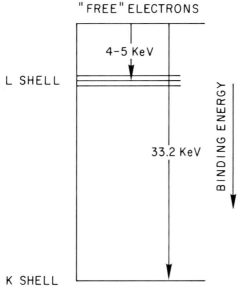

Fig. 1-2.   Electron energy level diagram for an iodine atom. Vertical axis represents energy required to remove orbital electrons from different shells (binding energy). Removing an electron from the atom, or going from an inner (e.g., K) to an outer (e.g., L) shell, requires an energy input, whereas an electron moving from an outer to an inner shell results in an emission of energy from the atom.

is symbolized by the notation K_B for the K shell,† L_B for the L shell (L_{IB}, L_{IIB}, L_{IIIB} for the L shell substates), and so forth. Binding energy is greatest for the innermost shell; i.e., $K_B > L_B > M_B$. . . . . Binding energy also increases with the positive charge (atomic number Z) of the nucleus, since a greater positive charge exerts a greater force of attraction on an electron. Therefore binding energies are greatest for the heaviest elements. Values of K shell binding energies for the elements are listed in Appendix A.

The energy required to move an electron from an inner to an outer shell is exactly equal to the difference in binding energies between the two shells. Thus the energy required to move an electron from the K shell to the L shell in an atom is $K_B - L_B$ (with slight differences for different L shell substates).

Binding energies and energy differences are sometimes displayed on an *energy level diagram*. Figure 1-2 shows such a diagram for the K and L shells of the element iodine. The top line represents an electron

† Sometimes the notation K_{ab} is also used.

completely separated from the parent atom ("unbound" or "free" electron). The bottom line represents the most tightly bound electrons, i.e., the K shell. Above this are lines representing substates of the L shell. (The M shell and other outer shell lines would be just above the L shell lines.) The distance from the K shell to the top level represents the K shell binding energy for iodine, i.e., 33.2 keV. To move a K shell electron to the L shell requires about $33 - 5 = 28$ keV of energy.

3. Atomic Emissions

When an electron is removed from one of the inner shells of an atom, an electron from an outer shell promptly moves in to fill the vacancy, and energy is released in the process. The energy released when an electron drops from an outer to an inner shell is exactly equal to the difference in binding energies between the two shells. The energy may appear as a photon of electromagnetic radiation (Figure 1-3). Electron binding energy differences have exact characteristic values for different elements; therefore the photon emissions are called *characteristic radiation* or *characteristic x rays*. The notation used to identify characteristic x rays from various electron transitions is summarized in Table 1-4. Note that some transitions are not allowed.

As an alternative to characteristic x-ray emission, the atom may undergo a process known as the *Auger* (pronounced oh-zhay') *effect*. In the Auger effect, an electron from an outer shell again fills the vacancy,

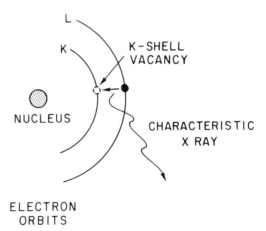

Fig. 1-3. Emission of characteristic x rays occurs when orbital electrons move from an outer shell to fill an inner-shell vacancy. (K_α x-ray emission illustrated.)

Table 1-4
Some Notation Used for Characteristic X Rays

Shell With Vacancy	Shell From Which Filled	Notation
K	L_I	Not allowed
K	L_{II}	$K_{\alpha 2}$
K	L_{III}	$K_{\alpha 1}$
K	M_I	Not allowed
K	M_{II}	$K_{\beta 3}$
K	M_{III}	$K_{\beta 1}$
K	N_I	Not allowed
K	$N_{II,III}$	$K_{\beta 2}$
L_{II}	M_{IV}	$L_{\beta 1}$
L_{III}	M_{IV}	$L_{\alpha 2}$
L_{III}	M_V	$L_{\alpha 1}$

but the energy released in the process is transferred to another orbital electron. This electron is then emitted from the atom instead of characteristic radiation. The process is shown schematically in Figure 1-4. The emitted electron is called an *Auger electron*.

The kinetic energy of an Auger electron is equal to the difference between the binding energy of the shell containing the original vacancy and the sum of the binding energies of the two shells having vacancies at the end. Thus the kinetic energy of the Auger electron emitted in Figure 1-4 is $K_B - 2L_B$ (ignoring small differences in L-substate energies).

Two orbital vacancies exist after the Auger effect occurs. These are

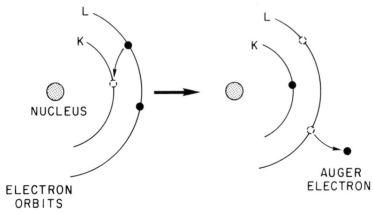

Fig. 1-4. Emission of an Auger electron as an alternative to x-ray emission. No x ray is emitted.

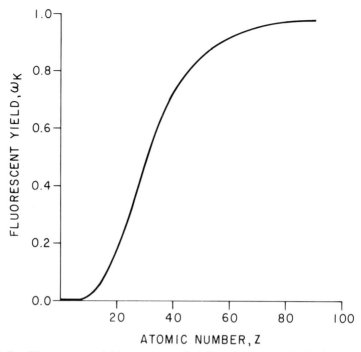

Fig. 1-5. Fluorescent yield ω_K, or probability that an orbital electron shell vacancy will yield characteristic x rays rather than Auger electrons, versus atomic number Z of the atom.

filled by electrons from the other outer shells, resulting in the emission of additional characteristic x rays or Auger electrons.

Whether a particular vacancy will result in emission of a characteristic x ray or an Auger electron is a matter of probabilities. The probability that it will yield characteristic x rays is called the *fluorescent yield,* symbolized by ω_K for the K shell, ω_L for the L shell, and so forth. Figure 1-5 is a graph of ω_K versus Z. Both characteristic x rays and Auger electrons are emitted by all elements, but heavy elements are more likely to emit x rays (large ω), whereas light elements are more likely to emit electrons (small ω).

The notation used to identify the shells involved in Auger electron emission is e_{abc}, where a identifies the shell with the original vacancy, b the shell from which the electron dropped to fill the vacancy, and c the shell from which the Auger electron was emitted. Thus the electron emitted in Figure 1-4 is a *KLL* Auger electron, symbolized by e_{KLL}. In the notation e_{Kxx}, the symbol x is arbitrary, referring to all Auger electrons produced from initial K shell vacancies.

Table 1-5
Basic Properties of Nucleons and Electrons

Particle	Charge†	Mass (u)	Mass (MeV)
Proton	+1	1.007277	938.211
Neutron	0	1.008665	939.505
Electron	−1	0.000549	0.511

†One unit of charge is equivalent to 1.602×10^{-19} coulombs.

D. THE NUCLEUS

1. Composition

The atomic nucleus is comprised of *protons* and *neutrons*. Collectively these particles are known as *nucleons*. The properties of nucleons and electrons are summarized in Table 1-5.

Nucleons are much more massive than electrons (by nearly a factor of 2000). On the other hand, nuclear diameters are very small in comparison to atomic diameters (10^{-13} cm versus 10^{-8} cm). Thus it can be deduced that the density of nuclear matter is very high ($\sim 10^{14}$ g/cm^3) and that the rest of the atom (electron cloud) is mostly empty space.

2. Terminology and Notation

An atomic nucleus is characterized by the number of neutrons and protons it contains. The number of protons determines the *atomic number* of the atom, Z. As mentioned earlier, this determines also the number of orbital electrons in the electrically neutral atom and therefore the *chemical element* to which the atom belongs.

The total number of nucleons is the *mass number* of the nucleus, A. The difference, $A - Z$, is the *neutron number, N*. The mass number A is approximately equal to, but not the same as, the *atomic weight* (AW) used in chemistry. The latter is the average weight of an atom of an element in its natural abundance (Appendix A).

The notation now used to summarize atomic and nuclear composition is $^A_Z X_N$, where X represents the chemical element to which the atom belongs. For example, an atom comprised of 53 protons, 78 neutrons (and thus 131 nucleons), and 53 orbital electrons represents the element iodine and is symbolized by $^{131}_{53}I_{78}$. Since all iodine atoms have atomic number 53, either the "I" or the "53" is redundant, and the "53" can be omitted. The neutron number, 78, can be inferred from the difference $131 - 53$ and also can be omitted. Therefore a shortened but still complete notation for this atom is ^{131}I. An acceptable alternative in terms of medical terminology is

I-131. Obsolete forms (often found in older texts) include I^{131}, $_{131}I$, and I_{131}.

3. Nuclear Families

Nuclear species are sometimes grouped into families having certain common characteristics. A *nuclide* is characterized by an exact nuclear composition, including the mass number A, atomic number Z, and arrangement of nucleons within the nucleus. To be classified as a nuclide, the species must have a "measurably long" existence, which for current technology means a lifetime greater than about 10^{-12} sec. For example, ^{12}C, ^{16}O, and ^{131}I are nuclides.

Nuclides that have the same atomic Z are called *isotopes*. Thus ^{125}I, ^{127}I, and ^{131}I are isotopes of the element iodine. Nuclides with the same mass number A are *isobars*—e.g., ^{131}I, ^{131}Xe, ^{131}Cs. Nuclides with the same neutron number N are *isotones*—e.g., $^{131}_{53}I_{78}$, $^{132}_{54}Xe_{78}$, $^{133}_{55}Cs_{78}$. A mnemonic device for remembering these relationships is that isoto*p*es have the same number of protons, isoto*n*es the same number of neutrons, and iso*bar*s the same mass number (A).

4. Nuclear Forces and Energy Levels

Nucleons within the nucleus are subject to two kinds of forces. Repulsive *coulombic* or *electrical forces* exist between positively charged protons. These are counteracted by very strong forces of attraction, called *exchange forces*, between any two nucleons. Exchange forces are effective only over very short distances, and their effects are seen only when nucleons are very close together, as they are in the nucleus. Exchange forces hold the nucleus together against the repulsive coulombic forces between protons.

Nucleons move about within the nucleus in a very complicated way under the influence of these forces. One model of the nucleus, called the *shell model*, portrays the nucleons as moving in "orbits" about one another in a manner similar to that of orbital electrons moving about the nucleus in the Bohr atom. Only a limited number of motions are allowed, and these are determined by a set of nuclear quantum numbers.

The most stable arrangement of nucleons is called the *ground* state. Other arrangements of the nucleons fall into two categories:

1. *Excited states* are arrangements that are so unstable that they have only a transient existence before transforming into some other state.

2. *Metastable states* also are unstable, but they have relatively long lifetimes before transforming into another state. These are also called *isomeric states*.

The dividing line for lifetimes between excited and metastable states is about 10^{-12} sec. This is not a long time according to everyday standards, but it is "relatively long" by nuclear standards. Some metastable states are quite long-lived, i.e., average lifetimes of several hours. (The prefix *meta* derives from the Greek word for "almost.") Because of this, metastable states are considered to have separate identities and are classified themselves as nuclides. Two nuclides that differ from one another in that one is a metastable state of the other are called *isomers*.

In nuclear notation, excited states are identified by an asterisk($^{A}X^{*}$) and metastable states by the letter m (^{Am}X or X-Am).† Thus ^{99m}Tc (or Tc-99m) represents a metastable state of ^{99}Tc, and ^{99m}Tc and ^{99}Tc are isomers.

Nuclear transitions between different nucleon arrangements involve discrete and exact amounts of energy, as do the rearrangements of orbital electrons in the Bohr atom. A *nuclear energy level diagram* is used to identify the various excited and metastable states of a nuclide and the energy relationships among them. Figure 1-6 shows a partial diagram for ^{131}Xe.‡ The bottom line represents the ground state, and other lines represent excited or metastable states. Metastable states usually are indicated by somewhat heavier lines. The vertical distances between lines are proportional to the energy differences between levels. A transition from a lower to a higher state requires an energy input of some sort, e.g., a photon or particle striking the nucleus. Transitions from higher to lower states result in the release of energy, which is given to emitted particles or photons.

5. Nuclear Emissions

The energy released in a nuclear transformation to a more stable state may appear as a photon of electromagnetic radiation. Photons of nuclear origin are called γ *rays* (gamma rays). The energy difference between the states involved in the transition determines the γ-ray energy. For example, in Figure 1-6 a transition from the level marked 0.364 MeV to the ground state would produce a 0.364 MeV γ ray. A transition from the 0.364 MeV level to the 0.080 MeV level would produce a 0.284 MeV γ ray.

As an alternative to emitting a γ ray, the nucleus may transfer the energy to an orbital electron and emit the electron instead of a photon. This process, which is similar to the Auger effect in x-ray emission

---

† The notation $^{A}X^{m}$ is common in Europe (e.g., $^{99}Tc^{m}$).

‡ Actually, these are the excited and metastable states formed during radioactive decay by β⁻ emission of ^{131}I (Chapter 2, Section D).

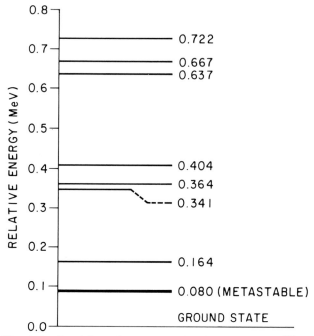

Fig. 1-6.   Partial nuclear energy level diagram for ^{131}Xe nucleus. Vertical axis represents energy differences between nuclear states (or "arrangements"). Going up the scale requires energy input. Coming down the scale results in the emission of nuclear energy. Heavier lines indicate metastable states.

(Section C.3), is called *internal conversion*. It is discussed in detail in Chapter 2, Section E.

6. Nuclear Binding Energy

When the mass of an atom is compared to the sum of the masses of its individual components (protons, neutrons, and electrons), it is always found to be less by some amount, Δm. This mass deficiency, expressed in energy units, is called the *binding energy* E_B of the atom:

$$E_B = \Delta mc^2 \tag{1-4}$$

For example, consider an atom of ^{12}C. This atom is comprised of six protons, six electrons, and six neutrons, and its mass is precisely 12.0 u (by definition of the universal mass unit u). The sum of the masses of its components is

electrons	6×0.000549 u	=	0.003294 u
protons	6×1.007277 u	=	6.043662 u
neutrons	6×1.008665 u	=	6.051990 u
			12.099006 u

Thus $\Delta m = 0.09906$ u. Since 1 u = 931.5 MeV, the binding energy of a ^{12}C atom is $0.09906 \times 931.5 = 92.22$ MeV.

The binding energy is the minimum amount of energy required to overcome the forces holding the atom together in order to separate it completely into its individual components. Some of this represents the binding energy of orbital electrons, i.e., the energy required to strip the orbital electrons away from the nucleus; however, comparison of the total binding energy of a ^{12}C atom with the K shell binding energy of carbon (Appendix A) indicates that most of this energy is *nuclear binding energy*, i.e., energy required to separate the nucleons.

Nuclear processes that result in the release of energy (e.g., γ-ray emission) always *increase* the binding energy of the nucleus. Thus a nucleus emitting a 1 MeV γ ray would be found to weigh *less* (by the mass equivalent of 1 MeV) after the γ ray was emitted than before. In essence, mass is converted to energy in the process.

7. Characteristics of Stable Nuclei

Not all combinations of protons and neutrons produce stable nuclei. Some are unstable, even in their ground states. An unstable nucleus emits particles and/or photons to transform itself into a more stable nucleus. This is the process of *radioactive disintegration* or *radioactive decay*, discussed in Chapter 2. A survey of the general characteristics of naturally occurring *stable nuclides* provides clues to the factors that contribute to nuclear instability and thus to radioactive decay.

A first observation is that there are favored neutron-to-proton ratios among stable nuclides. Figure 1-7 is a plot of the stable nuclides according to their neutron and proton numbers. For example, the nuclide $^{12}_{6}$C is represented by a dot at the point $Z = 6$, $N = 6$. The stable nuclides are clustered around an imaginary line called the *line of stability*. For light elements, the line corresponds to $N \approx Z$, i.e., about equal numbers of protons and neutrons. For heavy elements, it corresponds to $N \approx 1.5Z$, i.e. about 50 percent more neutrons than protons. The line of stability ends at ^{209}Bi. All heavier nuclides are unstable.

In general, there is a tendency toward instability in systems com-

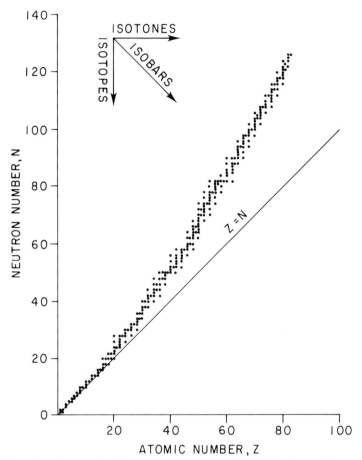

Fig. 1-7. Atomic number Z versus neutron number N for the stable nuclides. They are clustered around an imaginary line called the line of stability, $N \approx Z$ for light elements; $N \approx 1.5Z$ for heavy elements.

prised of large numbers of identical particles confined in a small volume. This explains the instability of very heavy nuclei. It also explains why, for light elements, stability is favored by more or less equal numbers of neutrons and protons rather than grossly unequal numbers. A moderate excess of neutrons is favored among heavier elements because neutrons provide only exchange forces (attraction), whereas protons provide both exchange forces and coulombic forces (repulsion). Exchange forces are effective over very short distances and thus affect only "close neighbors" in the nucleus, whereas the repulsive coulombic forces are effective over much greater distances. Thus an excess of neutrons is required in heavy nuclei to overcome the long-range repulsive Coulombic forces between a large number of protons.

Nuclides that are not close to the line of stability are likely to be unstable. Unstable nuclides lying above the line of stability are said to be "proton deficient," while those lying below the line are "neutron deficient." Unstable nuclides generally undergo radioactive decay processes that transform them into nuclides lying closer to the line of stability, as discussed in Chapter 2.

From Figure 1-7 it can be seen that there are often many stable isotopes of an element. Isotopes fall on vertical lines in the diagram. For example, there are ten stable isotopes of tin (Sn,† $Z = 50$). There may also be several stable isotones. These fall along horizontal lines. In relatively few cases, however, is there more than one stable isobar (isobars fall along descending 45° lines on the graph), reflecting the existence of several modes of "isobaric" radioactive decay that permit nuclides to transform along isobaric lines until the most stable isobar is reached. This will be discussed in detail in Chapter 2.

One also notes among the stable nuclides a tendency to favor even numbers. For example, there are 165 stable nuclides with both even numbers of protons and even numbers of neutrons. Examples are ${}^{4}_{2}\text{He}$ and ${}^{12}_{6}\text{C}$. There are 109 "even-odd" nuclides, with even numbers of protons and odd numbers of neutrons or vice versa. Examples are ${}^{9}_{4}\text{Be}$ and ${}^{11}_{5}\text{B}$. However, there are only four stable "odd-odd" nuclides: ${}^{2}_{1}\text{H}$, ${}^{6}_{3}\text{Li}$, ${}^{10}_{5}\text{B}$, and ${}^{14}_{7}\text{N}$. The stability of even numbers reflects the tendency of nuclei to achieve stable arrangements by the "pairing up" of nucleons in the nucleus.

Another measure of relative nuclear stability is nuclear binding energy, since this represents the amount of energy required to break the nucleus up into its separate components. Obviously, the greater the number of nucleons, the greater the total binding energy. Therefore a more meaningful parameter is the *binding energy per nucleon, E_B/A*. Higher values of E_B/A are indicators of greater nuclear stability.

Figure 1-8 is a graph of E_B/A versus A for the stable nuclides. Binding energy is greatest (~8 MeV/nucleon) for nuclides of mass number $A \approx 60$. It decreases slowly with increasing A, indicating the tendency toward instability for very heavy nuclides. Finally, there are a few peaks in the

---

† While most element symbols are simply one- or two-letter abbreviations of their (English) names, 11 symbols derive from Latin or Greek names of metals known for over two millennia: antimony (stibium, Sb); copper (cuprum, Cu); gold (aurum, Au); iron (ferrum, Fe); lead (plumbum, Pb); mercury (hydrargyrum, Hg); potassium (kalium, K); silver (argentum, Ag); sodium (natrium, Na); tin (stannum, Sn); tungsten (wolfram, W).

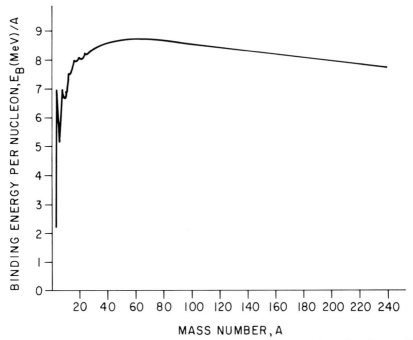

Fig. 1-8. Binding energy per nucleon versus mass number for the stable nuclides. [Adapted with permission from Evans RD, The Atomic Nucleus. New York, McGraw-Hill, 1972, p. 299].

curve representing very stable light nuclides, including $^4_2$He, $^{12}_6$C, and $^{16}_8$O. Note that these are all "even-even" nuclides.

REFERENCES

Basic mathematics and physics are reviewed in many textbooks, including the following:

Boyd CM, Dalrymple GV: Basic Science Principles of Nuclear Medicine. St. Louis, C. V. Mosby, 1974

Kemp LAW: Mathematics for Radiographers. Philadelphia, F. A. Davis, 1964

Kemp LAW, Oliver R: Basic Physics in Radiology (ed 2). Oxford, Blackwell Scientific, 1970

Nave CR, Nave BC: Physics for the Health Sciences. Philadelphia, W. B. Saunders, 1975

Recommended texts for in-depth discussions of topics in atomic and nuclear physics are the following:

Evans RD: The Atomic Nucleus. New York, McGraw-Hill, 1972

Johns HE, Cunningham JR: The Physics of Radiology (4th Ed.) Springfield, IL, Charles C Thomas, chap 1

Lapp RE, Andrews, HL: Nuclear Radiation Physics (ed 4). Englewood Cliffs, N.J., Prentice-Hall, 1972

Rollo FD: Atomic and nuclear physics, in Rollo FD (ed): Nuclear Medicine—Physics, Instrumentation, and Agents. St. Louis, C. V. Mosby, 1977, chap 1

2

Modes of Radioactive Decay

Radioactive decay is a process in which an unstable nucleus transforms into a more stable one by emitting particles and/or photons and releasing nuclear energy. Atomic electrons may become involved in some types of radioactive decay, but it is basically a *nuclear* process caused by *nuclear* instability. In this chapter we discuss the general characteristics of various modes of radioactive decay and their general importance in nuclear medicine.

A. GENERAL CONCEPTS

It is common terminology to call an unstable radioactive nucleus the *parent* and the more stable product nucleus the *daughter*. In many cases, the daughter also is radioactive and undergoes further radioactive decay. Radioactive decay is *spontaneous* in that the exact moment at which a given nucleus will decay cannot be predicted, nor is it affected to any significant extent by events occurring outside the nucleus.

Radioactive decay results in the release of nuclear energy. The energy released in a decay event is called the *transition energy*, sometimes designated *Q*. Most of this energy is imparted to emitted particles and photons, with a small (usually insignificant) fraction being imparted to the recoiling nucleus. The source of the energy released is a conversion of mass into energy. If all of the products of a particular decay event were gathered up and weighed, they would be found to weigh less than the original radioactive atom. Thus radioactive decay results not only in the transformation of one nuclear species into another but also in the transformation of mass into energy.

Each radioactive nuclide has a set of characteristic properties. These properties include the mode of radioactive decay and type of emissions, the transition energy, and the average lifetime of a nucleus of the radionuclide before it undergoes radioactive decay. Because these basic properties are characteristic of the nuclide, it is common to refer to a radioactive species, such as ^{131}I, as a *radionuclide*. The term *radioisotope* also is used but, strictly speaking, should be used only when specifically identifying a member of an isotopic family as radioactive—e.g., ^{131}I is a radioisotope of iodine.

B. CHEMISTRY AND RADIOACTIVITY

Radioactive decay is a process involving primarily the nucleus, whereas chemical reactions involve primarily the outermost orbital electrons of the atom. Thus the fact that an atom has a radioactive nucleus does not affect its chemical behavior, and the chemical state of an atom does not affect its radioactive characteristics. For example, an atom of the radionuclide ^{131}I exhibits the same chemical behavior as an atom of ^{127}I, a naturally occurring stable nuclide, and ^{131}I has the same radioactive characteristics whether it exists as iodide ion (I^-) or incorporated into a large protein molecule as a radioactive label. Independence of radioactive and chemical properties is of great significance in tracer studies with radioactivity—a radioactive *tracer* behaves in chemical and physiologic processes exactly the same as its stable, naturally occurring counterpart, and, further, the radioactive properties of the tracer do not change as it enters into chemical or physiologic processes.

There are two minor exceptions to these generalizations. The first is that chemical behavior can be affected by atomic mass differences. Since there are always mass differences between the radioactive and the stable members of an isotopic family (e.g., ^{131}I is heavier than ^{127}I), there may also be chemical differences. This is called the *isotope effect*. Note that this is a *mass* effect and has nothing to do with the fact that one of the isotopes is radioactive. The chemical differences are small unless the relative mass differences are large—e.g., ^{12}C versus ^{14}C, ^{3}H versus ^{1}H. While they are important in some experiments, such as measurements of chemical bond strengths, they are, fortunately, of no practical consequence in nuclear medicine.

A second exception is that the average lifetimes of radionuclides that decay by processes involving orbital electrons (e.g., internal conversion, Section E, and electron capture, Section F) can be changed very slightly by altering the chemical (orbital electron) state of the atom. The differences are so small that they cannot be detected except in elaborate nuclear physics experiments and again are of no practical consequence in nuclear medicine.

C. DECAY BY β⁻ EMISSION

Radioactive decay by β^- emission is a process in which, essentially, a neutron in the nucleus is transformed into a proton and an electron. Schematically, the process is

$$n \rightarrow p^+ + e^- + \nu + \text{energy} \qquad (2\text{-}1)$$

The electron (e^-) and the neutrino (ν) are ejected from the nucleus and carry away the energy released in the process as kinetic energy.† The electron is called a *beta particle* $(\beta^-$ particle). This neutrino is a "particle" having no mass or electrical charge. It undergoes virtually no interactions with matter and therefore is essentially undetectable. Its only practical consequence is that it carries away some of the energy released in the decay process.

Decay by β^- emission may be represented in standard nuclear notation as

$$^A_Z X \xrightarrow{\beta^-} {}^A_{Z+1} Y \qquad (2\text{-}2)$$

The parent radionuclide (X) and daughter product (Y) represent different chemical elements because atomic number increases by one. Thus β^- decay results in a *transmutation* of elements. Mass number A does not change because the total number of nucleons in the nucleus does not change. This is therefore an *isobaric* decay mode—i.e., the parent and daughter are isobars.

Radioactive decay processes are often represented by a *decay scheme*. Figure 2-1 shows such a diagram for ^{14}C, a radionuclide that decays solely by β^- emission. The line representing ^{14}C (the parent) is drawn above and to the left of the line representing ^{14}N (the daughter). Decay is "to the right" because atomic number *increases* by one (reading Z values from left to right). The vertical distance between the lines is proportional to the total amount of energy released, i.e., transition energy, for the decay process ($Q = 0.156$ MeV for ^{14}C).

---

† Actually in β^- emission an antineutrino, ν, is emitted, whereas in β^+ emission and electron capture, a neutrino, ν, is emitted. For simplicity, no distinction will be made in this text.

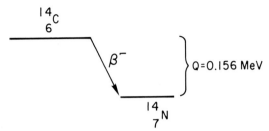

Fig. 2-1. Decay scheme diagram for ^{14}C, a β^- emitter. Q is the transition energy.

The energy released in β^- decay is shared between the β^- particle and the neutrino. This sharing of energy is more or less random from one decay to the next. Figure 2-2 shows the distribution, or *spectrum,* of β^--particle energies resulting from the decay of ^{14}C. The maximum possible β^--particle energy (i.e., the transition energy for the decay process) is denoted by E_β^{max} (0.156 MeV for ^{14}C). From the graph it is apparent that the β^- particle usually receives something less than half of the available energy. Only rarely does the β^- particle carry away all of the energy ($E_\beta \approx E_\beta^{max}$). The *average* energy of the β^- particle is denoted by $\overline{E}_\beta$. This varies from one radionuclide to the next but has a characteristic value for any given radionuclide. Typically, $E_\beta \approx \frac{1}{3}E_\beta^{max}$. For ^{14}C, $E_\beta = 0.0493$ MeV ($0.32E_\beta^{max}$).

Beta particles themselves present special detection and measurement

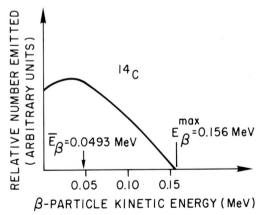

Fig. 2-2. Energy spectrum (number emitted versus energy) for β particles emitted by ^{14}C. Maximum β^- particle energy E_β^{max} is Q, the transition energy (Figure 2-1). Average energy $\overline{E}_\beta$ is 0.0493 MeV, about $\frac{1}{3}E_\beta^{max}$.

problems for nuclear medicine applications. These arise from the fact that they can penetrate only relatively small thicknesses of solid materials (Chapter 8, Section B.2). For example, the thickness is at most only a few millimeters of soft tissues. Therefore it is difficult to detect β^- particles originating from inside the body with a detector that is located outside the body. For this reason, radionuclides emitting only β^- particles rarely are used when measurement in vivo is required. Special types of detector systems are also needed to detect β^- particles because they will not penetrate even relatively thin layers of metal or other outside protective materials that are required on some types of detectors. The implications of this are discussed in Chapter 4.

The properties of various radionuclides of medical interest are presented in Appendix B. Radionuclides decaying solely by β^- emission listed there include ^3H, ^{14}C, and ^{32}P.

D. DECAY BY (β^-, γ) EMISSION

In some cases, decay by β^- emission results in a daughter nucleus that is in an excited or metastable state rather than in the ground state. If an excited state is formed, the daughter nucleus promptly decays to a more stable nuclear arrangement by the emission of a γ ray (Chapter 1, Section D.5). This sequential decay process is called (β^-, γ) decay. In standard nuclear notation, it may be represented as

$$\underset{Z}{\overset{A}{X}} \xrightarrow{\beta^-} \underset{Z+1}{\overset{A}{Y^*}} \xrightarrow{\gamma} \underset{Z+1}{\overset{A}{Y}} \qquad (2\text{-}3)$$

Note that γ emission does not result in a transmutation.

An example of (β^-, γ) decay is the radionuclide ^{133}Xe, which decays by β^- emission to one of three different excited states of ^{133}Cs. Figure 2-3 is a decay scheme for this radionuclide. The daughter nucleus decays to the ground state or to another, less energetic excited state by emitting a γ ray. If it is to another excited state, additional γ rays may be emitted before the ground state is finally reached. Thus in (β^-, γ) decay more than one γ ray may be emitted before the daughter nucleus reaches the ground state—e.g., β_2 followed by γ_1 and γ_2 in ^{133}Xe decay.

The number of nuclei decaying through the different excited states is determined by relative probability values that are characteristic of the particular radionuclide. For example, in ^{133}Xe decay (Figure 2-3) 98.3 percent of the decay events are by β_3 decay to the 0.081 MeV excited state, followed by emission of the 0.081 MeV γ ray. Only a very small number of the other β particles and γ rays of other energies are emitted.

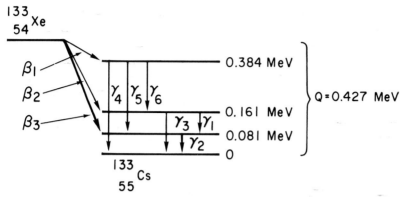

Fig. 2-3.   Decay scheme diagram for ^{133}Xe, a (β^-, γ) emitter. More than one γ ray may be emitted per disintegrating nucleus. Heavier lines indicate most probable decay modes.

The data presented in Appendix B include the relative number of emissions of different energies for each radionuclide listed.

In contrast to β^- particles, which are emitted with a continuous distribution of energies (up to E_β^{max}), γ rays are emitted with a discrete series of energy values. The spectrum of emitted radiation energies is therefore a series of discrete lines at energies that are characteristic of the radionuclide, rather than a continuous distribution of energies (Figure 2-4). In (β^-, γ) decay, the transition energy between the parent radionu-

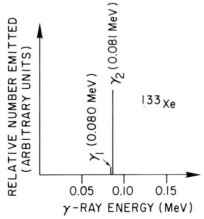

Fig. 2-4.   Emission for 0.080 and 0.081 MeV γ rays emitted in the decay of ^{133}Xe (γ_1 and γ_2 in Figure 2-3; higher-energy emissions omitted). Compare with Figure 2-2 for β particles.

clide and the ground state of the daughter has a fixed characteristic value. The distribution of this energy among the β^- particle, the neutrino, and the γ rays may vary from one nuclear decay to the next, but the sum of their energies in any decay event is always equal to the transition energy.

Gamma rays are much more penetrating than β^- particles. Therefore they do not present some of the measurement problems associated with β^- particles that were mentioned earlier, and they are suitable for a wider variety of applications in nuclear medicine. Some (β^-, γ) radionuclides of medical interest listed in Appendix B include ^{131}I, ^{133}Xe, and ^{137}Cs.

E. ISOMERIC TRANSITION (IT) AND INTERNAL CONVERSION (IC).

The daughter nucleus of a radioactive parent may be formed in a "long-lived" metastable or isomeric state, as opposed to an excited state. The decay of the metastable or isomeric state, by the emission of a γ ray is called an *isomeric transition* (Chapter 1, Section D.4). Except for their average lifetimes, there are no differences in decay by γ emission of metastable or excited states.

An alternative to γ-ray emission that is especially frequent among metastable states is decay by internal conversion. In this process, the nucleus decays by transferring energy to an orbital electron, which is ejected instead of the γ ray. It is as if the γ ray were "internally absorbed" by collision with an orbital electron (Figure 2-5). The ejected electron is called a *conversion electron*. These electrons usually originate from one of the inner shells (K or L), provided that the γ-ray energy is

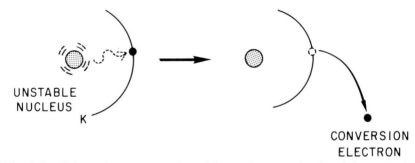

UNSTABLE
NUCLEUS
K

CONVERSION
ELECTRON

Fig. 2-5. Schematic representation of internal conversion involving a K shell electron. Unstable nucleus transfers its energy to an orbital electron rather than emitting a γ ray. Kinetic energy of conversion electron is γ-ray energy minus electron binding energy ($E_\gamma - K_\beta$).

sufficient to overcome the binding energy of that shell. The energy excess above the binding energy is imparted to the conversion electron as kinetic energy. The orbital vacancy created by internal conversion is subsequently filled by an outer shell electron, with the emission of characteristic x rays or Auger electrons (Chapter 1, Section C.3).

Whether a γ ray or a conversion electron is emitted is a matter of probabilities, which have characteristic values for different radionuclides. These probabilities are expressed in terms of the ratio of conversion electrons emitted to γ rays emitted (e/γ) and denoted by α (or α_K = e/γ for K shell conversion electrons emitted, etc.).

Internal conversion, like β⁻ decay, results in the emission of electrons. The important differences are that (1) in β⁻ decay the electron originates from the nucleus, whereas in internal conversion it originates from an electron orbit, and (2) β⁻ particles are emitted with a continuous spectrum of energies, whereas conversion electrons have a discrete series of energies determined by the differences between the γ-ray energy and orbital electron binding energies.

Metastable radionuclides are of great importance in nuclear medicine. Because of their relatively long lifetimes, it is possible to separate them from their radioactive parent and thus obtain a relatively "pure" source of γ rays. The separation of the metastable daughter from its radioactive parent is accomplished by chemical means in a radionuclide "generator" (Chapter 7, Section E). Metastable nuclides always emit a certain number of conversion electrons, and thus they are not really "pure" γ-ray emitters; however, the ratio of photons to electrons emitted is greater usually than for (β⁻, γ) emitters, and this is a definite advantage for studies requiring detection of γ rays from internally administered radioactivity.

A metastable nuclide of medical interest listed in Appendix B is ^{99m}Tc. Technetium-99m is currently by far the most popular radionuclide for nuclear medicine imaging studies.

F. ELECTRON CAPTURE (EC) AND (EC, γ) DECAY

Electron capture decay looks like, and in fact is sometimes called, "inverse β⁻ decay." An orbital electron is "captured" by the nucleus and combines with a proton to form a neutron:

$$p^+ + e^- \rightarrow n + \nu + \text{energy} \tag{2-4}$$

The neutrino is emitted from the nucleus and carries away some of the transition energy. Additional energy appears in the form of characteristic

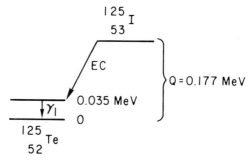

Fig. 2-6. Decay scheme diagram for ^{125}I, an (EC, γ) emitter.

x rays and Auger electrons, which are emitted by the daughter product when the resulting orbital electron vacancy is filled. Usually, the electron is captured from orbits that are closest to the nucleus, i.e., the K and L shells. The notation EC (K) is used to indicate capture of a K shell electron, EC (L) an L shell electron, and so forth.

Electron capture decay may be represented as

$$_{Z}^{A}X \xrightarrow{EC} \,_{Z-1}^{A}Y \tag{2-5}$$

Note that like β^- decay it is an isobaric decay mode leading to a transmutation of elements.

The characteristic x rays emitted by the daughter product after electron capture may be suitable for external measurement if they are sufficiently energetic to penetrate a few centimeters of body tissues. There is no precise energy cutoff point, but 25 keV is probably a reasonable value, at least for shallow organs, e.g., the thyroid. For elements with $Z \geq 50$, the energy of K–x rays exceeds 25 keV. The K–x rays of lighter elements and all L–x rays are of lower energy and generally are not suitable for external measurements. These lower-energy radiations introduce measurement problems similar to those encountered with β^- particles.

Electron capture decay results frequently in a daughter nucleus that is in an excited or metastable state. Thus γ rays (or conversion electrons) may also be emitted. This is called (EC, γ) decay. Figure 2-6 shows a decay scheme for ^{125}I, an (EC, γ) radionuclide finding application in thyroid and radioimmunoassay studies. Note that EC decay is "to the left" because electron capture *decreases* the atomic number by one. Medically important EC and (EC, γ) radionuclides listed in Appendix B include ^{57}Co, ^{67}Ga, ^{111}In, ^{123}I, ^{125}I, and ^{201}Tl.

G. POSITRON (β^+) AND (β^+, γ) DECAY

In radioactive decay by positron emission, a proton in the nucleus is transformed into a neutron and a positively charged electron. The positively charged electron — or *positron* (β^+) — and a neutrino are ejected from the nucleus. Schematically, the process is

$$p^+ \rightarrow n + e^+ + \nu + \text{energy} \qquad (2\text{-}6)$$

A positron is the antiparticle of an ordinary electron. After ejection from the nucleus, it loses its kinetic energy in collisions with atoms of the surrounding matter and comes to rest, usually within a few millimeters of the site of its origin in body tissues. This occurs within about 10^{-9} sec. The positron then combines with an ordinary electron in an *annihilation reaction*, in which its mass and that of the ordinary electron are converted into energy (Figure 2-7). The mass-energy equivalent of each particle is 0.511 MeV. This energy appears in the form of two 0.511 MeV *annihilation photons*, which leave the site of the annihilation in exact opposite directions (180° apart). Thus decay by β^+ emission ultimately results in the production of two 0.511 MeV photons.

Energy "bookkeeping" is somewhat more complicated in β^+ decay than in some of the previously discussed decay modes. The transition energy is divided among the kinetic energy of the positron, the neutrino, and the annihilation photons ($2 \times 0.511 = 1.022$ MeV). Thus there is a minimum transition energy requirement of 1.022 MeV before β^+ decay can occur. The excess transition energy above 1.022 MeV is shared between the positron (kinetic energy) and the neutrino. The positron

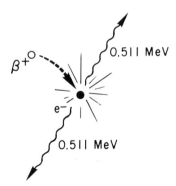

Fig. 2-7. Schematic representation of mutual annihilation reaction between a positron (β^+) and an ordinary electron. A pair of 0.511 MeV annihilation photons are emitted, "back to back" at 180° to each other.

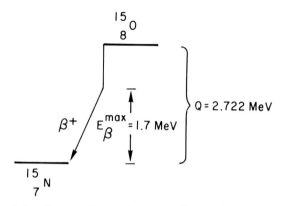

Fig. 2-8.   Decay scheme diagram for ^{15}O, a β^+ emitter. E_β^{max} is Q, the transition energy, minus 1.022 MeV, the energy of the annihilation photons.

energy spectrum is similar to that observed for β^- particles (Figure 2-2). The average β^+ energy also is denoted by $\overline{E}_\beta$ *and again is approximately* $\frac{1}{3}E_\beta^{max}$, where E_β^{max} is the transition energy minus 1.022 MeV.

In standard notation, β^+ decay is represented as

$$\begin{matrix} A \\ Z \end{matrix}X \xrightarrow{\beta^+} + \begin{matrix} A \\ Z-1 \end{matrix}Y \tag{2-7}$$

It is another isobaric decay mode, with a transmutation of elements. Figure 2-8 shows a decay scheme for ^{15}O, a β^+ emitter of medical interest. Decay is "to the left" because atomic number *decreases* by one. The vertical line represents the energy of the annihilation photons (1.022 MeV). The remaining energy (1.7 MeV) is E_β^{max}. With some radionuclides, β^+ emission may leave the daughter nucleus in an excited state, and thus additional γ rays may also be emitted [(β^+, γ) decay].

Positron emitters are useful in nuclear medicine because two photons are generated per nuclear decay event. The exact directional relationship between the annihilation photons is also useful because it permits the use of novel "coincidence counting" techniques (Chapter 20, Section D.1). Medically important β^+ radionuclides listed in Appendix B include ^{11}C, ^{13}N, and ^{15}O.

H. COMPETITIVE β^+ AND EC DECAY

Positron emission and electron capture have the same effect on the parent nucleus. Both are isobaric decay modes that decrease atomic number by one. They are alternative means for reaching the same

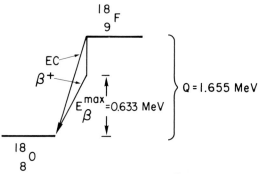

Fig. 2-9. Decay scheme diagram for ^{18}F, which decays by both EC and β^+ emission competitively.

endpoint (Equations 2-5 and 2-7, Figures 2-6 and 2-8). Among the radioactive nuclides, one finds that β^+ decay occurs more frequently among lighter elements (assuming the minimum 1.022 MeV transition energy requirement is met), whereas electron capture is more frequent among heavier elements, since in heavy elements orbital electrons tend to be closer to the nucleus and are more easily captured.

There are also radionuclides that can decay by either mode. An example is ^{18}F, the decay scheme for which is shown in Figure 2-9. for this radionuclide, 3 percent of the nuclei decay by (EC, γ) and 97 percent by (β^+, γ). Radionuclides of medical interest that undergo competitive (β^+, EC) decay listed in Appendix B include ^{18}F and ^{68}Ga.

J. DECAY BY α EMISSION AND BY NUCLEAR FISSION

Decay by α-particle emission and decay by nuclear fission are of relatively little importance in nuclear medicine but will be described here for the sake of completeness. Both of these decay modes occur primarily among very heavy elements that are of little interest as physiologic tracers.

In decay by α-particle emission, the nucleus ejects an α particle, which consists of two neutrons and two protons (essentially a $_2^4$He nucleus). In standard notation this is represented as

$$_Z^A X \xrightarrow{\alpha} {}_{Z-2}^{A-4}Y \qquad (2\text{-}8)$$

The α particle is emitted with kinetic energy usually between 4 and 8 MeV. Although quite energetic, α particles have *very* short ranges in solid

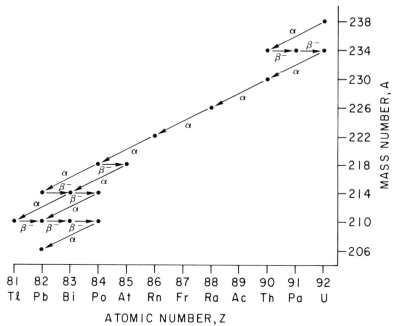

Fig. 2-10.   Illustration of series decay, starting from ^{238}U and ending with stable ^{206}Pb. [Adapted with permission from Hendee WR, Medical Radiation Physics. Chicago, Year Book Medical Publishers, Inc., 1970, p. 501.]

materials—e.g., about 0.03 mm in body tissues. Thus they present very difficult detection and measurement problems.

    Decay by α-particle emission results in a transmutation of elements, but is not isobaric. Atomic mass is decreased by four; therefore this process is common among very heavy elements that must lose mass to achieve nuclear stability. Heavy, naturally occurring radionuclides such as ^{238}U and its daughter products, undergo a series of decays involving α-particle and β$^-$-particle emission to transform into lighter, more stable nuclides. Figure 2-10 illustrates the "decay series" of ^{238}U → ^{206}Pb. The radionuclide ^{226}Ra in this series is of some medical interest, used in encapsulated form for implantation into tumors in radiation therapy. Note that there are "branching points" in the series where either α or β$^-$ emission may occur. Only every fourth atomic number value appears in this series because α emission results in atomic number differences of four units. The ^{238}U → ^{206}Pb series is called the "4n + 2" series. Others are ^{235}U → ^{207}Pb (4n + 3) and ^{232}Th → ^{208}Pb (4n). These three series are found in nature because in each case the parent is a very long-lived radionuclide (half-lives ~ 10^8 − 10^{10} yr) and small amounts remain from the creation of the elements. The fourth series, 4n + 1, is not found naturally because all of its members have much shorter lifetimes and have disappeared from nature.

An (α, γ) radionuclide of interest in nuclear medicine is ^{241}Am. It is used in encapsulated form as a source of 60 keV γ rays (Chapter 17, Section D).

Nuclear fission is the spontaneous fragmentation of a very heavy nucleus into two lighter nuclei. In the process a few (two or three) *fission neutrons* also are ejected. The distribution of nuclear mass between the two product nuclei varies from one decay to the next. Typically it is split in about a 60:40 ratio. The energy released is very large, often amounting to hundreds of MeV per nuclear fission, and is imparted primarily as kinetic energy to the recoiling nuclear fragments *(fission fragments)* and the ejected neutrons. Nuclear fission is the source of energy from nuclear reactors. The fission process is of interest in nuclear medicine because the fission fragment nuclei usually are radioactive, and, if chemically separable from the other products, can be used as medical tracers. Also, the neutrons may be used to produce radioactive materials by neutron activation, as discussed in Chapter 7, Section A.2. The fission nuclides themselves are of no use as tracers in nuclear medicine.

K. DECAY MODES AND THE LINE OF STABILITY

In Chapter 1, Section D.7 it was noted that on a graph of neutron versus proton numbers the stable nuclides tend to be clustered about an imaginary line called the line of stability (Figure 1-7). Nuclides lying off the line of stability generally are radioactive. The type of radioactive decay that occurs usually is such as to move the nucleus closer to the line. A radionuclide that is proton deficient (above the line) usually decays by β^- emission, since this transforms a neutron into a proton, moving the nucleus closer to the line of stability. A neutron-deficient radionuclide (below the line) usually decays by electron capture or β^+ emission, since these modes transform a proton into a neutron. Heavy nuclides frequently decay by α emission or by fission, since these are modes that reduce mass number.

It is also worth noting the β^-, β^+, and EC decay all can transform an "odd-odd" nucleus into an "even-even" nucleus. There are in fact a few "odd-odd" nuclides lying on or near the line of stability that decay both by β^- emission and by electron capture and β^+ emission. An example is ^{40}K (89 percent β^-, 11 percent EC or β^+). In this case, the instability created by odd numbers of protons and neutrons is sufficient to cause decay in both directions *away* from the line of stability; this, however, is an exception rather than the rule.

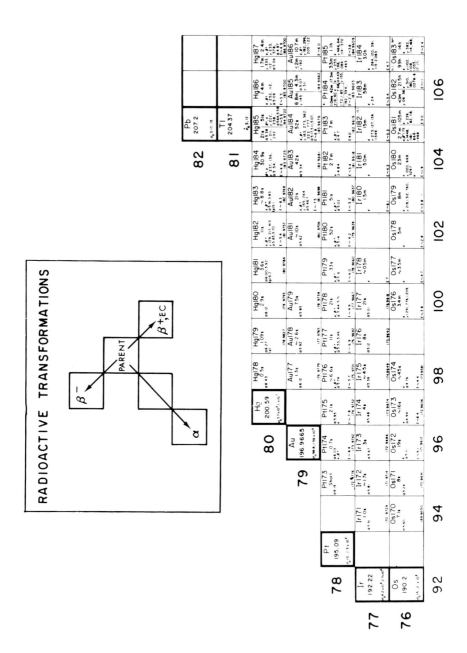

RADIOACTIVE TRANSFORMATIONS

L. SOURCES OF INFORMATION ON RADIONUCLIDES

There are several sources of information providing useful summaries of the properties of radionuclides. One is a chart of the nuclides, a portion of which is shown in Figure 2-11. Every stable or radioactive nuclide is assigned a square on the diagram. Isotopes occupy horizontal rows, and isotones occupy vertical columns. Isobars fall along descending 45° lines. Basic properties of each nuclide are listed in the boxes. Also shown in Figure 2-11 is a diagram indicating the transformations that occur for various decay modes. A chart of the nuclides is particuarly useful for tracing through a radioactive series.

Perhaps the most useful sources of data for radionuclides of interest in nuclear medicine are the MIRD publications, compiled by the Medical Internal Radiation Dosimetry committee of the Society of Nuclear Medicine.[1] Data from these tables for a few of the more important radionuclides are presented in Appendix B. Also presented are basic data for internal dosimetry, which will be discussed in Chapter 10.

REFERENCES

1. Dillman LT, Von der Lage FC: Radionuclide Decay Schemes and Nuclear Parameters for Use in Radiation-Dose Estimation. New York, The Society of Nuclear Medicine, 1975

Additional discussion of the modes of radioactive decay may be found in the following:
Hendee WR: Medical Radiation Physics (ed 2). Chicago, Yearbook Medical, 1979, Chap 2
Lapp RE, Andrews HL: Nuclear Radiation Physics (ed 4). Englewood Cliffs, N.J., Prentice-Hall, 1972, Chap 8
Rollo FD: Radioactivity and properties of nuclear radiation, in Rollo FD (ed): Nuclear Medicine Physics, Instrumentation, and Agents. St. Louis, C. V. Mosby, 1977, Chap 2

Fig. 2-11 (*left*). Portion of a chart of the nuclides. Vertical axis, atomic number; horizontal axis, neutron number. Also listed are atomic weights, thermal neutron capture cross sections (Chapter 7, Section D), half-lives of radioactive nuclides, and other data. [Reprinted by courtesy of Knolls Atomic Power Laboratory, Schenectady. Operated By The General Electric Company For The United States Department Of Energy Naval Reactors Branch.]

3

Decay of Radioactivity

Radioactive decay is a spontaneous process; that is, there is no way to predict with certainty the exact moment at which an unstable nucleus will undergo its radioactive transformation into another, more stable nucleus. Mathematically, radioactive decay is described in terms of probabilities and average decay rates. In this chapter we discuss these mathematical aspects of radioactive decay.

A. ACTIVITY

1. The Decay Constant

If one has a sample containing N radioactive atoms of a certain radionuclide, the average decay rate $\Delta N/\Delta t$ for that sample is given by

$$\Delta N/\Delta t = -\lambda N \qquad (3-1)$$

where λ is the *decay constant* for the radionuclide. The decay constant has a characteristic value for each radionuclide. It is the fraction of the atoms in a sample of that radionuclide undergoing radioactive decay per unit of time during a time period that is so short that only a small fraction decay during that interval. The units of λ are $(time)^{-1}$. Thus $\lambda = 0.01$ sec^{-1} means that, on the average, 1 percent of the atoms undergo radioactive decay each second. In Equation 3-1 the minus sign indicates that $\Delta N/\Delta t$ is negative; that is, N is decreasing with time.

Equation 3-1 is valid only as an estimate of the *average* rate of decay for a radioactive sample. From one moment to the next, the actual decay rate may differ from that predicted by Equation 3-1. These *statistical fluctuations* in decay rate are described in Chapter 6.

Some radionuclides can undergo more than one type of radioactive decay (e.g., ^{18}F: 97 percent β^+, 3 percent EC). For such types of "branching" decay, one can define a value of λ for each of the possible decay modes, e.g., λ_1, λ_2, λ_3, etc., where λ_1 is the fraction decaying per unit time by decay mode 1, λ_2 by decay mode 2, etc. The total decay constant for the radionuclide is sum of the branching decay constants:

$$\lambda = \lambda_1 + \lambda_2 + \lambda_3 + \ldots \qquad (3\text{-}2)$$

2. Definition and Units of Activity

The quantity $\Delta N/\Delta t$, the average decay rate, is the *activity* of the sample. It has dimensions decays per second (dps) or decays per minute (dpm) and is essentially a measure of "how radioactive" the sample is.

The basic unit of activity is the curie (Ci). A sample has an activity of one curie if it is decaying at a rate of 3.7×10^{10} dps (2.22×10^{12} dpm). Subunits and multiples of the curie are the millicurie ($1 \text{ mCi} = 10^{-3}$ Ci), the microcurie ($1 \text{ }\mu\text{Ci} = 10^{-3} \text{ mCi} = 10^{-6}$ Ci), the nanocurie ($1 \text{ nCi} = 10^{-9}$Ci), and the kilocurie ($1 \text{ kCi} = 1000$ Ci). Equation 3-1 may be modified for these units of activity:

$$A(\text{Ci}) = \lambda N/(3.7 \times 10^{10}) \qquad (3\text{-}3)$$

The curie was defined originally as the activity of 1 g of ^{226}Ra; however, this value "changed" from time to time as more accurate measurements of the ^{226}Ra decay rate were obtained. For this reason, the ^{226}Ra standard was abandoned in favor of a fixed value of 3.7×10^{10} dps. This is not too different from the currently accepted value for ^{226}Ra(3.656×10^{10} dps/g).

The SI unit of activity is the *bequerel* (Bq). A sample has an activity of 1 Bq if it decays at a rate of 1 sec^{-1} (one disintegration per second). Thus $1 \text{ Ci} = 3.7 \times 10^{10}$ Bq and $1 \text{ Bq} \approx 0.27 \times 10^{-10}$ Ci. Multiples of the bequerel are the kilobequerel ($1 \text{ kBq} = 10^3 \text{sec}^{-1}$), megabequerel ($1 \text{ MBq} = 10^6 \text{sec}^{-1}$), and gigabequerel ($1 \text{ GBq} = 10^9 \text{sec}^{-1}$). Equation 3-1 with λ in units of sec^{-1} gives sample activity in bequerels.

The transition from traditional to SI units for activity is still in progress in the U.S., and in day-to-day practice traditional units still are more commonly used. For these reasons we use traditional units followed in some cases by SI units in parentheses for illustration purposes. A nomogram is provided in Appendix F to further facilitate translations between traditional and SI units.

The amounts of activity used for nuclear medicine studies typically are in the μCi-mCi (37 kBq-37 MBq) range. Occasionally, Ci (37 GBq) amounts may be acquired for long-term supplies. External beam radiation sources (e.g. ^{60}Co therapy units) utilize kCi (37 × 10^3GBq) source strengths. At the other extreme, the most sensitive measuring systems used in nuclear medicine can detect activities at the nCi (37 Bq) level.

B. EXPONENTIAL DECAY

1. The Decay Factor

With the passage of time, the number N of radioactive atoms in a sample decreases. Therefore the activity A of the sample also decreases (Equation 3-3). Figure 3-1 will be used to illustrate radioactive decay with

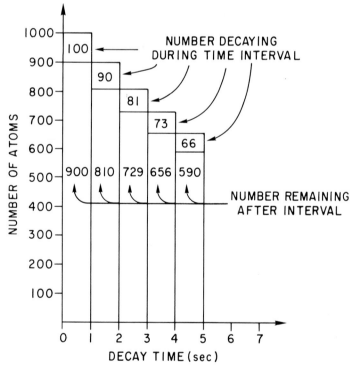

Fig. 3-1.   Decay of radioactive sample during successive 1 sec increments of time, starting with 1000 atoms, for λ = 0.1 sec^{-1}. Both number of atoms remaining and activity (decay rate) decrease with time.

the passage of time. Suppose one starts with a sample containing $N(0) = 1000$ atoms† of a radionuclide having a decay constant $\lambda = 0.1$ sec^{-1}. During the first 1 sec time interval, the approximate number of atoms decaying is $0.1 \times 1000 = 100$ atoms (Equation 3-1). The activity is therefore 100 dps, and after one second there are 900 radioactive atoms remaining. During the next second, the activity is $0.1 \times 900 = 90$ dps, and after two seconds 810 radioactive atoms remain. During the next second the activity is 81 dps, and after three seconds 729 radioactive atoms remain. Thus both the activity and the number of radioactive atoms remaining in the sample are decreasing continuously with time. A graph of either of these quantities is a curve that gradually approaches zero.

An exact mathematical expression for $N(t)$ can be derived using methods of calculus.‡ The result is

$$N(t) = N(0)e^{-\lambda t} \tag{3-4}$$

Thus $N(t)$, the number of atoms remaining after a time t, is equal to $N(0)$, the number of atoms at time $t = 0$, multiplied by the factor $e^{-\lambda t}$. This factor $e^{-\lambda t}$, the fraction of radioactive atoms remaining after a time t, is called the *decay factor* (DF). It is a *number* equal to e—the base of natural logarithms $(2.718. . .)$—raised to the power $-\lambda t$. For given values of λ and t, the decay factor can be determined by various methods as described in Section C. Note that since activity A is proportional to the number of atoms N (Equation 3-3), the decay factor also applies to activity versus time:

$$A(t) = A(0)e^{-\lambda t} \tag{3-5}$$

The decay factor $e^{-\lambda t}$ is an *exponential function* of time t. Exponential decay is characterized by the disappearance of a *constant fraction* of activity or number of atoms present per unit time interval. For example if $\lambda = 0.1$ sec^{-1}, the fraction is 10 percent per second. Graphs of $e^{-\lambda t}$ versus time t for $\lambda = 0.1$ sec^{-1} are shown in Figure 3-2. On linear graph paper, it is a curve gradually approaching zero; on *semilogarithmic* graph paper, it is a straight line. It should be noted that there are other processes besides radioactive decay that can be described by exponential functions. Examples are the absorption of x- and γ-ray beams (Chapter 9, Section B)

---

† $N(t)$ is symbolic notation for the number of atoms present as a function of time t. $N(0)$ is the number N at a specific time $t = 0$, i.e., at the starting point.

‡ The derivation is as follows:

$$dN/dt = -\lambda N \tag{3-4a}$$
$$dN/N = -\lambda dt \tag{3-4b}$$
$$\int dN/N = -\int \lambda dt \tag{3-4c}$$

from which follows Equation 3-4.

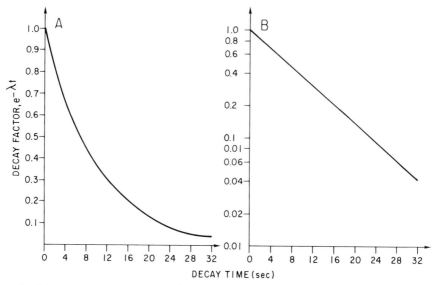

Fig. 3-2. Decay factor versus time shown on (A) linear and (B) semilogarithmic graph paper, for radionuclide with $\lambda = 0.1$ sec^{-1}.

and the clearance of certain tracers from organs by physiologic processes (Chapter 10, Section B.2).

When the exponent in the decay factor is "small," i.e., $\lambda t \lesssim 0.1$, the decay factor may be approximated by $e^{-\lambda t} \approx 1 - \lambda t$. This form may be used as an approximation in Equations 3-4 and 3-5.

2. Half-Life

As indicated in the preceding section, radioactive decay is characterized by the disappearance of a constant fraction of the activity present in the sample during a given time interval. The *half-life* ($T_{1/2}$) of a radionuclide is the time required for it to decay to 50 percent of its initial activity level. The half-life and decay constant of a radionuclide are related as†

---

† The relationships are derived as follows:

$$\tfrac{1}{2} = e^{-\lambda T_{1/2}} \tag{3-6a}$$

$$2 = e^{\lambda T_{1/2}} \tag{3-6b}$$

$$\ln 2 = \lambda T_{1/2} \tag{3-6c}$$

ln2, the natural logarithm of 2, has a value of approximately 0.693, from which follow Equations 3-6 and 3-7.

$$T_{1/2} = 0.693/\lambda \qquad (3\text{-}6)$$

$$\lambda = 0.693/T_{1/2} \qquad (3\text{-}7)$$

Usually, tables or charts of radionuclides list the half-life of the radionuclide rather than its decay constant. Thus it is more convenient to write the decay factor (DF) in terms of half-life rather than decay constant,

$$\mathrm{DF} = e^{-0.693t/T_{1/2}} \qquad (3\text{-}8)$$

3. Average Lifetime

The lifetimes of individual radioactive atoms in a sample range anywhere from "very short" to "very long." Some atoms decay almost immediately, whereas a few do not decay for a relatively long time (Figure 3-2). The *average lifetime* τ of the atoms in a sample has a value that is characteristic of the nuclide and is related to the decay constant λ by†

$$\tau = 1/\lambda \qquad (3\text{-}9)$$

Combining Equations 3-7 and 3-9, one obtains

$$\tau = 1.44T_{1/2} \qquad (3\text{-}10)$$

The average lifetime for the atoms of a radionuclide is therefore somewhat longer than its half-life.

The concept of average lifetime is of importance in radiation dosimetry calculations (Chapter 10, Section B.2).

C. METHODS FOR DETERMINING DECAY FACTORS

1. Tables of Decay Factors

It is essential that an individual working with radionuclides know how to determine decay factors. Perhaps the simplest and most straightforward approach is to use tables of decay factors, which are available

---

† The equation from which Equation 3-9 is derived is

$$\tau = \int_0^\infty e^{-\lambda t}\, dt \left/ \int_0^\infty dt \right. \qquad (3\text{-}9a)$$

Table 3-1
Decay Factors for ^{99m}Tc

Hours	Minutes			
	0	*15*	*30*	*45*
0	1.000	0.972	0.944	0.917
1	0.891	0.866	0.841	0.817
2	0.794	0.771	0.749	0.727
3	0.707	0.687	0.667	0.648
4	0.630	0.612	0.595	0.578
5	0.561	0.545	0.530	0.515
6	0.500	0.486	0.472	0.459
7	0.445	0.433	0.420	0.408
8	0.397	0.385	0.375	0.364
9	0.354	0.343	0.334	0.324
10	0.315	0.306	0.297	0.289
11	0.281	0.273	0.264	0.257
12	0.250	0.243	0.236	0.229

from vendors of radiopharmaceuticals, instrument manufacturers, etc. A sample page from such a table for ^{99m}Tc is shown in Table 3-1.

Example 3-1.
A vial containing ^{99m}Tc is labeled "2 mCi/ml @ 8 a.m." What volume should be withdrawn at 4 p.m. on the same day to prepare an injection of 1.5 mCi for a patient?

Answer.
From Table 3-1 the decay factor for ^{99m}Tc after 8 hours is found to be 0.397. Therefore the concentration of activity in the vial is 0.397 × 2 mCi/ml = 0.794 mCi/ml. The volume required for 1.5 mCi is 1.5 mCi ÷ 0.794 mCi/ml = 1.89 ml.

Tables of decay factors cover only limited time periods; however, they can be extended by employing principles based on the properties of exponential functions (Appendix C). For example, suppose that the desired time t does not appear in the table but that it can be expressed as a sum of times, $t = t_1 + t_2 + \ldots$, that do appear in the table. Then

$$DF(t_1 + t_2 + \ldots) = DF(t_1) \times DF(t_2) \times \ldots \quad (3\text{-}11)$$

Example 3-2.
What is the decay factor for ^{99m}Tc after 16 hours?

Answer.
Express 16 hours as 6 hours + 10 hours. Then, from Table 3-1, DF(16 hr) = DF(10 hr) × DF(6 hr) = 0.315 × 0.5 = 0.1575. Other combinations of times totaling 16 hours will provide the same result.

Occasionally, radionuclides are shipped in *precalibrated* quantities. A precalibrated shipment is one for which the activity calibration is given for some *future* time. To determine its present activity it is therefore necessary to calculate the decay factor for a time preceding the calibration time, i.e., a "negative" value of time. One can make use of tables of decay factors by employing another of the properties of exponential functions (Appendix C).

$$DF(-t) = 1/DF(t) \qquad (3\text{-}12)$$

Example 3-3.
A vial containing ^{99m}Tc is labeled "3 mCi @ 3 p.m." What is the activity at 8 a.m. on the same day?

Answer.
The decay time is $t = -7$ hours. From Table 3-1, DF(7 hr) = 0.445. Thus DF(−7 hr) = 1/0.445 = 2.247. The activity at 8 a.m. is therefore 2.247 × 3 mCi = 6.741 mCi.

2. Tables of Exponential Functions

Decay factors also can be determined by the use of tables of exponential functions. These are found in mathematical and scientific reference books, e.g., *The Handbook of Chemistry and Physics*. An abbreviated table is provided in Appendix C. To use these tables, one must first determine the value of the exponent $(0.693t/T_{1/2})$ in the decay factor and locate this value under the column labeled x in the table of exponential functions. The decay factor is then found under the column e^{-x} for positive values of time or under the column e^{+x} for "negative" values of time (i.e., precalibrated shipments). Linear interpolation is sufficiently accurate for values of x between those listed in the table. The table can be extended using the rules for exponential functions discussed in Section C.1 (Equations 3-11 and 3-12).

Many pocket calculators have capabilities for calculating exponential functions. The same rules as outlined above are used. First compute the exponent, $x = (0.693t/T_{1/2})$, then press the appropriate keys to obtain e^{-x}.

Example 3-4.
Use tables of exponential functions or a pocket calculator to determine the decay factor after 8 hours for ^{99m}Tc.

Answer.
The half-life of ^{99m}Tc is 6 hours. Therefore the exponent in the decay factor is $(0.693 \times 8/6) = 0.924$. From the table in Appendix C, for $x = 0.92$, $e^{-x} = 0.399$, and for $x = 0.94$, $e^{-x} = 0.391$. Interpolating between these values, one obtains DF(8 hr) ≈ 0.397. (Compare to Example 3-1; the answers agree within the limits of accuracy of the tables used.)

3. Graphical Methods

Exponential functions are straight lines on semilogarithmic graph paper (Figure 3-2). This useful property allows one to construct a "universal" decay curve on a sheet of semilogarithmic graph paper. The horizontal (linear) axis is labeled in terms of number of half-lives elapsed and the vertical (logarithmic) axis is labeled in terms of the decay factor. A straight line can be drawn by connecting any two points on the curve. These could be, for example, $(t = 0$, DF $= 1.0)$; $(t = T_{1/2}$, DF $= 0.5)$, $(t = 2T_{1/2}$, DF $= 0.25)$, etc. The graph can be used for any radionuclide provided that the elapsed time is expressed in terms of number of radionuclide half-lives elapsed. An example of a universal decay curve is shown in Figure 3-3.

Example 3-5.
Use the decay curve in Figure 3-3 to determine the decay factor for ^{99m}Tc after 8 hours.

Answer.
The half-life of ^{99m}Tc is 6 hours. Therefore the elapsed time is $8/6 = 1.33$ half-lives. From Figure 3-3, the decay factor is approximately 0.40. (Compare to Examples 3-1 and 3-4.)

D. SPECIFIC ACTIVITY

A radioactive sample may contain stable isotopes of the element represented by the radionuclide of interest. For example, a given ^{131}I sample may also contain the stable isotope ^{127}I. When stable isotopes of the radionuclide of interest are present in the sample, they are called *carrier,* and the sample is said to be *with carrier.* A sample that does not

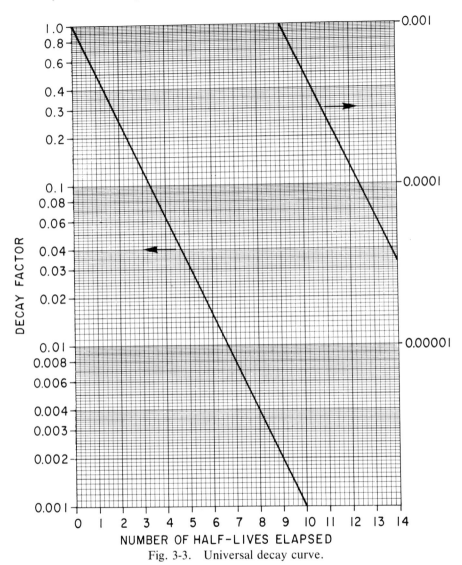

Fig. 3-3.   Universal decay curve.

contain stable isotopes of the element represented by the radionuclide is called *carrier-free*. Radionuclides may be produced carrier-free or with carrier, depending on the production method (Chapter 7).

The radio of radioisotope activity to total mass of the element present is called the *specific activity* of the sample. Specific activity has units of Ci/g, μCi/g, etc. The highest possible specific activity of a radionuclide is its *carrier-free specific activity* (CFSA). This can be calculated in a straightforward manner from the basic properties of the radionuclide.

Suppose a carrier-free sample contains 1 g of a radionuclide ^{A}X, having a half-life $T_{1/2}$ (sec). The atomic weight of the radionuclide is approximately equal to A, its mass number (Chapter 1, Section A.2). A sample containing A g of the radionuclide has approximately 6.023×10^{23} atoms (Avogadro's number); therefore a 1-g sample has $N \approx 6.023 \times 10^{23}/A$ atoms. The decay rate of the sample is $\Delta N/\Delta t$ (dps) $= \lambda N = 0.693 N/T_{1/2}$. Therefore its activity is

$$A(\text{Ci}) \approx (0.693 \times 6.023 \times 10^{23})/(A \times T_{1/2} \times 3.7 \times 10^{10}) \quad (3\text{-}13)$$

Since the sample contains 1 g of the radioisotope, this is also its specific activity in Ci/g. When the equation is normalized for the half-life in days (1 day = 86,400 sec), the result is

$$\text{CFSA (Ci/g)} \approx 1.3 \times 10^{8}/(AT_{1/2}) \quad (3\text{-}14)$$

where $T_{1/2}$ is given in days. Equation 3-14 also applies for specific activity in mCi/mg of μCi/μg.

In SI units, the equation for carrier-free specific activity is

$$\text{CFSA(Bq/g)} \approx 4.8 \times 10^{18}/AT_{1/2} \quad (3\text{-}15)$$

where $T_{1/2}$ again is in days.

Example 3-7.
What are the carrier-free specific activities of ^{131}I and ^{99m}Tc?

Answer.
For ^{131}I, $A = 131$ and $T_{1/2} = 8$ days. Using Equation 3-15,
$$\text{CFSA}(^{131}\text{I}) \approx (1.3 \times 10^{8})/(1.31 \times 10^{2} \times 8)$$
$$\approx 1.24 \times 10^{5} \text{ Ci/g}$$

For ^{99m}Tc, $A = 99$ and $T_{1/2} = 6$ hours $= 0.25$ days. Thus
$$\text{CFSA }(^{99m}\text{Tc}) \approx (1.3 \times 10^{8})/(0.99 \times 10^{2} \times 0.25)$$
$$\approx 5.3 \times 10^{6} \text{ Ci/g}$$

In SI units (Equation 3-15) the answers are
$$\text{CFSA}(^{131}\text{I}) \approx 4.8 \times 10^{18}/(1.31 \times 10^{2} \times 8)$$
$$\approx 4.6 \times 10^{15} \text{ Bq/g}$$
$$\text{CFSA}(^{99m}\text{Tc}) \approx 4.8 \times 10^{18}/(0.99 \times 10^{2} \times 0.25)$$
$$\approx 1.94 \times 10^{17} \text{ Bq/g}$$

Carrier-free specific activities for radionuclides having half-lives of days or weeks are very high. Most of the radionuclides used in nuclear medicine are in this category.

In most instances, a high specific activity is desirable because then a moderate amount of activity contains only a very small mass of the element represented by the radioisotope and can be administered to a patient without causing a pharmacologic response to that element. This is an essential requirement of a "tracer study." For example, a capsule containing 10μCi ($\sim$0.4MBq) of carrier-free ^{131}I contains only about 10^{-10} g of elemental iodine (mass = activity/specific activity), which is well below the amount necessary to cause any "iodine reaction." Even radionuclides of highly toxic elements, such as arsenic, have been given to patients in a carrier-free state. It is not possible to obtain carrier-free ^{99m}Tc because it cannot be separated from its daughter product, ^{99}Tc, a very long-lived and essentially stable isotope of technetium. Nevertheless, the mass of technetium in most ^{99m}Tc preparations is very small and has no physiological impact when administered to a patient.

Not all production methods result in carrier-free radionuclides. Also, in some cases carrier may be added to promote certain chemical reactions in radiochemistry procedures. When a preparation is supplied with carrier, usually the packaging material indicates specific activity. If the radioactivity exists as a label attached to some complex molecule, e.g., a protein molecule, the specific activity may be expressed in terms of the activity per unit mass of labeled substance, e.g., Ci/g protein. Specific activities of labeled compounds are sometimes expressed in dps/g of labeled material. Methods of calculating the specific activities of radionuclides produced in a non-carrier-free state are discussed in Chapter 7.

Radioactive preparations that are not carrier-free or that are attached as labels to complex molecules may present problems if the carrier or labeled molecule is toxic or has undesired pharmacologic effects. Two examples are ^{42}K in K^+ solution (intravenous K^+ injections may cause cardiac arrhythmia) and ^{131}I-labeled serum albumin (serum albumin may cause undesirably high protein levels when injected into intrathecal spaces for CSF studies). In situations such as these, the amount of material that can be administered safely to a patient may be limited by the amount of carrier or labeled molecule present rather than by the amount of radioactivity and associated radiation hazards.

E. DECAY OF A MIXED RADIONUCLIDE SAMPLE

The equations and methods presented in Sections B and C apply only to samples containing a single radionuclide species. When a sample contains a mixture of *unrelated* species (i.e., no parent–daughter relation-

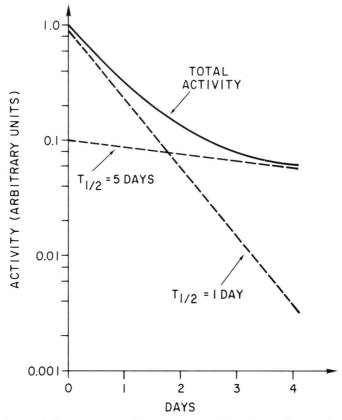

Fig. 3-4.   Activity versus time for a mixed sample of two radionuclides. Sample
contains initially ($t = 0$) 0.9 units of activity with half-life of 1 day and 0.1 units
of activity with half-life of 5 days.

ships) the total activity A_t is just the sum of the individual activities of the
various species:

$$A_t(t) = A_1(0)e^{-0.693t/T_{1/2,1}} + A_2(0)e^{-0.693t/T_{1/2,2}} + \dots \qquad (3\text{-}16)$$

where $A_1(0)$ is the initial activity of the first species and $T_{1/2,1}$ is its
half-life, and so forth.

Figure 3-4 shows total activity versus time for a sample containing
two unrelated radionuclides. A characteristic of such a curve is that it
always assumes eventually the slope of the curve for the radionuclide
having the longest half-life. Once the final slope has been established it
can be extrapolated as a straight line on semilogarithmic graph paper back

to time zero. This curve can then be subtracted from the total curve to give the net curve for the other radionuclides present. If more than two radionuclide species are present, the "curve stripping" operation can be repeated for the next-longest-lived species and so forth.

Curve stripping can be used to determine the relative amounts of various radionuclides present in a mixed sample, and their half-lives. It is especially useful for detecting and quantifying long-lived contaminants in radioactive preparations (e.g., ^{99}Mo in ^{99m}Tc).

F. PARENT-DAUGHTER DECAY

1. The Bateman Equations

A more complicated situation occurs when a sample contains radionuclides having parent-daughter relationships (Figure 3-5). The equation for the activity of the parent is simply that for a single radionuclide species (Equation 3-5), however, the equation for the activity of a daughter is complicated by the fact that the daughter product is being formed (by decay of the parent) at the same time it is decaying. The equation is†

$$A_d(t) = A_p(0) \frac{\lambda_d}{\lambda_d - \lambda_p} (e^{-\lambda_p t} - e^{-\lambda_d t}) + A_d(0)e^{-\lambda_d t} \qquad (3\text{-}17)$$

----

† The differential equations from which Equation 3-17 is derived are

$$dN_p/dt = -\lambda_p N_p \qquad (3\text{-}17a)$$
$$dN_d/dt = -\lambda_d N_d + \lambda_p N_p \qquad (3\text{-}17b)$$

These equations provide

$$N_d(t) = N_p(0) \frac{\lambda_p}{\lambda_d - \lambda_p} (e^{-\lambda_p t} - e^{-\lambda_d t}) + N_d(0)e^{-\lambda_d t} \qquad (3\text{-}17c)$$

Multiplying Equation 3-17c by λ_d and substituting $A_d = \lambda_d N_d$, $A_p = \lambda_p N_p$, one obtains Equation 3-17.

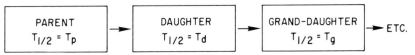

Fig. 3-5. Schematic representation of series decay. Activities of daughter, granddaughter, etc. are described by the Bateman equations.

where A_p and A_d are the activities of the parent and daughter radionuclides, respectively, and λ_p and λ_d are their respective decay constants. The second term, $A_d(0)e^{-\lambda_d t}$, in Equation 3-17 is just the residual daughter product activity remaining from any that might have been present at the starting time, $t = 0$. In the rest of this discussion, it will be assumed that $A_d(0) = 0$, and only the first term in Equation 3-17 will be considered.

Equation 3-17 is the *Bateman equation* for a simple parent–daughter mixture. Bateman equations for sequences of three or more radionuclides in a sequential decay scheme are found in other texts.[1] Equation 3-17 will be analyzed for three general situations.†

2. Secular Equilibrium

The first situation applies when the half-life of the parent, T_p, is so long that the decrease of parent activity is negligible over the course of the observation period. An example is ^{226}Ra $(T_p = 1620$ yr$) \rightarrow {}^{222}$Rn $(T_d = 4.8$ days). In this case, $\lambda_p \approx 0$; thus Equation 3-17 can be written

$$A_d(t) \approx A_p(0)(1 - e^{-\lambda_d t}) \qquad (3\text{-}18)$$

Figure 3-6 illustrates the buildup of daughter product activity versus time. After one daughter product half-life, $e^{-\lambda_d t} = \frac{1}{2}$ and $A_d \approx \frac{1}{2}A_p$. After two half-lives, $A_d \approx \frac{3}{4}A_p$, and so forth. After a "very long" time, $e^{-\lambda_d t} \approx 0$, and the activity of the daughter equals that of the parent. When this occurs $(A_d \approx A_p)$ the parent and daughter are said to be in *secular equilibrium*.

3. Transient Equilibrium

The second situation occurs when the parent half-life is longer than the daughter half-life, but is not "infinite." An example of this case is ^{99}Mo $(T_{1/2} = 66$ hr$) \rightarrow {}^{99m}$Tc $(T_{1/2} = 6$ hr$)$. When there is a significant decrease in parent activity over the course of the observation period, one can no longer assume $\lambda_p \approx 0$, and Equation 3-17 cannot be simplified. Figure 3-7 shows the buildup and decay of daughter product activity for a hypothetical parent-daughter pair with $T_p = 10T_d$. The activity increases and eventually exceeds that of the parent, reaches a maximum

---

† An unusual situation occurs when $\lambda_p = \lambda_d = \lambda$, i.e., parent and daughter have the same half-life. In this case, Equation 3-17 reduces to

$$A_d(t) = A_p(0)te^{-\lambda t} + A_d(0)e^{-\lambda t} \qquad (3\text{-}17d)$$

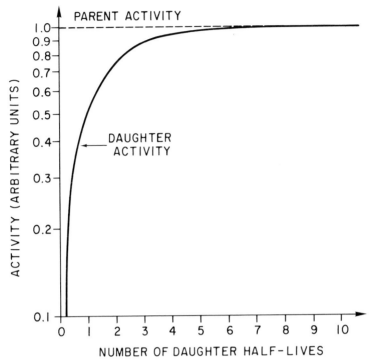

Fig. 3-6. Buildup of daughter activity when $T_d \ll T_p \approx \infty$. Eventually, secular equilibrium is achieved.

value, and then decreases and follows the decay of the parent. When this stage of "parallel" decay rates has been reached—i.e., parent and daughter activities decreasing but *ratio* of parent to daughter activities constant—the parent and daughter are said to be in *transient equilibrium*. The ratio of daughter activity to parent activity in transient equilibrium is

$$A_d/A_p = T_p/(T_p - T_d) \tag{3-19}$$

The time at which maximum daughter activity is available is determined using the methods of calculus† with the result

$$t_{max} = [1.44 T_p T_d/(T_p - T_d)] \ln(T_p/T_d) \tag{3-20}$$

where T_p and T_d are the half-lives of the parent and daughter, respectively.

† Set $dA_d/dt = 0$ and solve for t_{max}.

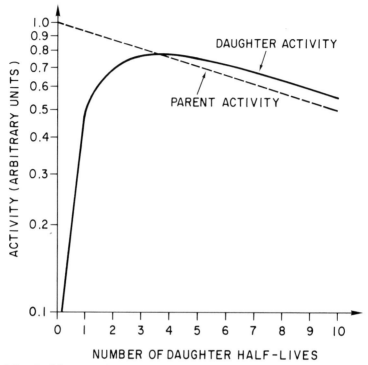

Fig. 3-7.   Buildup and decay of activity for $T_p = 10T_d$. Eventually, transient equilibrium is achieved when parent and daughter decay curves are parallel.

Figure 3-7 is similar to that for ^{99}Mo ($T_p = 66$ hr) $\rightarrow$ ^{99m}Tc ($T_d = 6$ hr); however, the time-activity curve for ^{99m}Tc is complicated by the fact that only a fraction (0.924) of the parent ^{99}Mo atoms decay to ^{99m}Tc. The remainder bypass the ^{99m}Tc metastable state and decay to the ground state of ^{99m}Tc. Thus the ^{99m}Tc activity is given by Equation 3-17 multiplied by 0.924 and the ratio of ^{99m}Tc/^{99}Mo activity in transient equilibrium by Equation 3-19 multiplied by the same factor; however, t_{max} remains as given by Equation 3-20.

4. No Equilibrium

When the daughter half-life is longer than the parent half-life, there is no equilibrium between them. An example of this combination is ^{131m}Te ($T_{1/2} = 30$ hr) $\rightarrow$ ^{131}I ($T_{1/2} = 8$ days). Figure 3-8 shows the buildup and decay of the daughter product activity for a hypothetical parent-daughter pair with $T_p = 1/10T_d$. It increases, reaches a maximum (Equation 3-20 still applies for t_{max}), and then decreases. Eventually, when the parent

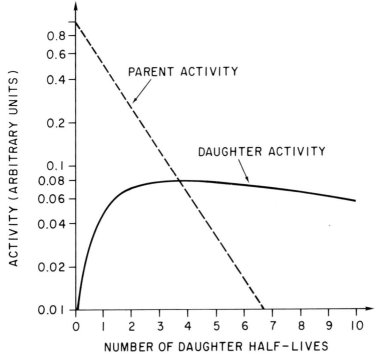

Fig. 3-8.   Buildup and decay of activity for $T_p = 1/10\ T_d$. There is no equilibrium relationship established between the parent and daughter decay curves.

activity is essentially zero, the remaining daughter activity decays with its own characteristic half-life.

REFERENCES

1.   Lapp RE, Andrews HL: Nuclear Radiation Physics (ed 4). Englewood Cliffs, N.J., Prentice-Hall, 1972, pp 189–191

4

Radiation Detectors

When radiations from a radioactive material pass through matter, they interact with atoms and molecules and transfer energy to them. The transfer of energy has two effects: *ionization* and *excitation*. Ionization occurs when the energy transferred is sufficient to cause an orbital electron to be stripped away from its parent atom or molecule, thus creating an *ion pair* (a negatively charged electron and a positively charged atom or molecule). Excitation occurs when electrons are perturbed from their normal arrangement in an atom or molecule, thus creating an atom or molecule in an *excited state*. Both of these processes are involved in the detection of radiation events; however, ionization is the primary event, and hence the term "ionizing radiation" is used frequently when referring to the emissions from radioactive material. Radiation interactions are discussed in detail in Chapters 8 and 9. In this chapter, we describe the basic principles of radiation detectors used in nuclear medicine.

A. GAS-FILLED DETECTORS

1. Basic Principles

Most gas-filled detectors belong to a class of detectors called *ionization detectors*. These detectors respond to radiation by means of ionization-induced electrical currents. The basic principles are illustrated in Figure 4-1. A volume of gas is contained between two electrodes having

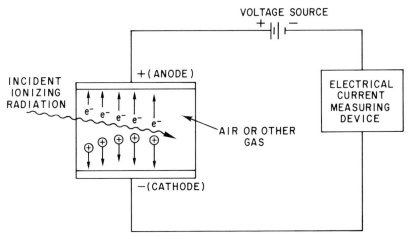

Fig. 4-1. Basic principles of a gas-filled detector. Electrical charge liberated by ionizing radiation is collected by positive and negative electrodes.

a voltage difference (and thus an electric field) between them. The negative electrode is called the *cathode*, the positive electrode the *anode*. The electrodes are shown as parallel plates, but they may be a pair of wires, concentric cylinders, etc. Under normal circumstances, the gas is an insulator and no electrical current flows between the electrodes; however, when the gas is ionized—e.g., by radiations from a radioactive material—the electrons are attracted to the positive electrode and ionized atoms to the negative electrode, causing a momentary flow of a small amount of electrical current.

Gas-filled detectors include *ionization chambers, proportional counters,* and *Geiger–Müller (GM) counters.* The use of these detectors in nuclear medicine is somewhat limited because their stopping power and detection efficiency for x and γ rays is quite low; however, they find some use for applications in which detection efficiency is not a major factor, and for detection and measurement of nonpenetrating, particle-type radiations. Some of their applications are discussed in Chapters 14 and 23.

2. Ionization Chambers

In most ionization chambers, the gas between the electrodes is air. The chamber may or may not be sealed from the atmosphere. Many different designs have been used for the electrodes in an ionization chamber, but usually they consist of a wire inside of a cylinder, or a pair of concentric cylinders.

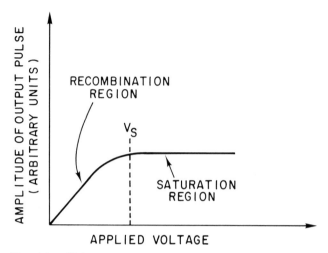

Fig. 4-2. Voltage response curve (charge collected versus voltage applied to the electrodes) for a typical ionization chamber. In usual operation, applied voltage exceeds saturation voltage V_s to ensure complete collection of liberated charge.

For maximum efficiency of operation, the voltage between the electrodes must be sufficient to ensure complete collection of ions and electrons produced by radiation within the chamber. If the voltage is too low, some of the ions and electrons simply recombine with one another without contributing to electrical current flow. Figure 4-2 shows the effect of voltage difference between the electrodes on the electrical current recorded by an ionization chamber per ionizing radiation event detected. Recombination occurs at low voltages (*recombination region* of the curve). As the voltage increases there is less recombination, and the response (electrical current) increases. When the voltage becomes sufficient to cause complete collection of all of the charges produced, the curve enters a plateau called the *saturation region*. The voltage at which the saturation region begins is called the *saturation voltage*, V_s. Typically, $V_s \approx$ 50–300 volts, depending on the design of the chamber. Ionization chambers are operated at voltages in the saturation region. This ensures a maximum response to radiation and also that the response will be relatively insensitive to instabilities in the voltage applied to the electrodes.

The amount of electrical charge released in an ionization chamber by a single ionizing radiation event is very small. For example, the energy

expended in producing a single ionization event in air is about 34 eV.†
Thus a 1 MeV β particle, for example, causes about $(10^6/34) \approx 3 \times 10^4$
ionizations and releases a total amount of electrical charge of only about
3×10^{-15} coulombs.

Because of the small amount of electrical charge or current involved,
ionization chambers generally are not used to record or count individual
radiation events. Instead, the total amount of current passing through the
chamber caused by a beam of radiation is measured. Alternatively, the
electrical charge released in the chamber by the radiation beam may be
collected and measured.

Small amounts of electrical current are measured using sensitive
current-measuring devices called *electrometers*. Two devices consisting
of ionization chambers and electrometers in nuclear medicine are *survey
meters* and *dose calibrators*. A typical ionization chamber survey meter is
shown in Figure 4-3. The survey meter is battery-operated and portable.
The ionization chamber consists of an outer cylindrical electrode (metal
or graphite-coated plastic) with a wire electrode running down its center.
A protective cap on the end of the chamber is left in place for most
measurements; however it is removed for measurement of nonpenetrating
radiations such as α particles, β particles, and low-energy (≤10 keV)
photons. Ionization current is displayed on a front-panel meter. Usually
the meter is calibrated to read *exposure rate* (R/hr or mR/hr; Chapter 23,
Section A.3). Survey meters are used to monitor radiation levels for
radiation protection purposes (Chapter 23, Section E). A typical survey
meter can measure exposure rates down to about 1 mR/hr.

Dose calibrators are used to assay activity levels in syringes, vials,
etc. containing materials that are to be administered to patients. Unlike
the other types of ionization chambers discussed in this section, dose
calibrators generally have sealed chambers. Dose calibrators are discussed in detail in Chapter 14, Section C.1.

A device that records total charge collected over a period of time is
the *pocket dosimeter*. The basic principles are illustrated in Figure 4-4.
The ionization chamber electrodes are a central charging electrode and
the outside case of the dosimeter. They are insulated electrically from one
another, and they form an electrical capacitor. The capacitor is first
charged to a reference voltage V by connecting the charging rod to a
separate charging unit. If the capacitance between the charging electrode

---

† The average energy expended in producing a single ionization event is symbolized by
W. This is not the same as the average energy required to ionize an air molecule, but is the
average energy expended per ionization by the ionizing particle, including both ionization
and excitation effects. This is discussed in detail in Chapter 8, Section A.4. Values of W for
some detector materials are listed in Table 4-1.

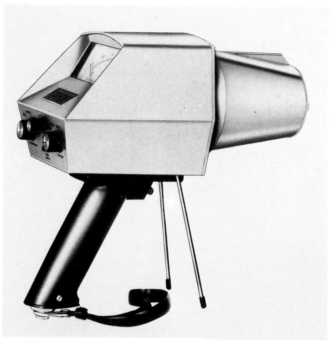

Fig. 4-3.   Radiation survey meter employing an ionization chamber detector. Voltage source is provided by batteries. Meter at left indicates radiation level. Switches are used to select different scale factors. The ion chamber at right is covered by a protective cap that can be removed to detect radiations with low penetrating power. [Courtesy Victoreen Instruments.]

and the case is C, the charge stored on the capacitor is $Q = V \times C$. When the chamber is exposed to radiation, electrical charge ΔQ is collected by the electrodes, discharging the capacitor. The voltage change across the capacitor is measured and is related to the amount of electrical charge collected by the ionization chamber electrodes ($\Delta Q = \Delta V \times C$).

Pocket dosimeters are used in nuclear medicine to monitor radiation

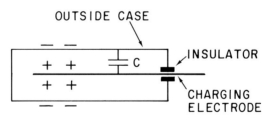

Fig. 4-4.   Schematic representation of a pocket dosimeter.

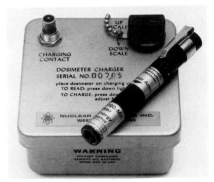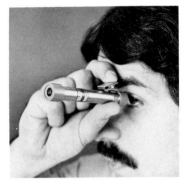

Fig. 4-5. Left: Pocket dosimeter with charging system. Right: Technique for reading pocket dosimeter. [Courtesy Victoreen Instruments.]

levels for radiation protection purposes. A typical system is shown in Figure 4-5. The ionization chamber is contained in a small metal or plastic cylinder (~1.5 cm diam × 10 cm long) that can be clipped to a shirt pocket or collar. Electrodes recessed into one end of the chamber are used to connect the dosimeter to a separate charger unit to charge up the capacitor to the reference voltage. Voltage on the capacitor causes a fine wire within the chamber to be deflected. The position of the wire changes as the voltage on the capacitor changes. The wire is observed through a viewing window at one end of the chamber. Its position is read against a scale that has been calibrated in terms of the total radiation recorded by the chamber, usually in R or mR of exposure (Chapter 23, Section A.3). Pocket dosimeters are suitable for measuring radiation exposures down to about 10 mR to an accuracy of about 20 percent.

A basic problem with ionization chambers is that they are quite inefficient as detectors for x and γ rays. Only a very small percentage (<1 percent) of x or γ rays passing through the chamber actually interact with and cause ionization of air molecules. Indeed, most of the electrical charge released in an ionization chamber by photon radiations comes from secondary electrons knocked loose from the walls of the chamber by the incident radiations rather than by direct ionization of air molecules. The relatively low detection efficiency of ionization chambers is not a serious limitation in the applications described above.

Two additional problems with ionization chambers should be noted. The first is that for x and γ rays, their response changes with photon energy because photon absorption in the gas volume and in the chamber walls (i.e., detection efficiency) and relative penetration of photons through the chamber walls are both energy-dependent processes. Figure 4-6 shows a typical energy-response curve for a survey meter. A second

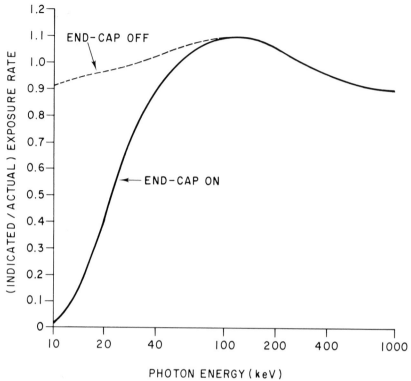

Fig. 4-6.   Energy response curve for a typical ionization chamber survey meter having a removable protective end cap.

problem is that in *unsealed* chambers the density of the air in the chamber, and hence its absorption efficiency, changes with atmospheric pressure ($\rho \propto P$) and temperature ($\rho \propto 1/T$). Most chambers are calibrated to read accurately at sea-level pressure ($P_{ref} = 1.013 N/m^2 = 760$ mm Hg) and average room temperature ($T_{ref} = 22°C = 295°K$). For other temperatures T and pressures P the chamber reading must be corrected (multiplied) by a temperature–pressure correction factor

$$C_{TP} = (P_{ref} \times T) / (P \times T_{ref}) \qquad (4\text{-}1)$$

Temperature must be expressed on the Kelvin scale in this equation ($°K = °C + 273$). The correction is significant in some cases, e.g., at higher elevations ($P \approx 0.85 N/m^2 \approx 640$ mmHg at 1600 meter elevation). Note that temperature–pressure corrections are *not* required with sealed chambers, e.g., most dose calibrators. A defective seal on such an instrument obviously could lead to erroneous readings.

3. Proportional Counters

In an ionization chamber, the voltage between the electrodes is sufficient only to collect those charges liberated by direct action of the ionizing radiations; however, if the voltage is increased to a sufficiently high value, the electrons liberated by radiation gain such high velocities and energies when accelerated toward the positive electrode that they cause additional ionization. This process is called *gas amplification* of charge. The factor by which ionization is increased is called the *gas amplification factor*. This factor increases rapidly with applied voltage, as shown in Figure 4-7. The gas amplification factor may be as high as 10^6, depending on the chamber design and the applied voltage.

Detectors that operate in the ascending portion of the curve shown in Figure 4-7 are called *proportional counters*. In this region, the ionization caused by an incident radiation event is multiplied (amplified) by the gas amplification factor. The total amount of charge produced is equal to the number of ionizations caused by the primary radiation event (at 34 eV/ionization in air) multiplied by the gas amplification factor. Thus the total charge produced is proportional to the total amount of energy deposited in the detector by the detected radiation event.

Actually, proportional counters are not simply ionization chambers operated at high voltages, but are specially constructed chambers designed to optimize the gas amplification effect. A typical design is

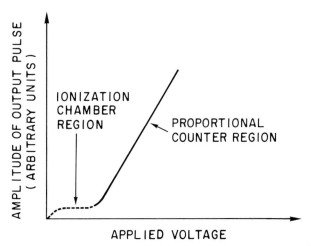

Fig. 4-7. Voltage response curve for a proportional counter. With increasing applied voltage, charge collected increases because of gas amplification effect.

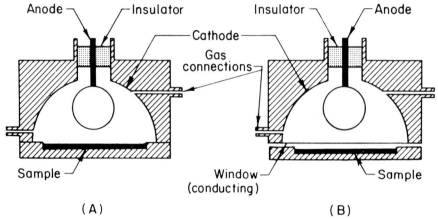

Fig. 4-8.   Typical proportional counter designs. Special gas mixtures for proportional counters are introduced through the gas connections. (A) Sample is placed directly within counting chamber ("windowless" chamber). (B) Sample is separated from counting chamber by a thin radiation entrance window. [From Robinson CV: Geiger-Müller and proportional counters, in Hine GJ (ed): Instrumentation in Nuclear Medicine (vol 1). New York, Academic Press, 1967, p 66. Used by permission of author and Academic Press.]

illustrated in Figure 4-8. The wire loop is the anode around which the gas amplification occurs. In the example shown in Figure 4-8A, the sample is actually placed inside the counter chamber ("windowless" chamber), whereas in Figure 4-8B it is separated from the chamber volume by a thin radiation entrance window. Proportional counters are filled with special gas mixtures, e.g., 90 percent argon and 10 percent methane, or xenon at high pressure.

The major advantage of proportional counters over ionization chambers is that the size of the electrical signal produced by an individual ionizing radiation event is much larger. They are, in fact, useful for detecting and *counting* individual radiation events. Furthermore, since the size of an individual current pulse is proportional to the amount of energy deposited by the radiation event in the detector, proportional counters can be used for energy-sensitive counting, i.e., to discriminate between radiation events of different energies on the basis of electrical pulse size (Chapter 11). They are still inefficient detectors for x and γ rays, however. Consequently, they find very limited use in nuclear medicine. Proportional counters are used mostly in research applications for measuring nonpenetrating radiations such as α particles and β particles. Some applications are discussed in Chapter 14, Section C.2.

4. Geiger–Müller Counters

A *Geiger–Müller counter* (or GM counter) is a gas-filled detector designed for maximum gas amplification effect. The principles of a GM counter are shown in Figure 4-9. The center wire (anode) is maintained at a high positive voltage relative to the outer cylindrical electrode (cathode). The outer electrode may be a metal cylinder or a metallic film sprayed on the inside of a glass or plastic tube. Some GM counters have a thin radiation *entrance window* at one end of the tube. The cylinder or tube is sealed and filled with a special gas mixture, typically argon plus a quenching gas (discussed below).

When ionization occurs in a GM counter, electrons are accelerated toward the center wire. Gas amplification occurs in the GM counter as in a proportional counter. In addition, when electrons strike the center wire, they do so with such energy that ultraviolet (UV) photons are emitted. Some of the UV photons travel to and liberate additional electrons from the outer wall of the chamber. These electrons are accelerated toward the center wire, where they cause more UV radiation to be emitted, and so forth (Figure 4-9). In this way, an *avalanche ionization* is propagated throughout the gas volume and along the entire length of the center wire.

As the avalanche progresses, the electrons, being relatively light, are quickly collected, but the heavy, slow-moving positive ions are not. Eventually, a "hose" of slow-moving positive charges is formed around

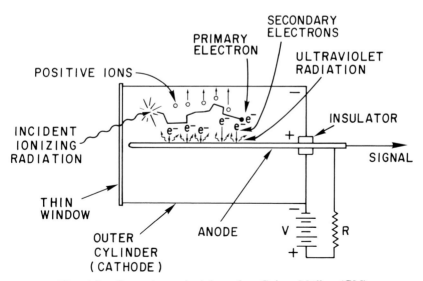

Fig. 4-9. Operating principles of a Geiger-Müller (GM) counter.

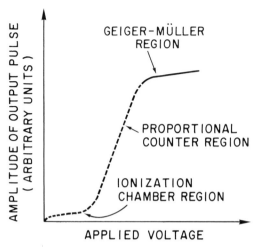

Fig. 4-10. Voltage response curve (pulse amplitude versus applied voltage) for a GM counter.

the center wire. The avalanche then terminates because electrons in this region find themselve in a heavy cloud of positive ions and are captured by them before they reach the center wire.

The avalanche ionization in a GM tube releases a large and essentially constant quantity of electrical charge, regardless of voltage applied to the tube (Figure 4-10) and the energy of the ionizing radiation event. (The gas amplification factor may be as high as 10^{10}.) The large electrical signal is easily detected with electronic circuits. Thus a GM counter, like a proportional counter, can be used to detect and count individual ionizating radiation events; however, because the size of the electrical signal output is constant, regardless of the energy of the radiation detected, a GM counter cannot be used to distinguish between radiation events of different energies.

Once the avalanche has terminated in a GM counter, an additional problem arises. The positive ion cloud moves toward the outer electrode. When the ion cloud is very close to the outer electrode, electrons are pulled out from it to neutralize the positive ions. Some of these electrons enter higher-energy orbits of the positive ions; when they eventually drop into the lower-energy orbits, UV radiation is emitted. This can cause the release of more electrons from the outer wall and set off another avalanche. Thus if no precautions are taken, a single ionizing radiation event causes the GM counter to go into a pulsating series of discharges. This is prevented by a process known as *quenching*.

In an older and now virtually obsolete technique, quenching was accomplished electrically by momentarily reducing the voltage between the counter electrodes when the counting electronics first sensed that an avalanche had occurred. The voltage was reduced to a point where it was insufficient to sustain a second avalanche, even if additional ionizations were to occur (see below, Figure 4-11). The reduced voltage was maintained until the positive ion cloud had been neutralized, typically in a few tenths of a millisecond. Normal voltage was then restored and the detector was ready for the next radiation event.

A more practical solution is to introduce a *quenching gas* into the counter gas mixture. Such GM counters are called *self-quenched*. Effective quenching gases have three properties: First, they tend to give up electrons easily. When the positive ion cloud is formed, molecules of the quenching gas neutralize other ions by donating electrons to them. The ion cloud is thus converted into ionized molecules of quenching gas. Second, when the quenching gas molecules are neutralized by electrons entering higher-energy orbits, they deenergize themselves by dissociating into molecular fragments rather than by emitting UV photons. Third, the quenching gas molecules are strong absorbers of UV radiation. Thus the few UV photons that are released during neutralization of the positive ion cloud are quickly absorbed before they can set off another avalanche.

Commonly used quenching gases include heavy organic vapors (e.g., alcohol) and halogen gases (e.g., Cl_2). The organic vapors are more effective quenching agents but have the disadvantage that their molecular fragments do not recombine after dissociation. Thus an organic quenching gas eventually is used up, typically after about 10^{10} radiations have been detected. Halogen gas molecules recombine after dissociation and thus have an essentially unlimited lifetime in a GM counter.

A certain minimum voltage is required between the electrodes of a GM counter to sustain an avalanche ionization. This voltage can be determined by exposing the GM counter to a constant source of radiation and observing the counting rate as a function of voltage applied to the counter electrodes. Figure 4-11 shows the results of such an experiment. This curve is called the *voltage characteristic* of the GM counter.

At low voltages no avalanches occur since electrons do not strike the center wire with sufficient energy to release UV photons. No avalanches occur until the *threshold* voltage is reached. Then the counting rate increases rapidly to a *plateau region* beyond which it remains essentially constant. The point at which the plateau begins is called the *knee* of the curve. In the plateau region, all of the radiation events causing ionization also cause avalanches and are counted. Since the radiation source is constant, the counting rate is constant.†

---

† Actually, for most GM counters the counting rate increases by 1–2 percent per 100 volts in the plateau region. This is of no practical consequence in nuclear medicine.

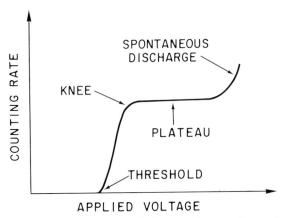

Fig. 4-11. Voltage characteristic (counting rate from a fixed radiation source versus applied voltage) for a GM counter. When the applied voltage is less than the threshold voltage, avalanche effect does not occur, and no radiation events are recorded. At very high voltages, spontaneous discharge events occur within the chamber. These are not caused by radiation events.

When the voltage is increased to a very high value, the counting rate again begins to increase. This happens when the voltage is so high that spontaneous ionization begins to occur in the chamber. The curve then enters the *spontaneous discharge* region. GM counters should not be operated in the spontaneous discharge region because no useful information can be obtained there. Furthermore, if the counter contains an organic quenching gas, it is rapidly used up by the spontaneous discharges, thus shortening the life of the counter. The proper operating voltage is the plateau region, about one-third the distance from the knee to the spontaneous discharge region.

GM counters are simple, rugged, and relatively inexpensive radiation detectors. Much of the early (pre-1950s) work in nuclear medicine was done with GM counters; however, they have since been replaced for most applications by other types of detectors. The major disadvantages of GM counters are low detection efficiency (<1%) for γ rays and x rays and inability to distinguish between radiation events of different energies on the basis of pulse size for energy-selective counting (because all pulses from a GM counter are of the same size).

GM counters are used mostly in survey meters for radiation protection purposes. An example is shown in Figure 4-12. The detector in this survey meter is of an *end-window* type. The entrance window at the end

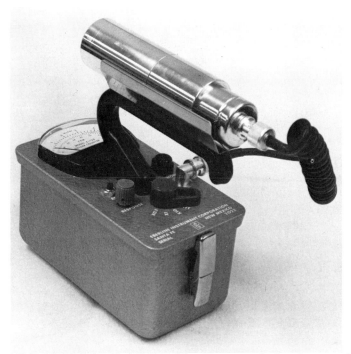

Fig. 4-12.   Radiation survey meter with GM counter radiation detector. [Courtesy Eberline Instruments Corp.]

of the counter tube is a thin layer of mica (0.01 mm thick) that is sufficiently thin to permit passage of particles and particles into the counter. The rather fragile window is protected by a wire screen. GM counters designed for counting only relatively penetrating radiations, such as γ rays and high-energy β particles, have thicker, sturdier windows, e.g., 0.1 mm thick aluminum or stainless steel. Many GM counters are provided with removable covers on the entrance window which can be used to distinguish between penetrating and nonpenetrating radiations by observing the difference between counting rates with and without the cover in place. GM survey meters are more sensitive than ionization chamber survey meters, typically by about a factor of 10.

B. SEMICONDUCTOR DETECTORS

Semiconductor detectors are essentially solid-state analogs of gas-filled ionization chambers. Because the solid detector materials used in semiconductor detectors are 2000–5000 times more dense than gases

(Table 4-1), they have much better stopping power and are much more efficient detectors for x and γ rays.

Semiconductor detectors normally are poor electrical conductors; however, when they are ionized by an ionizing radiation event, the electrical charge produced can be collected by an external applied voltage, as it is with gas-filled detectors. This principle could not be applied using a conducting material for the detector (e.g., a block of metal) because such a material would conduct a large amount of current even without ionizing events. Insulators (e.g., glass) are not suitable detector materials either, because they do not conduct even in the presence of ionizing radiation. Hence only semiconductor materials can function as "solid ionization chambers."

The most commonly used semiconductor detector materials are silicon (Si) and germanium (Ge). Some of their characteristics are listed in Table 4-1. One ionization is produced per (approximately) 3 eV of radiation energy absorbed. By comparison, this value for gases (air) is about 34 eV/ionization. Thus a semiconductor detector not only is a more efficient absorber of radiation but produces about a ten times larger electrical signal (per unit of radiation energy absorbed) than a gas-filled detector. The signal is large enough to permit detection and counting of individual radiation events. Furthermore, the size of the electrical signal is proportional to the amount of radiation energy absorbed; therefore semiconductor detectors can be used for energy-selective radiation counting. For reasons to be discussed in Chapter 11, they are in fact the preferred type of detector for this application.

In spite of their apparent advantages, semiconductor detectors have a number of problems that have limited their use in nuclear medicine. The first is that both Si and Ge (especially Ge) conduct a significant amount of thermally induced electrical current at room temperature. This background current creates a "noise current" that interferes with detection of radiation-induced currents. Therefore Si detectors (usually) and Ge

Table 4-1
Some Properties of Detector Materials Used as
Ionization Detectors

	Si (Li)	Ge (Li) or Ge	Air
ρ (g/cm^3)	2.33	5.36	0.001297
Z	14	32	~7.6
W† (eV)	3.5	2.94	33.7

†Average energy expended per electron-hole pair created or per ionization.

detectors (always) must be operated at temperatures well below room temperature.

A second problem is the presence of impurities even in relatively pure crystals of Si and Ge. Impurities (atoms of other elements) enter into and disturb the regular arrangement of silicon and germanium atoms in the crystal matrix. These disturbances create "electron traps" and capture electrons released in ionization events. This results in a substantial reduction in the amount of electrical signal available.

Two approaches have been used to solve the impurity problem. One is to prepare very pure samples of the detector material. This has been accomplished only with germanium and is, unfortunately, quite expensive. Also, the size of pure crystals is limited to about 5 cm diameter by about 1 cm thick. Detectors made of high-purity germanium are sometimes called *intrinsic germanium* detectors. A second approach is to deliberately introduce into the crystal matrix "compensating" impurities that donate electrons to fill the electron traps created by other impurities. Lithium (Li) is commonly used in silicon and germanium detectors for this purpose. Detectors made of "lithium-doped" materials are called *lithium-drifted* detectors, or Si(Li) or Ge(Li) detectors. Unfortunately, the process of preparing Si(Li) or Ge(Li) crystals is time-consuming and expensive. Crystal sizes are limited to a few centimeters in diameter by about 1 cm thick for Si(Li) and about 5 cm diameter by about 5 cm thick for Ge(Li).

An additional problem is that lithium ions tend to "condense" within the crystal matrix at room temperature, especially in germanium. Therefore Si(Li) and Ge(Li) not only must be operated at low temperatures (to minimize thermally induced background currents) but Ge(Li) detectors must and Si(Li) detectors should also be *stored* at low temperatures. Liquid nitrogen ($T = 77°K$ or $-196°C$) is used for detector cooling. Ge(Li) detectors can be ruined by only an hour or so at room temperature. Si(Li) detectors can tolerate elevated temperatures, but they provide optimum performance if they also are stored at liquid nitrogen temperatures.

Figure 4-13 shows schematically a typical semiconductor detector assembly. The detector consists of a thin circular disc of the detector material [Si(Li), Ge(Li), or high-purity germanium] with electrodes attached to its opposite faces for charge collection. One electrode is a thin metal foil fastened to the front surface ("entrance window"), while the other is a wire or set of wires embedded in the opposite surface of the crystal. Other detector shapes and electrode configurations are also used.

Figure 4-13 also shows in cross section an apparatus used to cool the crystal with liquid nitrogen. A "cold finger" extends from the liquid nitrogen container (a Dewar flask) to cool the detector. Some of the

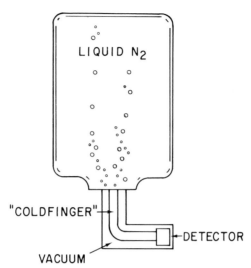

Fig. 4-13.   Schematic representation of a typical semiconductor detector assembly. "Coldfinger" is a thermal conduc-
tor for cooling the detector element.

preamplifier electronic circuitry is also cooled to reduce electronic noise
levels. Liquid nitrogen evaporates and the container needs periodic
refilling—typically every 2–3 days, depending on container size and
insulation characteristics.

Some applications of semiconductor detectors are discussed in
Chapter 14, Section A and Chapter 17, Section D.

C. SCINTILLATION DETECTORS

1. Basic Principles

As indicated earlier in this chapter, radiation from radioactive
materials interacts with matter by causing ionization and/or excitation of
atoms and molecules. When the ionized or excited products undergo
recombination or deexcitation, energy is released. Most of the energy is
dissipated as thermal energy, e.g., molecular vibrations in gases or liquids
or lattice vibrations in a crystal; however, in some materials a portion of
the energy is released as visible light.† These materials are called

---

† For simplicity, the term "visible light" will be used to describe scintillation emissions. In fact, the emissions from most scintillators extend into the UV portion of the
spectrum as well.

scintillators, and radiation detectors made from them are called *scintillation detectors.*

Scintillator materials are actually fairly common in everyday experience. Luminous dials on watches or clocks are painted with a mixture containing a scintillator material (usually zinc sulfide) and a small amount of radioactivity (e.g., ^{3}H, ^{147}Pm, or, at one time, ^{226}Ra). Dials containing ^{226}Ra are readily identified because they produce radiation levels at the face of the watch crystal that are measured easily with a survey meter (tens of mR/hour at the crystal face). Dials containing ^{3}H or ^{147}Pm produce much lower radiation levels because these radionuclides emit only low-energy particles that cannot penetrate the crystal face. Intensifying screens used in radiography also use scintillator materials.

The scintillator materials used for detectors in nuclear medicine are of two general types: inorganic substances in the form of solid crystals and organic substances dissolved in liquid solution. The scintillation mechanisms are different for these two types and will be described separately in later sections.

A characteristic common to all scintillators is that the amount of light produced by a single γ ray, β particle, etc. is very small. In the early days of nuclear physics, it was common to study the characteristics of particles by observing and counting, in a darkened room, the scintillations produced by these particles on a zinc sulfide scintillation screen. The obvious limitations on counting speed and accuracy with this system have been eliminated in modern applications with the introduction of ultrasensitive electronic light detectors called photomultiplier tubes.

2. Photomultiplier Tubes

Photomultiplier (PM) tubes (also called *multiplier phototubes* or just *phototubes* and sometimes abbreviated *PMT*) are electronic tubes that produce a pulse of electrical current when stimulated by very weak light signals, e.g., the scintillations produced by a γ ray or β particle in a scintillation detector. Their basic principles are illustrated in Figure 4-14.

The inside front surface of the glass *entrance window* of the PM tube is coated with a *photoemissive* substance. A photoemissive substance is one that ejects electrons when struck by photons of visible light. CsSb and other bialkali compounds are commonly used for this material. The photoemissive surface is called the *photocathode,* and electrons ejected from it are called *photoelectrons.* The conversion efficiency for visible light to electrons is typically one to three photoelectrons per ten visible light photons striking the photocathode.

A short distance from the photocathode is a metal plate called a

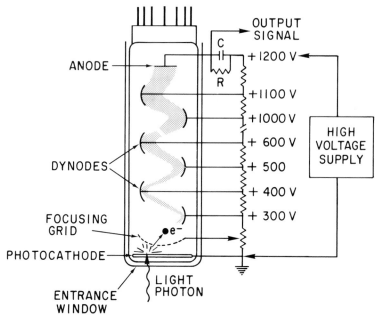

Fig. 4-14.   Basic principles of a photomultiplier (PM) tube. (Note: Three dynode stages omitted.)

dynode. The dynode is maintained at a positive voltage (typically 200–400 V) relative to the photocathode and attracts the photoelectrons ejected from it. A *focusing grid* directs the photoelectrons toward the dynode. The dynode is coated with a material having relatively high *secondary emission* characteristics. CsSb also can be used for this material. A high-speed photoelectron striking the dynode surface ejects several *secondary electrons* from it. The electron multiplication factor depends on the energy of the photoelectron, which in turn is determined by the voltage difference between the dynode and the photocathode.

Secondary electrons ejected from the first dynode are attracted to a second dynode, which is maintained at 50–150 V higher potential than the first dynode, and the electron multiplication process is repeated. This occurs through many additional dynode stages (typically 9–12 in all), until finally a shower of electrons is collected at the *anode*. Typical electron multiplication factors are $\times 3$ to $\times 6$ per dynode. The total electron multiplication factor is very large—e.g. 6^{10} ($\sim 6 \times 10^{7}$) for a ten-stage tube with average multiplication factor 6 at each dynode. Thus a relatively large pulse of current is produced when the tube is stimulated by even a relatively weak light signal. Note that the amount of current produced is proportional to the intensity of the light signal incident on the photocath-

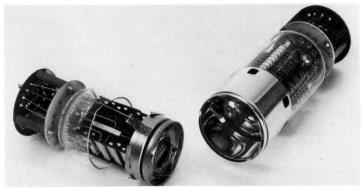

Fig. 4-15.   Two typical PM tubes. The glass envelope of the tube on the left has been removed to show the structures inside.

ode and thus also to the amount of energy deposited by the radiation event in the crystal.

Photomultiplier tubes require a high-voltage supply. For example, as shown in Figure 4-14, if the tube has nine dynodes, with the first at $+300$ V relative to the photocathode and the remaining eight dynodes and the anode at additional $+100$ V increments, a voltage of $+1200$ V is needed. Furthermore, the voltage supply must be very stable because the electron multiplication factor is very sensitive to dynode voltage changes. Typically a 1 percent increase in high voltage applied to the tube increases the amount of current collected at the anode by about 10 percent. This is of considerable importance in applications where pulse size is being measured, e.g., in pulse-height spectrometry to determine γ-ray energies (Chapter 11).

Photomultiplier tubes are sealed in glass and evacuated. Electrical connections to the dynodes, the photocathode, and the anode are made through pins in the tube base (Figure 4-15). The focusing of the electron beam from one dynode to the next can be affected by external magnetic fields. Therefore PM tubes often are wrapped in metal foil for magnetic shielding. "Mu-metal," an alloy comprised of iron, nickel, and small amounts of copper and chromium, is commonly used for this purpose. Photomultiplier tubes come in various sizes. Most of those used in nuclear medicine have photocathodes in the range 2.5–7.5 cm diameter.

3. Inorganic Scintillators [NaI(Tl)]

Inorganic scintillators are crystalline solids that scintillate because of characteristics of their crystal structure. Individual atoms and molecules of these substances do not scintillate. They are scintillators only in crystalline form.

Some inorganic crystals are scintillators in their pure state—e.g., pure NaI crystals are scintillators at liquid nitrogen temperatures. Most are "impurity activated," however. These are crystals containing small amounts of "impurity" atoms of other elements. Impurity atoms in the crystal matrix cause disturbances in its normal structure. Because they are responsible for the scintillation effect the impurity atoms in the crystal matrix are sometimes called *activator centers*. Some impurity-activated scintillators that have been used in radiation detectors include ZnS(Ag), NaI(Tl), and CdS(Ag). In each case, the element in parentheses is the impurity that is added to create activator centers in the crystal.

The most commonly used scintillator, by far, for detectors in nuclear medicine is NaI(Tl) (*thallium-activated sodium iodide*). Some basic properties of NaI(Tl) along with those of other scintillators of potential interest for nuclear medicine applications are summarized in Table 4-2.

Pure NaI crystals are scintillators only at liquid nitrogen temperatures. They become efficient scintillators at room temperatures with the addition of small amounts of thallium. Single crystals of NaI(Tl) for radiation detectors are "grown" from molten sodium iodide to which has been added a small amount of thallium (0.1–0.4 mole percent). Crystals of relatively large size are grown in ovens under carefully controlled temperature conditions. Crystal sizes of 5–15 cm diam × 1–5 cm thick are common for applications in nuclear medicine. Detectors for Anger cameras (Chapter 15) use NaI(Tl) crystals typically 30–50 cm diam × 1.25 cm thick.

Figure 4-16 shows the construction of a typical NaI(Tl) crystal and PM tube assembly. The crystal is sealed in an aluminum or stainless steel jacket with a transparent glass or plastic *optical window* at one end to permit the exit of scintillation light from the crystal to the PM tube. A transparent optical "coupling grease" is used between the crystal and the PM tube to minimize internal reflections at this interface. The crystal and PM tube are hermetically sealed in a light-tight jacket to keep out moisture and extraneous light and for mechanical protection. The inside surface of the radiation entrance window and sides of the crystal are coated with a reflective material that reflects light so that it can be collected by the photocathode. With efficient optical coupling, good reflective surfaces, and a crystal free of cracks or other opacifying defects, about 30 percent of the light emitted by the crystal actually reaches the cathode of the PM tube. Some NaI(Tl) detectors have very thin aluminum or beryllium foil "entrance windows" to permit detection of radiations having relatively low penetrating power, e.g., low-energy x rays and γ rays ($E \leq 10$ keV) and β particles; however, most NaI(Tl) detectors have thicker entrance windows of aluminum or stainless steel

Table 4-2
Properties of Some Scintillator Materials

Property			Material			
	NaI (Tl)	CsF	BGO‡	Plastic	GSO§	BaF₂
ρ (g/cm³)	3.67	4.61	7.13	1.03	6.71	4.89
Atomic numbers	11,53	55,9	83,32,8	6,1	58,64,14,8	56,9
Effective atomic number	50	53	74		59	54
Scintillation decay time (nsec)*	230	2.5	300	2	60	0.8‖ 620#
Photon yield† (per keV)	40	2.5	4.8	15	6.4	2.0 6.5
Index of refraction	1.85	1.48	2.15	1.58	1.9	1.56
Hygroscopic	Yes	Very	No	No	No	very little
Wavelength of maximum emission (Å)	4150	3900	4800	—	4300	2250‖ 3100#

Reprinted from Eriksson L, Bohn C, Kesselberg M, Litton J-E, Bergstrom M, Blomquist G: A high resolution positron camera. In *The Metabolism of the Human Brain Studied with Positron Emission Tomography*. Greitz T, Ingvan DH, Widen L (eds.), Raven Press, New York, 1985. pp. 33–46. With permission.

*Time required for emission of ~67% of the light.
†Average number of scintillation photons emitted per keV of ionizing radiation energy absorbed.
‡Bi₃Ge₄O₁₂.
§Ge₂SiO₅ (Ce).
‖Fast component.
#Slow component.

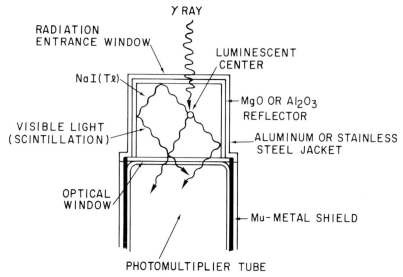

Fig. 4-16.   Arrangement of NaI(Tl) crystal and PM tube in a typical detector assembly.

and are not well suited for detecting these types of radiation. Figure 4-17 shows some typical integral NaI(Tl) crystal and PM tube assemblies.

Some reasons for the usefulness of NaI(Tl) include the following:

1. It is relatively dense (ρ = 3.67 g/cm^3) and contains an element of relatively high atomic number (iodine, Z = 53). Therefore it is a good absorber and efficient detector of penetrating radiations, such as x rays and γ rays.
2. It is a relatively efficient scintillator, yielding one visible light photon per approximately 30 eV of radiation energy absorbed.
3. It is transparent to its own scintillation emissions. Therefore there is little loss of scintillation light caused by self-absorption, even in NaI(Tl) crystals of relatively large size.
4. A NaI(Tl) detector provides an output signal (from the PM tube) that is proportional in amplitude to the amount of radiation energy absorbed in the crystal. Therefore it can be used for energy-selective counting.

Some disadvantages of NaI(Tl) detectors are the following:

1. The NaI(Tl) crystal is quite fragile and easily fractured by mechanical or thermal stresses (e.g., rapid temperature changes). Fractures in the crystal do not necessarily destroy its usefulness as a detector, but

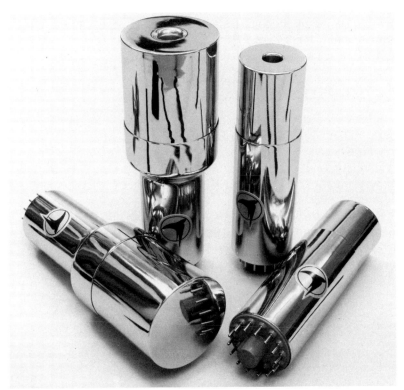

Fig. 4-17.   NaI(Tl) crystal and PM tube assemblies. (Courtesy of Bicron Corporation, Newbury, Ohio)

they create opacifications within the crystal that reduce the amount of scintillation light reaching the photocathode.

2. Sodium iodide is hygroscopic. Exposure to moisture or a humid atmosphere causes a yellowish surface discoloration that again impairs light transmission to the PM tube. Thus hermetic sealing is required.

3. Sodium iodide crystals of large size (e.g., 20–30 cm diam) are difficult to grow and quite expensive (i.e., several thousands of dollars).

Other types of detectors have advantages over NaI(Tl) detectors in certain areas—e.g., gas-filled detectors are cheaper, and semiconductor detectors have better energy resolution (Chapter 11). Bismuth germanate ($Bi_4Ge_3O_{12}$, also called BGO) and cesium fluoride (CsF) are other scintillators that find use in nuclear medicine (Table 4-2), particularly for applications involving positron emission tomography, or PET scanning

(Chapter 20, Section D). However, the overall advantages of NaI(Tl) have made it the detector of choice for nearly all routine applications in nuclear medicine, and it seems likely that this situation will prevail for some time into the future.

4. Organic Liquid Scintillators

In contrast to inorganic scintillators, the scintillation process in organic scintillators is an inherent molecular property. The scintillation mechanism is one of molecular excitation (e.g., by absorbing energy from a γ ray or β particle) followed by a deexcitation process in which visible light is emitted. These substances are scintillators whether they are in solid, liquid, or gaseous forms.

Certain plastics (e.g., see Table 4-2) are organic scintillators; however, by far the most common application for organic scintillators is in liquid form for *liquid scintillation (LS) counting*. In these systems, the scintillator is dissolved in a solvent material in a glass or plastic vial, and the radioactive sample is added to this mixture. The vial is then placed in a light-tight enclosure between a pair of PM tubes to detect the scintillaton events (Figure 4-18).

Liquid scintillator solutions are comprised of four components:

1. An organic *solvent* comprises most of the solution. The solvent must dissolve not only the scintillator material but also the radioactive sample added to it. The solvent actually is responsible for most of the direct absorption of radiation energy from the sample. High-speed electrons generated by ionizing radiation events in the solvent then transfer energy to the scintillator molecules, causing the scintillation effect. Commonly used solvents include toluene, dioxane, and xylene.

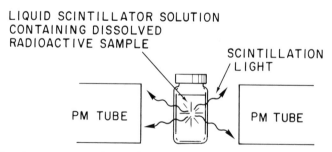

Fig. 4-18. Arrangement of sample and detector for liquid scintillation (LS) counting. Sample is dissolved in liquid scintillator solution in a glass or plastic vial.

Table 4-3
Some Liquid Scintillator Solutions

Solvent (ml)	Primary Solute (g/liter)	Secondary Solute (g/liter)
For nonaqueous soluble materials		
Toluene 1000	PPO (5.0)	POPOP (0.1)
Xylene 1000	PPO (4.0)	POPOP (0.05)
For carbon dioxide		
Toluene 1000 (add 1 ml hydroxide of hyamine 1 N in methanol to each 15 ml of solution)	PPO (4.0)	POPOP (0.05)
For aqueous solutions		
Toluene 500	PPO (4.0)	POPOP (0.01)
Ethanol 500		
Naphthalene 60 g	PPO (4.0)	Dimethyl POPOP (0.02)
Ethylene glycol 20 ml		
Methanol 100 ml		
Dilute with dioxane to 1 liter		

Adapted with permission from Karmen A: Liquid scintillation counting, in Wagner HN Jr (ed): Principles of Nuclear Medicine. Philadelphia, W.B. Saunders Co., 1968, p. 247.

2. The *primary solute* (or primary *fluor*) absorbs energy from the solvent and emits light. Usually, its emissions are in the UV or near-visible portion of the spectrum. Some common primary scintillators include *p*-terphenyl and PPO (2,5-diphenyloxazole).
3. The emissions of the primary solute usually are not well matched to the response characteristics of photomultiplier tubes. Therefore a *secondary solute,* or *waveshifter,* is added to the solution. The function of this material is to absorb emissions of the primary solute and reemit photons of longer wavelength, which are better matched to the PM tube response. POPOP (1,4-di-[2-5-phenyloxazole] benzene) is a commonly used secondary scintillator.
4. Liquid scintillator solutions frequently contain *additives* to improve some aspect of their performance, e.g., the efficiency of energy transfer from the solvent to the primary solute. *Solubilizers* (e.g., hyamine) are sometimes added to improve the dissolution of added samples such as blood.

Some typical liquid scintillator solutions are described in Table 4-3. Different solvents are used, depending on the type of sample to be measured.

Because of the intimate relationship between sample and detector, LS counting is the method of choice for efficient detection of particles, low-energy x and γ rays, and other nonpenetrating radiations. It is widely used for measurement of ^3H and ^{14}C. In medical applications, it is used primarily for sensitive assay of radioactivity in biologic specimens, e.g., blood, urine, etc.

Although well suited for counting nonpenetrating radiations in biologic samples, LS counters have numerous drawbacks as general purpose radiation detectors. They are inefficient detectors of penetrating radiations such as γ rays and x rays of moderate energy because the detector solution is comprised primarily of low-density, low-Z materials. Liquid scintillators generally have low light output, only about one-third that of NaI(Tl). This problem is worsened by the relatively inefficient light coupling from the scintillator vial to the PM tubes as compared to NaI(Tl) integral detectors.

For sample counting, special sample preparation may be required to dissolve the sample. Problems in sample preparation are discussed in Chapter 14, Section B.6. Also, the sample itself is "destroyed" when it is added to the scintillator solution.

Finally, all LS counting suffers from the problem of *quenching*. Quenching in this context refers to any mechanism that reduces the amount of light output from the sample (not to be confused with the type of quenching that occurs in Geiger–Müller tubes, Section A.4). There are basically three types of liquid scintillation quenching:

1. *Chemical quenching* is caused by substances that compete with the primary fluor for absorption of energy from the solvent but that are themselves not scintillators. Dissolved oxygen is one of the most troublesome chemical quenchers.
2. *Color quenching* is caused by substances that absorb the emissions of the primary or secondary solute. Blood and other colored materials are examples. Fogged or dirty containers can also produce a type of color quenching.
3. *Dilution quenching* occurs when a relatively large volume of sample is added to the scintillator solution. The effect is to reduce the concentraton of primary and secondary solutes in the final solution, thus reducing the scintillator output efficiency.

Quenching can be minimized in various ways—e.g., dissolved oxygen may be purged by ultrasound, hydrogen peroxide may be added for color bleaching, etc. However, there are no convenient ways to eliminate all causes of quenching; therefore, a certain amount must be accepted in all practical LS counting. Quenching becomes a serious problem when there are wide variations in its extent from one sample to the next. This causes unpredictable variations in light output, for the same amount of radiation energy absorbed, from one sample to the next. *Quench correction* methods are employed in liquid scintillation counters to account for this effect (Chapter 14, Section B.5).

REFERENCES

A general reference for radiation detectors is the following:
Ouseph PJ: Introduction to Nuclear Radiation Detectors. New York, Plenum Press, 1975

Additional references for specific types of detectors are as follows:
Armantrout GA: Principles of semiconductor detector operation, in Hoffer PB, Beck RN, Gottschalk A (eds): Semiconductor Detectors in the Future of Nuclear Medicine. New York, The Society of Nuclear Medicine, 1971, chap 2
Hine GJ: Sodium iodide scintillators, in Hine GJ (ed): Instrumentation in Nuclear Medicine (vol 1). New York, Academic Press, 1967, pp 95–117
Rapkin E: Preparation of samples for liquid scintillation counting, in Hine GJ (ed): Instrumentation in Nuclear Medicine (vol 1). New York, Academic Press, 1967, pp 182–226
Robinson CV: Geiger-Müller and proportional counters, in Hine GJ (ed): Instrumentation in Nuclear Medicine (vol 1). New York, Academic Press, 1967, pp 57–72
Takayanagi SI, Iio M: Miniature semiconductor radiation detectors, in Hine GJ, Sorenson JA (eds): Instrumentation in Nuclear Medicine (vol 2). New York, Academic Press, 1974, pp 485–508

A detailed reference for scintillation detectors is the following:
Birks JB: The Theory and Practice of Scintillation Counting. London, Pergamon Press, 1967

5

Electronic Instrumentation for Radiation Detection Systems

Most of the radiation detectors used in nuclear medicine are operated in a "pulse mode;" that is, they generate pulses of electrical charge or current that are counted to determine the number of radiation events detected. In addition, by analyzing the amplitude of pulses from the detector, it is possible with energy-sensitive detectors, such as scintillation and semiconductor detectors and proportional counters, to determine the energy of each radiation event detected. Selection of a narrow energy range for counting permits discrimination against events other than those of the energy of interest, such as scattered radiation and background radiation or the multiple emissions from a mixture of radionuclides.

Figure 5-1 shows in schematic form the basic electronic components of a nuclear radiation counting instrument. These components are present in systems ranging from the most simple sample counters to complex imaging instruments. The purpose of this chapter is to describe the basic principles of these components. The electronics for specific systems also are described in Chapters 11–17. Basic principles of electricity and electronics are reviewed in some of the references listed at the end of the chapter.

A. PREAMPLIFIERS

Table 5-1 summarizes the pulse output characteristics of detectors used in nuclear medicine. Most of them produce pulse signals of relatively small amplitude. In addition, all of the detectors listed have a relatively

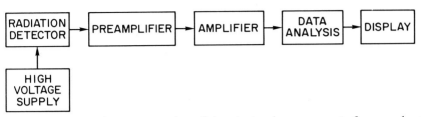

Fig. 5-1.   Schematic representation of the electronic components for a nuclear radiation counting system.

high output impedance, i.e., a high internal resistance to the flow of electrical current. In handling electronic signals, it is important that the impedance levels of successive components be matched to one another, or electronic interferences that distort the pulse signals may develop and system performance will be degraded.

The purposes of a *preamplifier* (or preamp) are threefold: (1) to amplify, if necessary, the relatively small signals produced by the radiation detector; (2) to match impedance levels between the detector and subsequent components in the system; and (3) to shape the signal pulse for optimal signal processing by the subsequent components.

Figure 5-2A shows a simplified diagram of a typical preamplifier. The symbol—$\boxed{A}$—represents the signal (pulse) amplifying component. The resistor (R) and capacitor (C) provide pulse shaping. The signal from the detector is typically a sharply rising pulse of electrical current of relatively short duration (≤ 1 μsec, except for Geiger–Müller counters; Table 5-1). Electrical charge Q is deposited on capacitor of capacitance C,

Table 5-1
Typical Signal Output and Pulse
Duration of Various Radiation Detectors

Detector	Typical Signal (volts)	Typical Pulse Duration (microseconds)
Sodium iodide scintillation with phototube	0.5–2V	0.25†
Liquid scintillation with phototube	0.05–0.2V	10^{-2}†
Plastic scintillation with phototube	0.5–0.2V	10^{-3}†
Semiconductor	10^{-3}V	10^{-1}–1
Gas proportional	10^{-3}–10^{-2}V	10^{-1}–1
Geiger–Müller	0.5–10V	50–300

†Mean decay time.

A.

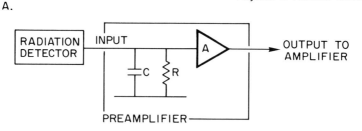

B.

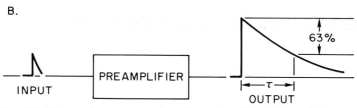

Fig. 5-2.   (A) Schematic representation of a preamplifier for a radiation counting system. The symbol —[A⟩— represents a voltage or current amplifying element. C and R form a pulse-shaping circuit. (B) Input and output pulse signals for the preamplifier. $\tau = (R \times C)$ is the time constant of the pulse-shaping circuit.

causing a voltage $V_0 = Q/C$ to appear across it and at the input to the amplifier element. With energy-sensitive detectors, the amount of charge, Q, and thus the amplitude of the voltage V_0 are proportional to the energy of the radiation event detected. The electrical charge leaks off the capacitor through the resistor of resistance R, causing the voltage on the capacitor and at the input to the amplifier element to decrease exponentially with time t according to

$$V = V_0\, e^{-t/RC} \tag{5-1}$$

The product $R \times C$ is called the *time constant* τ of the pulse-shaping circuit. The voltage decreases exponentially, dropping by 63 percent of its initial value during one time constant (Figure 5-2B). When R is given in ohms and C in farads, the time constant is given in seconds. Typical preamplifier time constants for nuclear medicine detectors are 20–200 μsec.

The amount of amplification provided by the amplifier element of the preamplifier varies with the type of detector. With scintillation detectors, the photomultiplier tube already provides a considerable degree of amplification (10^5–10^{10}); thus relatively little additional amplification may be needed. Typically, a *gain factor* (ratio of output to input amplitudes) of 5–20 is used for these detectors; however, some NaI(Tl) systems employ no preamplifier gain (gain factor of 1).

Detectors producing very small signals, e.g., semiconductor detectors, may require a relatively high degree of preamplifier gain, perhaps in the range 10^3–10^4. It is not a trivial problem to design an amplifier that provides this amount of gain without introducing noise "signals" and temperature-related gain instabilities. Most of the modern high-gain preamplifiers employ *field-effect transistors* (FETs), which provide the desired low-noise and temperature-stability characteristics.

For energy-sensitive detectors, the preamplifier must operate in a *linear* fashion; that is, the amplitude of the signal out must be directly proportional to the amount of charge delivered to it by the detector. This preserves the relationship between pulse amplitude and energy of the radiation event detected, so that subsequent energy analysis may be applied to the pulse signals.

For the best results, the preamplifier component should be located as close as possible to the detector component. This maximizes the electronic signal-to-noise ratio (S/N) by amplifying the signal before additional noise or signal distortion can occur in the long cable runs that frequently separate the detector from the rest of the signal-processing components. This is particularly critical for detectors with small output signals (e.g., semiconductor detectors or scintillation detectors used for detecting low-energy radiations). It is also important for applications in which energy resolution is critical (Chapter 11). Frequently, detectors and preamplifiers are sold as single units. Scintillation cameras use the same close arrangement of detector and preamplifier to optimize spatial resolution and image sharpness (Chapter 15, Section B.2).

B. AMPLIFIERS

1. Amplification and Pulse-shaping Functions

The amplifier component of a nuclear counting instrument has two major functions: (1) to amplify the still relatively small pulses from the preamp (usually millivolts) to sufficient amplitude (volts) to drive auxiliary equipment (pulse-height analyzers, scalers, etc.), and (2) to reshape the slow decaying pulse from the preamp into a narrow one to avoid the problem of pulse pileup at high counting rates and to improve the electronic signal-to-noise ratio.

The gain factor on an amplifier may range from $\times 1$ to $\times 1000$. Usually it is adjustable, first by a coarse adjustment ($\times 2$, $\times 4$, $\times 8$, etc.), and then by means of a fine gain adjustment providing gain factors between the coarse steps. The coarse gain adjustment permits amplification of pulses over a wide range of amplitudes from different detectors and

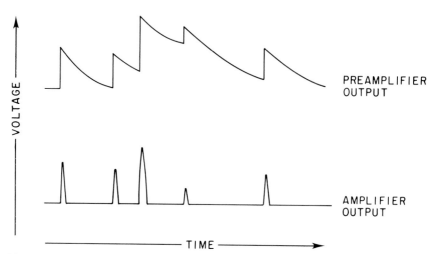

Fig. 5-3. Sequence of pulse signals in a radiation counting system. Top:
Relatively long preamplifier time constant results in overlapping of pulse signals.
Bottom: Amplifier output pulses have been shortened but without significant loss
of amplitude or timing information.

preamplifiers to the maximum output capability of the amplifier. The fine
gain adjustment permits precise calibration of the relationship between
amplifier output pulse amplitude (volts) and radiation energy absorbed
(keV or MeV). For example, a convenient ratio might be 10 V of pulse
amplitude per 1 MeV of radiation energy absorbed in the detector. This
calibration is discussed further in Chapter 13, Section A.6.

Pulse shaping—specifically, pulse shortening—is an essential function of the amplifier. The output of the preamp is a sharply rising pulse
that decays with a time constant of about 50 μsec, returning to baseline
after about 500 μsec. Thus if a second pulse occurs within 500 μsec, it
rides on the tail of the previous pulse, providing incorrect amplitude
information (Figure 5-3). The system could not operate at counting rates
exceeding a few hundred events per second without introducing this type
of amplitude distortion.

The pulse-shaping circuits of the amplifier must provide an output of
cleanly separated pulses (Figure 5-3), even though the output pulses from
the preamp overlap. It must do this without distorting the information in
the preamplifier signal, which is, mainly, (1) pulse amplitude (proportional
to the energy of radiation event for energy-sensitive detectors) and (2) rise
time (time at which the radiation event was detected). An additional
function of the pulse-shaping circuits is to discriminate against electronic

noise signals, such as microphonic pickup, 60–120 Hz power line frequency, etc.

The most common methods for amplifier pulse shaping are resistor-capacitor, Gaussian, and delay-line methods. The resistor-capacitor technique, commonly referred to as *RC shaping,* will be described to illustrate the basic principles. More detailed circuit descriptions are found in references at the end of this chapter.

2. RC Shaping

Basic RC pulse-shaping circuits are shown in Figure 5-4. When a sharply rising pulse of relatively long duration (e.g., preamplifier output pulse) is applied to the CR, or *differentiation circuit* (Figure 5-4A), the output is a rapidly rising pulse that decays with a time constant τ_d determined by the RC product of the circuit components (Equation 5-1). The amplitude of the output pulse depends on the amplitude of the sharply rising portion of the input pulse and is insensitive to the "tail" of any preceding pulse. Note that a CR differentiation circuit is also used for pulse shaping in the preamplifier; however, the time constants used in the preamplifier circuits are much longer than those used in the amplifier. Figure 5-4A also illustrates how the CR circuit discriminates against low-frequency noise signals.

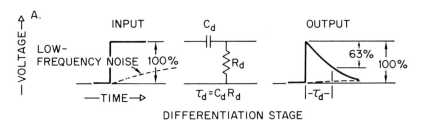

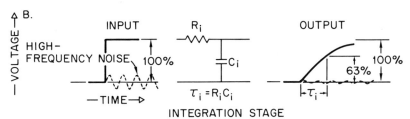

Fig. 5-4.   Basic RC pulse-shaping circuits. (A) Differentiation provides a sharply rising output signal that decays with time constant τ_d and discriminates against low-frequency noise. (B) Integration circuit provides an output pulse that rises with time constant τ_i and discriminates against high-frequency noise.

A.

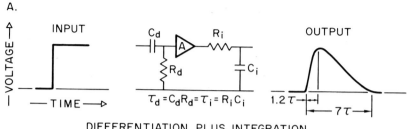

DIFFERENTIATION PLUS INTEGRATION

B.

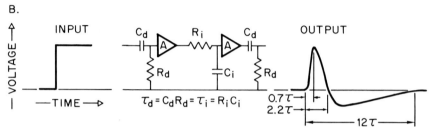

DOUBLE DIFFERENTIATION PLUS INTEGRATION

Fig. 5-5. RC pulse-shaping circuits combining differentiation and integration stages. (A) Differentiation followed by integration. (B) Differentiation–integration–differentiation circuit.

Figure 5-4B shows an RC, or *integration* circuit. (Note that differentiation and integration differ only by the interchange of R and C.) When a sharply rising pulse is applied to this circuit, the output is a pulse with a shape described by

$$V = V_0 (1 - e^{-t/RC}) \tag{5-2}$$

where V_0 is the amplitude of the input pulse and $RC = \tau_i$ is the integration time constant of the circuit. This circuit discriminates effectively against high-frequency noise, as illustrated in Figure 5-4B.

Figure 5-5A shows a pulse-shaping circuit combining differentiation and integration stages. When the time constants of the two circuits are equal ($\tau = \tau_i = \tau_d$), the output is a pulse that rises to a maximum value in a time equal to 1.2τ and then decays to approximately zero in 7τ. The maximum amplitude of the output pulse is determined by the amplitude of the input pulse. For scintillation and semiconductor detectors, a time constant in the range $\tau \sim 0.25–5.0$ μsec usually is chosen. Thus the output pulse is shortened considerably relative to the pulse from the preamplifier (50–500 μsec) and is suitable for high counting rate applications. Except for a very small negative overshoot at the end of the pulse, the output pulse from this circuit has only one polarity (positive in Figure 5-5A) and is called a *unipolar* output.

Figure 5-5B illustrates another type of shaping, called *double differential* shaping. The output pulse from this circuit has both positive and negative components and therefore is a *bipolar* pulse. For equal time constant values, the bipolar output pulse has a shorter rise time and positive portion and a longer total duration than the unipolar output pulse. Unipolar pulses are preferred for signal-to-noise characteristics and are used where energy resolution is important. Bipolar pulses are preferred for high counting rate applications.

Research-grade amplifiers generally are provided with adjustable pulse-shaping time constants. A longer time constant provides better pulse amplitude information and is preferred in applications requiring optimal energy resolution, e.g., with Si(Li) or Ge(Li) detectors (Chapter 11, Section C.3). A shorter time constant is preferred in applications requiring more precise event timing and higher counting rate capabilities, e.g., scintillation cameras (Chapters 15–16) and coincidence detection of positron annihilation photons (Chapter 20, Section D.1).

3. Baseline Shift and Pulse Pileup

Baseline shift and *pulse pileup* are two practical problems that occur in all amplifiers at high counting rates. Baseline shift is caused by the negative component that occurs at the end of the amplifier output pulse. A second pulse occurring during this component will be slightly depressed in amplitude (Figure 5-6A). Inaccurate pulse amplitude and an apparent shift (decrease) in energy of the detected radiation event are the result (See Figure 11-10).

Special circuitry has been developed to minimize baseline shift. This is called *pole zero cancellation, or baseline restoration.* This type of circuitry is employed in modern scintillation cameras to provide a high counting rate capability for cardiac studies. These circuits are described in the references listed at the end of this chapter.

At high counting rates, amplifier pulses can occur so close together that they fall on top of each other. This is referred to as pulse pileup (Figure 5-6B). When this happens two pulses sum together and produce a single pulse with an amplitude that is not representative of either. Pulse pileup distorts energy information and also contributes to counting losses (deadtime) of the detection system, since two pulses are counted as one (Chapter 12, Section C).

Both baseline shift and pulse pileup can be decreased by decreasing the width of the amplifier pulse, i.e., the time constant of the amplifier; however, shortening of the time constant usually produces poorer signal-

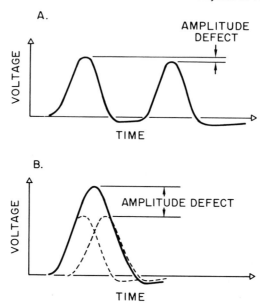

Fig. 5-6. (A) Schematic representation of baseline shift, caused by a pulse riding on the "tail" of a preceding pulse. (B) Pulse pileup effects for two pulses occurring very close together in time.

to-noise ratio and energy resolution. It is generally true that all the factors that provide high count rate capabilities in amplifiers also degrade energy resolution (Chapter 11, Section B.6).

Generally, amplifiers with double differentiation or double delay-line bipolar outputs are employed with NaI(Tl) detectors. In addition, short time constants of 0.025–0.5 μsec are used. The relatively poor inherent energy resolution of NaI(Tl) detectors is not affected significantly by this type of amplifier, and a high counting rate capability is provided. Semiconductor detectors usually require much more sophisticated amplifiers, with unipolar pulse shaping, longer time constants (0.5–8 μsec), and circuits for stabilizing the baseline to maintain their exceptionally good energy resolution at high counting rates (Chapter 11, Section C.3).

C. PULSE-HEIGHT ANALYZERS (PHAs)

1. Basic Functions

When an energy-sensitive detector is used [e.g., NaI(Tl) or a semi-conductor detector], the amplitude of the voltage pulse from the amplifier is proportional to the amount of energy deposited in the detector by the detected radiation event. By examining the amplitudes of amplifier output pulses, it is possible to determine the energies of detected radiation events. Selective counting of only those pulses within a certain *amplitude* range makes it possible to restrict counting to a selected *energy* range and to discriminate against background, scattered radiation, etc. outside the desired energy range (see Figure 11-6).

A device used for this purpose is called a *pulse-height analyzer* (PHA). A PHA is used to select for counting only those pulses from the amplifier falling within selected voltage amplitude intervals or "channels." If this is done for only one channel at a time, the device is called a *single-channel analyzer* (SCA). A device that is capable of analyzing simultaneously within many different intervals or channels is called a *multichannel analyzer* (MCA). Basic principles of these instruments are discussed in the following sections. The procedures for calibrating and using PHAs in practical counting measurements are discussed in Chapter 13, Section A.6.

2. Single-Channel Analyzers (SCAs)

A single channel analyzer (SCA) is used to select for counting only those pulses from the amplifier that fall within a selected voltage amplitude range. Since at this stage in the system voltage amplitude is proportional to radiation energy deposited in the detector, it is equivalent to selecting an energy range for counting. Modern amplifiers produce output pulses with amplitudes in the range 0–10 volts. Therefore the voltage selection provided by most SCAs is also in the 0–10 V range.

An SCA has three basic circuit components (Figure 5-7): a *lower level discriminator* (LLD), an *upper level discriminator* (ULD), and an *anticoincidence* circuit. The LLD sets a threshold voltage amplitude V (or energy E) for counting. The ULD sets an upper voltage limit $V + \Delta V$ (or $E + \Delta E$). The difference between these voltages (or energies), ΔV (or ΔE), is called the *window width*. Usually the LLD and ULD voltages are selected by means of potentiometer controls that are adjusted to select some fraction of a 10 V reference voltage.

The LLD and ULD establish voltage levels in electronic circuits called *comparators*. As their name implies, these circuits compare the amplitude of an input pulse in the LLD and ULD voltages. They produce an output pulse only when these voltages are exceeded. Pulses from the comparator circuits are then sent to the anticoincidence circuit, which produces an output pulse when only one (LLD) but not both (ULD and LLD) pulses are present (Figure 5-7). Thus only those input pulses with amplitudes between V and $V + \Delta V$ (i.e., within the selected energy window) cause output pulses from the SCA.

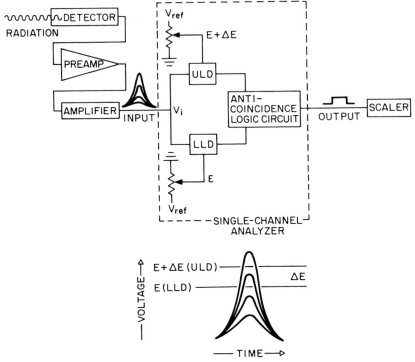

Fig. 5-7. Principles of a single-channel pulse-height analyzer. Top: Electronic components that are used to generate an output pulse only when pulse amplitude falls between voltages established by LLD and ULD circuits. These voltages are an adjustable portion of a reference voltage V_{ref}. Bottom: LLD and ULD voltages in effect establish an energy range (E to $E + \Delta E$) for counting because pulse voltage amplitude V is proportional to radiation event energy E. Only pulse signals within the ΔE bracket are counted.

The SCA output pulses are used to drive counters, ratemeters, and other circuits. The output pulses from the SCA are all of the same amplitude and shape (typically 4 V amplitude, 1 μsec duration). Their amplitudes no longer contain information about radiation energy, since this information has already been extracted by the SCA.

Commercially made SCAs frequently have two front-panel controls: a lower-level (voltage V or energy E) control and a window (ΔV or ΔE) control. The LLD control is also called the *base level* on some instruments. The upper-level voltage is determined by electronic summation of lower-level and window voltages on these instruments.

Some instruments include "percent window" selections. With these instruments, the window width voltage is selected as a certain percentage of the window center voltage. (The window center voltage is the lower level voltage V plus one-half of the window voltage, $\Delta V/2$.) For example, if one were to set the window center at 2 V with a 20 percent window, the window width would be 0.4 V (20 percent of 2 V), and the window would extend from 1.8 to 2.2 V.

On many nuclear medicine instruments, manufacturers have provided pushbuttons to select automatically the analyzer lower level and window voltages appropriate for commonly used radionuclides. In these systems, the pushbuttons insert calibrated resistance values into the SCA circuitry in place of the variable resistances shown in Figure 5-7.

Another possibility on some instruments is to remove the upper-level voltage limit entirely. Then all pulses with amplitudes exceeding the lower level voltage result in output pulses. An analyzer operated in this mode is sometimes called a *discriminator*. Many auxiliary counting circuits (scalers, ratemeters, etc.) have a built in discriminator at their inputs to reject low-level electronic noise pulses.

3. Timing Methods

Accurate time placement of the radiation event is important in some nuclear medicine applications. For example, in the scintillation camera (Chapter 15), accurate timing is required to identify the multiple phototubes involved in detecting individual radiation events striking the NaI(Tl) crystal (i.e., for determining the location of each event with the position logic of the camera). An even more critical timing problem occurs in coincidence counting of positron annihilation photons (Chapter 20, Section D.1) and in the liquid scintillation counter (Chapter 14, Section B).

Most SCAs used in nuclear medicine employ *leading-edge* timing. With this method, as shown in Figure 5-8A, the analyzer output pulse occurs at a fixed time T_D following the instant at which the rising portion of the input pulse triggers the lower level discriminator. This type of timing is adequate for many applications; however, it suffers a certain amount of inaccuracy [5–50 nsec with NaI(Tl)] because the timing of the output pulse depends on the amplitude of the input pulse (Figure 5-8A). This timing variation Δt is called *timing walk*.

More precise timing is obtained with analyzers employing *fast timing* techniques. One such method is called *zero-crossover* timing (Figure 5-8B). This method requires a bipolar input pulse to the SCA. The output pulse occurs at the time of crossover of the bipolar pulse from a positive to a negative voltage value. The zero-crossover method is much less sensitive to pulse amplitude than the leading-edge method and can provide timing accuracy to within ± 4 nsec with NaI(Tl) detectors. Other

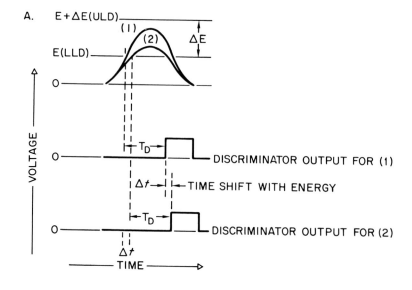

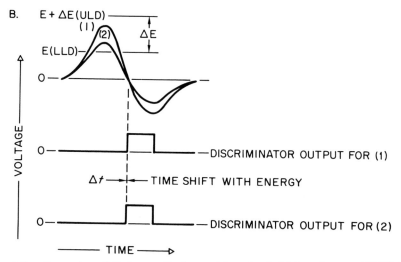

Fig. 5-8. Examples of timing methods used in pulse-height analyzers. (A) With leading-edge timing, output pulse occurs at a fixed time T_D after the leading edge of the pulse passes through the LLD voltage. (B) With zero-crossover timing, output pulse occurs when the bipolar input pulse passes through zero. The latter is preferred for precise timing because there is very little time shift with different pulse amplitudes (energy).

fast-timing methods include *peak detection* and *constant fraction* techniques. They are discussed in references listed at the end of this chapter.

4. Multichannel Analyzers (MCAs)

Some applications of pulse-height analysis require simultaneous recording of events in multiple voltage or energy windows. One approach is to use many SCAs, each with its own voltage window. For example, some imaging devices have two or three independent SCAs to record simultaneously the multiple γ-ray energies emitted by nuclides such as ^{67}Ga; however, this approach is unsatisfactory when tens or even thousands of different windows are required, as in some applications of pulse-height spectroscopy (Chapter 11). Multiple SCAs would be expensive, and the adjusting and balancing of many different analyzer windows would be a very tedious project.

A practical solution is provided by a *multichannel analyzer* (MCA). Figure 5-9 demonstrates the basic principles. The heart of the MCA is an *analog-to-digital converter* (ADC), which measures and sorts out the incoming pulses according to their amplitudes. The pulse amplitude range, usually 0–10 V, is divided by the ADC into a finite number of discrete intervals, or *channels,* which may range from 100 in small analyzers to as many as 8192 (2^{13}) in larger systems. Thus, for example, the ADC in a 1000-channel analyzer would divide the 0–10 V amplitude range into 1000 channels, each 10 V/1000 = 0.01 V wide: 0–0.01 V corresponding to channel 1, 0.01–0.02 V to channel 2, etc. The ADC converts an *analog* signal (volts of pulse amplitude), which has an essentially infinite number of possible different values, into a *digital* one (channel number), which has only a finite number of integer values (Figure 5-9). An ADC also is used in the interface between Anger cameras and computer systems (Chapter 21, Section A).

For each analyzer channel, there is a corresponding storage location in the MCA *memory*. The memory of an MCA is the same as the magnetic core or semiconductor memories found in digital computers. The MCA memory counts and stores the number of pulses recorded in each analyzer channel. The number of memory storage locations available determines the number of MCA channels. The sorting and storage of the energy information from radiation detectors with an MCA is used to record the *pulse-height spectrum* (counts/channel versus channel number, or energy) as shown in Figure 5-9B.

Finally, the number of events recorded per channel during the measurement period is shown on a *display device,* such as a television or CRT (cathode ray tube) display (Sections G and H of this chapter). Alternatively, they can be printed out sequentially by a line printer or teletypewriter.

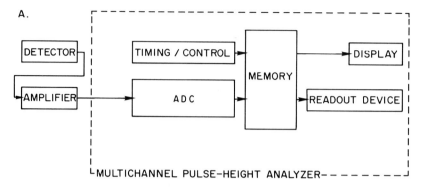

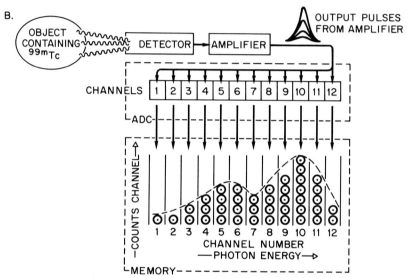

Fig. 5-9. Principles of a multichannel analyzer (MCA). (A) Basic components. (B) Example of pulse sorting according to amplitude for radiation events detected from an object containing ^{99m}Tc.

Two types of ADCs are commonly used in nuclear medicine for MCAs and for interfaces between scintillation cameras and computers. In the *Wilkinson,* or *ramp* converter (Figure 5-10), an input pulse from the radiation detector and amplifier causes an amount of charge to be deposited onto a capacitor at the ADC input. The amount of charge deposited depends on the pulse amplitude or energy. The capacitor discharges through a resistor, with a relatively long RC time constant. While the capacitor is discharging, a gate pulse activates a clock oscillator to produce a train of pulses that are counted in a counting circuit. When

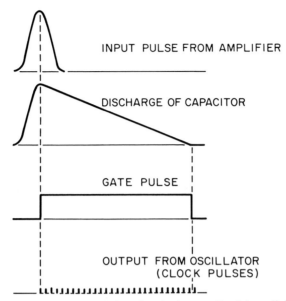

Fig. 5-10.   Principles of analog (pulse amplitude) to digital (channel number) conversion in the Wilkinson or ramp converter. Input pulse is used to charge a capacitor, and discharge time, which is proportional to pulse amplitude, is measured using a clock oscillator.

the capacitor has been discharged, the gate pulse is terminated and the clock oscillator is turned off. The number of clock pulses counted is determined by the capacitor discharge time, which in turn is determined by the initial amount of charge deposited on the capacitor and thus depends on the amplitude of the input pulse. The MCA control circuits increment by one count the memory channel corresponding to the number of clock pulses counted, then clear the input circuitry and prepare the MCA to accept the next input pulse.

In the *successive approximation* or *SA* converter, digitization occurs by comparing the pulse amplitude to a selected sequence of voltage levels. The first comparison level is equal to one-half of the full-scale (maximum) value. If the pulse amplitude is greater than this level the first digital "bit" is set to "1"; if not, it is set to "0." The comparison voltage level then is either increased or decreased by one-half of its initial level, (i.e., to 25% or 75% of full-scale) depending on whether the pulse amplitude did or did not exceed the initial level. The comparison is repeated and the second digital bit is recorded as "1" or "0," depending on whether the pulse amplitude is greater or smaller than the new comparison voltage level. The comparisons are repeated through several steps, each time decreasing the voltage increment by one-half. The final set of bits provides a binary (base 2) representation for the amplitude of the input pulse.

For both the ramp and successive approximation converters, the output is represented as a binary number between $0-2^n$. The value of n determines the number of possible digital levels into which the input pulse amplitude can be converted. For example, an 8-bit converter, for which n = 8, divides the input range into 256 digital levels (2^8 = 256), a 10-bit converter into 1024 levels (2^{10} = 1024), etc. The larger the number of bits, the more accurately the ADC can determine the pulse amplitude. Thus, an 8-bit converter can determine amplitude to an accuracy one part in 256, a 10-bit converter to one part in 1024, etc. Generally, a larger number bits is favored for accuracy, but the digital conversion process then requires somewhat more time and the digitized values for pulse amplitude require greater amounts of computer storage space. Most nuclear medicine studies can be performed with 8-bit converters, but 10- and 12-bit converters also are used where accuracy is a prime concern, e.g., high-resolution energy spectroscopy with semiconductor detectors (Chapter 11, Section C.3).

A finite amount of time is required for the digital conversion processes described above. For example, for a 10-bit (1024 channel) ramp converter with a 100 MHz (10^8 cycles/sec) clock, the capacitor discharge time required for an event in the 1000th channel (1000 clock pulses) is 1000 pulses $\div$ 10^8 pulses/sec = 10^{-5} sec or 10 μsec. For an SA converter, time is needed for each of the voltage comparisons, e.g., a 10-bit SA converter must perform a sequence of ten voltage comparisons, each requiring a fraction of a microsecond to complete.

In addition to the conversion process, time is required to increment the memory location, reset the clock pulse counter on comparison voltage levels, etc. The ADC can be a "bottleneck" in MCAs as well as in the digital conversion process for signals from an Anger camera (Chapter 21, Section A); however, with careful attention to design, this no longer is a limiting factor for applications involving NaI(Tl) detectors, for which the primary time limitation is the decay time of the individual scintillation events.

Most MCAs have additional capabilities, such as offset or expansion of the analyzer voltage range, time histogram capabilities, etc. These are discussed in detail in MCA operators' manuals. Some scintillation cameras, well counters, and liquid scintillation counters contain MCAs that are used to examine and select energy windows of interest.

D. DIGITAL COUNTERS AND RATEMETERS

1. Scalers and Timers

Digital counters are used to count output signals from radiation detectors after pulse-height analysis of the signals. A device that only counts pulses is called a *scaler*. An auxiliary device that controls the scaler counting time is called a *timer*. An instrument that incorporates both functions in a single unit is called a *scaler–timer*. The number of counts recorded and the elapsed counting time may be displayed on a visual readout or may be printed out by printer or teletypewriter.

Figure 5-11 shows the front panel of a scaler–timer and a printer. A

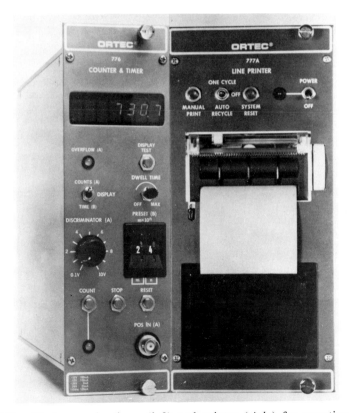

Fig. 5-11. Modern scaler-timer (*left*) and printer (*right*) for counting pulses (radiation events). These are also examples of NIM components (Section F). [Courtesy of EG&G ORTEC. Oak Ridge, Tennessee.]

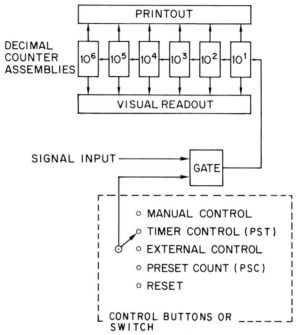

Fig. 5-12. Schematic representation of components and controls for a scaler–timer.

visual readout of counts and time is provided on the scaler by small light-emitting diodes (LEDs). The small size, low power requirements, and reliability of LEDs have resulted in their widespread use for digital readout displays of this type.

Figure 5-12 shows schematically the basic elements of a scaler–timer. The input pulse must pass through an electronic "gate" that is opened or closed by front-panel switches or pushbutton controls that select the mode of operation. When the gate is open, the pulses pass through to decimal counter assemblies (DCAs). Each DCA records from zero to nine events. The tenth pulse resets the counter assembly to zero and sends a pulse to the next DCA in the series. The number of counter assemblies determines the number of decades of scaler capacity. Thus a six-decade scaler has six DCAs and a counting capacity from 0 to 999,999 counts. (Usually the "one-millionth count" resets the scaler to "zero" and turns on an overflow light). Data from each DCA are transferred to the display for continuous visual readout of the number of counts recorded during the counting interval.

As shown in Figure 5-12, the scaler gate can be controlled in a number of different ways. In *preset-time* (PST) mode, the gate is controlled by a timer circuit (usually an oscillator-driven clock circuit) that opens the gate for a counting time selected by front-panel switches. The counting interval begins when a "start" button is depressed and is terminated automatically when the selected counting time has elapsed. In *preset-count* (PSC) mode, the counting interval ends when a preselected number of counts has been recorded. Preset-count mode is used when one wants to achieve the same degree of statistical reliability for all measurements in a series of counting measurements (Chapter 6). When PSC mode is used, a method must be available to determine the elapsed time for each counting measurement (e.g., a visual display or printout of elapsed counting time) so that counting rates for each measurement can be determined (preset counts/elapsed time).

External *control* of the scaler gate may be provided by an external timer or a sample-changer assembly. *Manual control* permits the operator to start and stop the counting interval by depressing front-panel "start" and "stop" buttons.

The maximum counting rate capability depends on the minimum time separation required between two pulses for the scaler to record them as separate events. A 20 MHz scaler (2×10^7 counts per second) can separate pulses that are spaced by 50 nsec, or 5×10^{-8} sec apart (2×10^7 counts/sec is equivalent to 1 count/5×10^{-8} sec). Most modern scalers are capable of 20–50 MHz counting rates, which means they can count at rates of several hundred thousand counts per second with losses of 1 percent or less due to pulse overlap or pileup (Chapter 12, Section C; Figure 5-6). Since pulse resolving times of most radiation detectors and their associated preamplifiers and amplifiers are on the order of 1 μsec, the counting rate limits of modern scalers are rarely of practical concern.

2. Analog Ratemeters

An *analog ratemeter* is used to determine the average number of events (e.g., SCA output pulses) occurring per unit of time. The average is determined continuously, rather than over discrete counting intervals, as would be the case with a scaler–timer. The output of a ratemeter is a continuously varying voltage level proportional to the average rate at which pulses are received at the ratemeter input. The output voltage can be displayed on a front-panel meter or recorded on a strip chart recorder calibrated to read in counts per minute or counts per second.

Figure 5-13 shows the basic components of an analog ratemeter. Input pulses pass through a pulse shaper, which shapes them to a constant amplitude and width. Each shaped pulse then causes a fixed amount of charge, Q, to be deposited on the capacitor C. The rate at which the

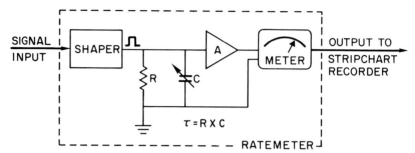

Fig. 5-13.   Schematic representation of an analog ratemeter. Adjustable capacitor C provides variable ratemeter time constant τ.

charge discharges through the resistor R is determined by the product
$R \times C$, which is called the *ratemeter time contant* τ.

Suppose that input pulses arrive at an average rate $\bar{n}$ pulses per
second. The capacitor discharge then produces an average current $\bar{I}$
through the resistor R_p given by

$$\bar{I} = \bar{n}Q \tag{5-3}$$

By Ohm's law, this causes an average voltage

$$\bar{V} = \bar{n}QR_p \tag{5-4}$$

to appear at the input to amplifier A. If the amplification factor of this
amplifier is k, the average output voltage $\bar{V_0}$ is given by

$$\bar{V_0} = k\bar{n}QR_p \tag{5-5}$$

Thus if k, Q, and R_p are constant factors for a given measurement,
average output voltage V_o is proportional to average input counting
rate $\bar{n}$.

The output voltage V_o can be used to drive a meter or a strip chart
recorder calibrated to read average counting rate. The calibration usually
is performed by adjusting the amplifier gain factor k. This factor is
adjusted to select different full-scale ranges for the readout device, e.g.,
0–1000 cpm, 0–10,000 cpm, etc.

A ratemeter that follows the relationship described by Equation 5-5 is
called a *linear* ratemeter. For some applications it is desirable to have a
logarithmic relationship:

$$\bar{V}_0 = k \log (\bar{n}QR_p) \tag{5-6}$$

The logarithmic conversion usually is performed by a logarithmic amplifier. *Logarithmic ratemeters* have the advantage of a very wide range of counting rate measurement, typically four or five decades, without the need to change range settings as with a linear ratemeter; however, it is more difficult to discern small changes in counting rate with a logarithmic ratemeter.

The voltage relationships described by Equations 5-5 and 5-6 apply to *average* values only. When the input pulse rate changes, the ratemeter output voltage does not respond instantaneously but responds over a period of time determined by the ratemeter time constant τ. Figure 5-14 illustrates the response characteristic of a linear ratemeter. The relationship between indicated counting rate R_i and the new average counting $\overline{R}_a$, following a change occurring at time $t = 0$ from a previous average value $\overline{R}_0$, is given by

$$R_i = \overline{R}_a - (\overline{R}_a - \overline{R}_0)e^{-t/\tau} \qquad (5\text{-}7)$$

The ratemeter reading (or output voltage) approaches its new average value exponentially with time t. Typically, three to five time constants are needed to reach a new stable value.

The ratemeter time constant is selected by a front panel switch (usually by adjusting the capacitor value C) and may range from hundredths of a second to tens of seconds. Figure 5-14 shows that a ratemeter actually provides a distorted representation of counting rate versus time (rounded edges and delayed response). This distortion can be minimized by choosing a very short time constant (Figure 5-14B). A long time constant has the advantage of smoothing out statistical fluctuations in counting rate, but it produces a more distorted representation of changes in counting rates (Figure 5-14A). These tradeoffs are discussed further in Chapter 6, Section D.9.

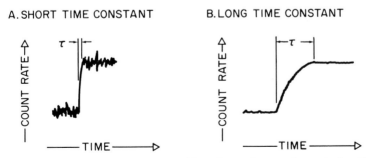

Fig. 5-14.   Ratemeter response to a sudden change in counting rate for different ratemeter time constants. A short time constant (A) reflects the change more accurately, but a long time constant (B) provides smaller statistical noise fluctuations (Chapter 6, Section D.9).

E. HIGH-VOLTAGE POWER SUPPLIES

The high-voltage power supply provides the charge collection voltage for semiconductor, gas proportional, and Geiger–Müller (GM) detectors and the accelerating voltage for electron multiplication in the PM tubes used with scintillation detectors such as NaI(Tl) and liquid scintillators. The high-voltage power supply converts the alternating (AC) voltage provided by the line source into a constant or direct (DC) voltage.

Whereas variation of the high voltage (HV) has little effect on the output pulse amplitude with semiconductor and GM detectors, changes in the HV with gas proportional or scintillation detectors strongly affect their output pulse amplitude. For example, a 1 percent change in the HV on a scintillation detector PM tube can change the output pulse amplitude by 10 percent or more because the HV on the PM tube (and on gas proportional counters) determines the multiplication factor for the number of electrons caused by an ionization event in those detectors.

Instabilities in HV power supplies can arise from a number of factors, such as time, temperature changes, variations in line voltage, and the amount of current drawn by the detector (commonly referred to as the output load). In a well-regulated HV power supply suitable for scintillation detectors, the effects of time and temperature are more important than the effects of line voltage and current loads (unless maximum current ratings are exceeded); however, the former problems are still relatively small, since modern HV supplies are very stable for long time periods and over wide temperature ranges.

The output current rating of the HV power supply must be sufficient for the particular detector system. Most scintillation detectors draw about one milliampere (mA) of current, for which the 0–10 mA rating of most commercial HV supplies is adequate. If the current load is inadvertently increased above this limit, it will affect the stability and may even damage the HV supply. Thus the current requirements of the detector or detectors should be within the specified limits for the HV supply. The current requirements need to be specified at the intended operating voltage of the detector, since the current load drawn by the detector will increase with the applied voltage. Many commercial HV supplies have an overload protection circuit that will shut off the unit if the recommended current load is exceeded.

Superimposed on the DC output of the high voltage supply is a time-varying component, usually of relatively small amplitude, referred to as "ripple." The amplitude of ripple ranges from 10 to 100 mV in most commercial units. Ripple in the HV supply can be a serious problem with high-resolution semiconductor detectors, since it produces noise in the detector output and reduces the energy resolution of the detector. HV supplies used in conjunction with high-resolution semiconductors usually have a ripple of <10 mV.

F. NUCLEAR INSTRUMENT MODULES (NIMs)

Most of the counting and imaging instruments used in nuclear medicine are dedicated to specific and well-defined tasks. Usually, they are designed as self-contained "hard-wired" units, with no capability for interchanging components, such as amplifiers, SCAs, or scalers, between different instruments. Although this generally results in an efficiently designed and attractively packaged instrument, there are some applications, especially in research, for which interchangeability of components is highly desirable. For example, most scaler, timers, and ratemeters can be used with any detector system, but different detectors may require different amplifiers, and different types of pulse-height analyzers may be desired for different pulse-timing requirements.

Flexibility and interchangeability of components are provided by the *nuclear instrument module,* or NIM. Individual NIM components (scalers, amplifiers, etc.) slide into slots in a master "bin" from which they draw their operating power. They have standard input and output signals and are interconnectable with standard cables and connectors.

A NIM system generally is more expensive than a dedicated system with the same capabilities; however, it has the advantage that it can be upgraded or applied to different counting problems by replacement of individual components rather than replacing the entire unit. A wide variety of component types and performance specifications are available in the NIM system. Examples of NIM components are shown in Fig. 5-11.

G. CATHODE RAY TUBE (CRT)

The *cathode ray tube* (CRT) is the most common display device employed in nuclear medicine. The CRT is an evacuated tube containing the basic components shown in Figure 5-15. Cathode ray tubes are used on scintillation cameras, scanners, computers, MCAs, well counters, and liquid scintillation counters. In all these applications the output signals of the instrument are transferred to the CRT, which presents a two-dimensional visual display of the data as points, lines, or characters on the output screen of the CRT. In this section, we will examine the basic features of the CRT and its major components.

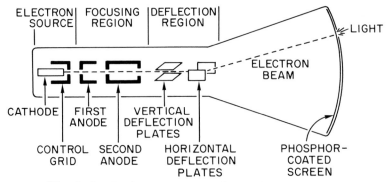

Fig. 5-15. Basic components of a cathode ray tube (CRT).

1. Electron Gun

The electron gun provides a focused source of electrons and consists of a *cathode, control grid,* an *accelerating* and *focusing anode* (Figure 5-16). Most CRTs use a hot or thermionic emission cathode. Electrons are boiled off the cathode by heating it with an electric current. This type of electron source is commonly referred to as a hot filament and is similar to that used in x-ray tubes. The cathode can be made of tungsten, thoriated tungsten (tungsten coated with a few percent of thorium), or nickel coated with oxides of barium and strontium. Most CRTs employ the last type because of low work function (energy required to remove electrons from the cathode surface).

The control grid is a cap that fits over the cathode. The electrons pass through a small hole in its center (Figure 5-16). A negative potential on the

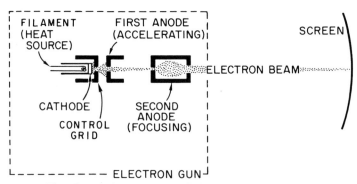

Fig. 5-16. Components of the electron gun in a CRT.

grid can be varied to control the number of electrons that are allowed to pass. The control of the grid is complete in that it can shut off completely the flow of electrons or allow large numbers of electrons to pass.

The accelerating anode is similar in shape to the grid except that its orientation is reversed (Figure 5-16). The flat end contains a small hole through which the electrons pass. This is the accelerating anode. It has a high positive potential that attracts the electrons and accelerates them to high velocities. Most of the electrons actually strike the front face of the first anode, but a small percentage pass through the opening and are accelerated down the CRT tube as a narrow beam.

The focusing anode further shapes the electron beam to focus it to a sharp point where it strikes the phosphor-coated screen (Figure 5-16). A negative potential on the second anode is used to both compress and focus the beam of electrons. The diameter of the electron beam striking the phosphor screen is usually about 0.1 mm.

Thus the electron gun provides a variable-intensity source of electrons and acts as an electrostatic lens to focus a narrow beam of electrons onto the phosphor-coated screen.

2. Deflection Plates

Deflection plates (Figures 5-15 and 5-17) are used to move the electron beam across the screen. Two different types of deflection are used in CRTs: *electrostatic* and *electromagnetic*. Electrostatic deflection employs two sets of plates mounted at right angles to each other. Voltages are applied to one pair to exert a force on the electron beam in the vertical direction and on the other pair for the horizontal direction (Figure 5-17) on the display screen. The amount of deflection is proportional to the voltage applied to the deflection plates.

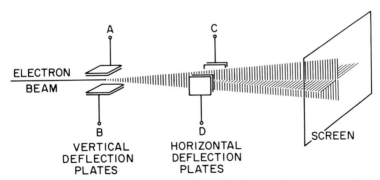

Fig. 5-17.   Deflection plates used to position the electron beam on the phosphor-coated screen of a CRT.

For electromagnetic deflection, the plates shown in Figure 5-17 are replaced by two sets of wire coils. Magnetic fields are produced by passing a current through the coils. Deflection of the electron beam is controlled by varying the current (i.e., strength of magnetic fields) through the two sets of coils.

Electrostatic deflection usually is employed in small displays (up to about 25 cm diam) and can display points at a rate of about 10^6 points/sec. Larger displays use electromagnetic deflection for better focusing and resolution, but are slower (up to about 10^5 points/sec).

3. Phosphor-coated Display Screens

The *display screen* is a glass screen having an inside surface coated with a phosphorescent material. The high-velocity electrons striking the phosphor cause it to give off *phosphorescent light*. The brightness of the phosphorescent light depends on the intensity and energy of the electron beam. The lifetime of the light emission from the phosphor is referred to as the *persistence* time and ranges from microseconds to minutes, depending on the phosphor material. If the persistence time is short, the data presented on the screen must either be refreshed from a memory device or be photographed with a camera using a continuous exposure as the data are displayed.

Some CRTs have very long persistence time (up to several minutes or longer). These CRTs are referred to as *persistence scopes*. In comparison to a conventional CRT (Figure 5-15), a persistence scope has two additional components: a fine mesh screen called the *storage mesh* located in the electron beam path directly behind the phosphor-coated display screen, and an additional electron source called the *flood gun* located just outside the deflection region. When the primary electron beam scans the phosphor-coated display screen, some of the high-energy electrons in the beam strike the storage mesh and release secondary electrons from it. These electrons are attracted to the display screen, leaving a positive-charge pattern on the storage mesh. The flood gun then generates a cloud of electrons that are acclerated toward the storage mesh and display screen. The number of these electrons passing through different regions of the storage mesh and striking the display screen is determined by the amount of positive charge on the storage mesh, which in turn is determined by the intensity of the primary electron beam as it scanned that region. The rate at which the charge pattern leaks from the storage mesh can be adjusted electronically in "variable persistence" scopes, permitting the rate of build up and decay of the displayed pattern to be varied. This type of CRT frequently is used as a visual monitor to facilitate patient positioning with the Anger camera (Chapter 15, Section

B.4); however, persistence scopes generally are not used for photographic image recording because of their limited grey scale and relatively large dot sizes.

4. Focus and Brightness Controls

The *focus* of the electrostatic-type CRT can be controlled, as discussed earlier, by varying the voltage on the second anode of the electron gun. By changing the anode voltage, the electron beam can be narrowed to a sharp spot on the display screen. The focus control is a potentiometer (variable resistor), which usually can be varied by means of a front panel knob.

The *intensity* or *brightness* control is a potentiometer that changes the voltage on the control grid of the CRT. Decreasing the (negative) voltage on the control grid causes an increased flow of electrons and increases the spot intensity. Conversely, increasing the (negative) control grid voltage results in a decrease in spot intensity. A knob for brightness (or intensity) control is provided on the front panel of most CRT displays.

5. Color Cathode Ray Tubes

A color CRT has three electron guns that focus three different electron beams onto arrays of individual phosphors in a cluster on the output display screen, as shown in Figure 5-18. The individual phosphors produce colors of red, green, and blue when struck by the electron beam. The electron guns are turned on individually or simultaneously to produce a range of colors from the single-phosphor colors to combinations or blends of colors. A total of about 64 different colors recognizable by the human eye can be produced with a three-electron-gun system.

H. OSCILLOSCOPES

The oscilloscope is an instrument that displays as a function of time the amplitude (voltage) and frequency of signals from such devices as EEGs and EKGs. It is also used for testing, calibrating, and repairing electronic equipment in nuclear medicine. A typical oscilloscope consists of a CRT, a signal amplifier for the vertical deflection plate of the CRT, and a time-sweep generator.

An amplifier is provided so that small voltage inputs can be amplified and applied to the vertical deflection plate to display the amplitude of the input signals. The time-sweep generator is connected to the horizontal deflection plates of the CRT to sweep the electron beam across the screen

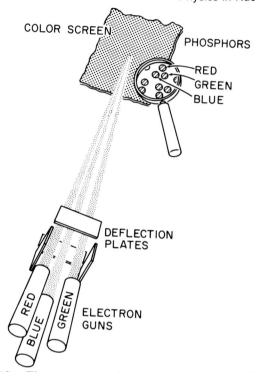

Fig. 5-18.   Electron guns and phosphors for a color CRT display.

at a constant speed and repetition rate. The horizontal sweep rate can usually be varied from nanoseconds (10^{-9} sec) to seconds per centimeter by a calibrated selector switch on the front panel of the oscilloscope. Thus the oscilloscope provides a visual display of time-varying electrical signals.

The most common nuclear medicine application of oscilloscopes is in cardiac studies. In this application the oscilloscope is not only used to display the EKG pattern but also for selection of multiple phases of the cardiac cycle for gating the scintillation camera (Chapter 21, Section A.3).

I. TELEVISION MONITORS

Television (TV) monitors are the most common type of display used with computers in nuclear medicine. They are basically CRTs in which the horizontal and vertical deflection plates are controlled by constant-frequency time-sweep generators. Thus the horizontal and vertical scan-

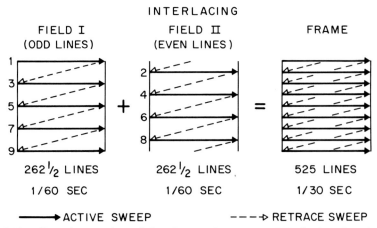

Fig. 5-19.   Scanning motion of the electron beam on a TV display. Interlaced lines of two fields (left) produce a frame (right).

ning motion of the electron beam is in a fixed sequence and at a fixed rate. The scanning sequence is as follows (Figure 5-19): The electron beam is first scanned in a horizontal direction across the phosphorescent screen. This is referred to as the *active sweep,* since the electron gun is on and the variation in the intensity (and energy) of the beam at each point along the scan represents the image data along a corresponding line. At the end of the first scan the beam is scanned back in the horizontal direction without transmitting information to the screen. This is called the *retrace sweep,* and is about five times faster than the active sweep. Each active sweep is displaced slightly below the preceding one. The number of active sweeps across the screen for the full image is usually 525 or 625, but may be as high as 1024 or more. Thus the image is divided into 525 or more horizontal lines on the output screen of the TV monitor.

Most TV monitors sweep through all the odd-numbered horizontal lines (1, 3, 5, etc.) and then return to the top of the screen (*vertical retrace*) to resweep the image for the even-numbered lines (2, 4, 6, etc.). This is called *interlacing.* The two sets of scan lines are called *fields* (Figure 5-19). The image produced by the two interlaced fields is called a *frame.* A frame is completed in 1/30 of a second with AC line frequencies of 60 cycles/sec (U.S.) and 1/25 of a second for 50 cycles/sec line frequencies (Europe). The frame rate (30 per second) is sufficient to maintain the appearance of continuous motion on moving images, without a "jerky" appearance: fields are repeated at a rate of 60 per second, which is beyond the temporal resolution of the human eye; thus the image does not appear to flicker.

The vertical resolution of TV monitors is determined by the number of horizontal lines; however, because of the time required for retrace sweeps and inaccuracies in line position, the full number of lines (i.e., 525) is not available for the final image.[1] Typically only 65 percent of the lines are actually used to define the resolution (i.e., a 525-line TV monitor has a vertical resolution of 343 lines).

The horizontal resolution is limited electronically by the rate at which the brightness signal can be varied during the horizontal sweep without significant distortion. This is referred to as the *bandpass* frequency or *bandwidth*. Usually the TV monitors have bandwidths that produce a horizontal resolution about equal to the vertical resolution.

REFERENCES

1. Templeton AW, Dwyer SJ, Jansen C, et al: Standard and high-scan line television systems. Radiology 91:725–730, 1968

    Basic electricity and electronics are discussed in the following:
Harris CC: Applied electronics, in Rollo FD (ed): Nuclear Medicine Physics, Instrumentation, and Agents. St. Louis, C. V. Mosby Co., 1977, pp 111–191
Prior RM: Electronics, in Boyd CM, Dalrymple GV (eds): Basic Science Principles of Nuclear Medicine. St. Louis, C. V. Mosby Co., 1974, chap 7
Rollo FD, Richardson RL: Basic electronics, In Rollo FD (ed): Nuclear Medicine Physics, Instrumentation, and Agents. St. Louis, C. V. Mosby Co., 1977, pp 72–110

    Useful descriptions of basic principles of detectors and counting system components are often published by instrument manufacturers. See, for example:
ORTEC Physical Science Division Catalog. ORTEC Inc., 100 Midland Road, Oak Ridge, TN 37830

    Other, more detailed references on nuclear counting electronics are as follows:
Kowalski E: Nuclear Counting Electronics. New York, Springer, 1970
Krugers J: Instrumentation in Applied Nuclear Chemistry. New York, Plenum Press, 1973

6

Nuclear Counting Statistics

All measurements are subject to measurement error. This includes physical measurements, such as radiation counting measurements used in nuclear medicine procedures, as well as biological and clinical studies, such as evaluation of the effectiveness of an imaging technique. In this chapter, we discuss the type of errors that occur, how they are analyzed, and how in some cases, they can be minimized.

A. TYPES OF MEASUREMENT ERROR

Measurement errors are of three general types:

Blunders are errors that are adequately described by their name. Usually they produce grossly inaccurate results and their occurrence is easily detected. Examples in radiation measurements include the use of incorrect instrument settings, incorrect labeling of sample containers, injecting the wrong radiopharmaceutical into the patient, etc. When a single data value seems to be grossly out of line with others in an experiment, statistical tests are available to determine whether the suspect value may be discarded (Section E.3). Apart from this there is no way to "analyze" errors of this type, only to avoid them by careful work.

Systematic errors produce results that differ consistently from the correct result by some fixed amount. The same result may be obtained in repeated measurements, but it is the wrong result. For example, length measurements with a "warped" ruler, or radiation counting measurements with a "sticky" timer or other persistent instrument malfunction, could contain systematic errors. Observer "bias" in the subjective interpretation of data (e.g., scan reading) is another example of systematic error, as would be the use for a clinical study of two population groups having underlying differences in some important characteristic, e.g., different average ages. Measurement results having systematic errors are said to be *inaccurate*.

It is not always easy to detect the presence of systematic error. Measurement results affected by systematic error may be very repeatable and not too different from the expected results, which may lead to a mistaken sense of confidence. One way to detect systematic error in physical measurements is by the use of measurement *standards*, which are known from previous measurements with a properly operating system to give a certain measurement result. For example, radionuclide standards, containing a known quantity of radioactivity, are used in various "quality assurance" procedures to test for systematic error in radiation counting systems. Some of these procedures are described in Chapter 12, Section D.

Random errors are variations in results from one measurement to the next, arising from physical limitations of the measurement system or from actual random variations of the measured quantity itself. For example, length measurements with an ordinary ruler are subject to random error because of inexact repositioning of the ruler and limitations of the human eye. In clinical or animal studies, random error may arise from differences between subjects, e.g., in uptake of a radiopharmaceutical. Random error always is present in radiation counting measurements because the quantity that is being measured—namely, the rate of emission from the radiation source—is itself a randomly varying quantity.

Random error affects measurement *reproducibility* and the ability to detect real differences in measured data. Measurements that are very reproducible—in that nearly the same result is obtained in repeated measurements—are said to be *precise*. It is possible to minimize random error by using careful measurement technique, refined instrumentation, etc; however, it is impossible to eliminate it completely. There is always *some* limit to the precision of a measurement or measurement system. The amount of random error present is sometimes called the *uncertainty* in the measurement.

It also is possible for a measurement to be precise (small random error) but inaccurate (large systematic error), or vice versa. For example, length measurements with a warped ruler may be very reproducible (precise); nevertheless, they still are inaccurate. On the other hand, radiation counting measurements may be imprecise (because of inevitable variations in radiation emission rates) but still they can be accurate, at least in an average sense.

Because random errors always are present in radiation counting and other measured data, it is necessary to be able to analyze them and to obtain estimates of their magnitude. This is done using methods of statistical analysis. (For this reason, they are also sometimes called *statistical errors*.) The remainder of this chapter describes these methods of analysis. The discussion will focus on applications involving nuclear radiation counting measurements; however, some of the methods to be described also are applicable to a wider class of experimental data as discussed in Section E.

B. NUCLEAR COUNTING STATISTICS

1. The Poisson Distribution

Suppose that a long-lived radioactive sample is counted repeatedly under supposedly identical conditions with a properly operating counting system. Because the disintegration rate of the radioactive sample undergoes random variations from one moment to the next, the numbers of counts recorded in successive measurements (N_1, N_2, N_3, etc.) are not the same. Given that different results are obtained from one measurement to the next, one might question if a "true value" for the measurement actually exists. One possible solution is to make a large number of measurements and use the average $\overline{N}$ as an estimate for the "true value":

$$\text{True Value} \approx \overline{N} \tag{6-1}$$

$$\overline{N} = (N_1 + N_2 + \cdots + N_n)/n \tag{6-2}$$

$$= \sum_{i=1}^{n} \frac{N_i}{n} \tag{6-3}$$

where n is the number of measurements taken. The notation Σ_i indicates that a sum is taken over values of the parameter with the subscript i.

Unfortunately, multiple measurements are impractical in routine practice, and one must usually be satisfied with taking only one measurement. The question then is, how good is the result of a single measurement as an estimate of the "true value," i.e., what is the uncertainty in this result? The answer to this depends on the *frequency distribution* of the measurement results. Figure 6-1 shows a typical frequency distribution curve for radiation counting measurements. The solid dots show the different possible results, (i.e., number of counts recorded) versus the probability of getting each result. The probability is peaked at a mean value m, which is the "true value" for the measurement. Thus if a large

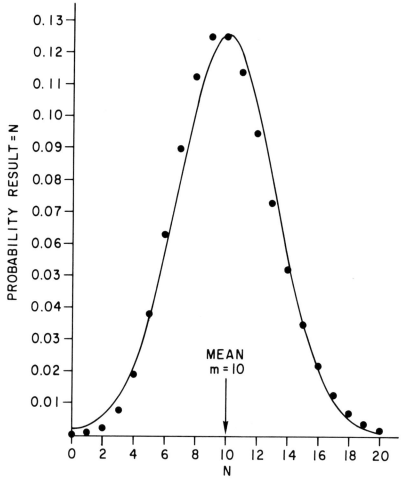

Fig. 6-1.   Poisson (●) and Gaussian (—) distributions for mean, m, and variance, σ^2, = 10.

number of measurements were made and their results averaged, one would obtain

$$\overline{N} \approx m \qquad\qquad (6\text{-}4)$$

The solid dots in Figure 6-1 are described mathematically by the *Poisson distribution*. For this distribution, the probability of getting a certain result N when the true value is m

$$P(N;m) = e^{-m}\, m^N/N! \qquad\qquad (6\text{-}5)$$

where e (= 2.718 . . .) is the base of natural logarithms and $N!$ (N *factorial*) is the product of all integers up to N (i.e., $1 \times 2 \times 3 \times \cdots \times N$). From Figure 6-1 it is apparent that the probability of getting the exact result $N = m$ is rather small; however, one could hope that the result would at least be "close to" m. Note that the Poisson distribution is defined only for non-negative integer values of N (0,1,2, . . .).

The probability that a measurement result will be "close to" m depends on the relative width, or dispersion, of the frequency distribution curve. This is related to a parameter called the *variance, σ^2*, of the distribution. The variance is a *number* such that 68.3 percent ($\sim \frac{2}{3}$) of the measurement results fall within $\pm \sigma$ (i.e. square root of the variance) of the true value m. For the Poisson distribution, the variance is given by

$$\sigma^2 = m \qquad (6\text{-}6)$$

Thus one expects to find approximately $\frac{2}{3}$ of the counting measurement results within the range $\pm \sqrt{m}$ of the true value m.

Given only the result of a single measurement, N, one does not know the exact value of m or of σ; however, one can reasonably assume that $N \approx m$, and thus that $\sigma \approx \sqrt{N}$. One can therefore say that if the result of the measurement is N, there is a 68.3 percent chance that the true value of the measurement m is within the range $N \pm \sqrt{N}$. This is called the "68.3 percent *confidence interval*" for m; i.e., one is 68.3 percent confident that m is in the range $N \pm \sqrt{N}$.

The range $\pm \sqrt{N}$ is the uncertainty in N. The *percentage uncertainty in N* is

$$V = (\sqrt{N}/N) \times 100\% \qquad (6\text{-}7)$$

$$= 100\%/\sqrt{N} \qquad (6\text{-}8)$$

Example 6-1.
  Compare the percentage uncertainties in the measurements N_1 = 100 counts and N_2 = 10,000 counts.

Answer.
  For N_1 = 100 counts, V_1 = $100\%/\sqrt{100}$ = 10% (Equation 6-8). For N_2 = 10,000 counts, V_2 = $100\%/\sqrt{10,000}$ = 1%. Thus the percentage uncertainty in 10,000 counts is only $\frac{1}{10}$ the percentage uncertainty in 100 counts.

Equation 6-8 and Example 6-1 indicate that *large numbers of counts have smaller percentage uncertainties and are statistically more reliable than small numbers of counts.*

Other confidence intervals can be defined in terms of σ or $\sqrt{N}$. They

Table 6-1
Confidence Levels in Radiation Counting Measurements

Range	Confidence Level for m (True Value) (%)
$N \pm 0.675\sigma$	50
$N \pm \sigma$	68.3
$N \pm 1.64\sigma$	90
$N \pm 2\sigma$	95
$N \pm 3\sigma$	99.7

are summarized in Table 6-1. The 50 percent confidence interval ($0.675\sqrt{N}$) is sometimes called the *probable error* (PE) in N.

2. The Standard Deviation

The variance σ^2 is related to a statistical index called the *standard deviation* (SD). The standard deviation is a number that is calculated for a series of measurements. If n counting measurements are made, with results $N_1, N_2, N_3, \ldots, N_n$, and a mean value $\overline{N}$ for those results is found, the standard deviation is

$$SD = \left(\sum_{i=1}^{n} \frac{(N_i - \overline{N})^2}{n - 1} \right)^{1/2} \tag{6-9}$$

(recall that raising a quantity to the ½ power is the same as taking its square root). The standard deviation is a measure of the dispersion of measurement results about the mean and is in fact an estimate of σ, the square root of the variance. For radiation counting measurements one therefore should obtain

$$SD \approx \sqrt{N} \tag{6-10}$$

This can be used as a test to determine if the random error observed in a series of counting measurements is consistent with that predicted from random variations in source decay rate, or if there are additional random errors present, e.g., from faulty instrument performance. This is discussed further in Section E.

3. The Gaussian Distribution

When the mean value m is "large" the Poisson distribution can be approximated by the *Gaussian distribution* (also called the *normal distribution*). The equation describing the Gaussian distribution is

$$P(x;m,\sigma) = (1/\sqrt{2\pi\sigma^2})\, e^{-(x-m)^2/2\sigma^2} \qquad (6\text{-}11)$$

where m and σ^2 are again the mean and variance. Equation 6-11 describes a symmetric "bell-shaped" curve. As shown by Figure 6-1, the Gaussian distribution is very similar to the Poisson distribution for $m = 10$. For $m \gtrsim 20$, the distributions are virtually indistinguishable. Two important differences are that the Poisson distribution is defined only for non-negative integers, whereas the Gaussian distribution is defined for any value of x, and that for the Poisson distribution, the variance σ^2 is equal to the mean, m, whereas for the Gaussian distribution, it can have any value.

The Gaussian distribution with $\sigma^2 = m$ is a useful approximation for radiation counting measurements when the only random error present is that due to random variations in source decay rate. When additional sources of random error are present—e.g., a random error or uncertainty of ΔN counts due to variations in sample preparation technique, counting system variations, etc.—the results are described by the Gaussian distribution with variance given by

$$\sigma^2 \approx m + (\Delta N)^2 \qquad (6\text{-}12)$$

The resulting Gaussian distribution curve would be wider than a Poisson curve with $\sigma^2 = m$. The confidence intervals given in Table 6-1 may be used for the Gaussian distribution with this modified value for the variance. For example, the 68.3 percent confidence interval for a measurement result N would be $\pm (N + (\Delta N)^2)^{1/2}$ (assuming $N \approx m$).

Example 6-2.
  A 1 ml radioactive sample is pipetted into a test tube for counting. The precision of the pipette is specified as "± 2 percent," and 5000 counts are recorded from the sample. What is the uncertainty in sample counts per ml?

Answer.
  The uncertainty in counts arising from pipetting precision is 2% × 5000 counts = 100 counts. Therefore $\sigma^2 = 5000 + (100)^2 \approx 15{,}000$, and the uncertainty is $\sqrt{15{,}000} \approx 122$ counts. Compare this to the uncertainty of $\sqrt{5000} \approx 71$ counts that would be obtained without the pipetting uncertainty.

C. PROPAGATION OF ERRORS

The preceding section described methods for estimating the random error or uncertainty in a single counting measurement; however, most nuclear medicine procedures involve multiple counting measurements, from which ratios, differences, and so on are used to compute the final result. If a set of independent counting measurements, N_1, N_2, N_3, ... are used in the calculations, the uncertainty in the final result can be calculated using the following rules.

    1. Sums and Differences

$$\sigma(N_1 \pm N_2 \pm N_3 \pm ..) = \sqrt{N_1 + N_2 + N_3 + \cdots} \qquad (6\text{-}13)$$

    2. Constant Multipliers
If a counting measurement N is multiplied by a constant k,

$$\sigma(kN) = k\sigma_N = k\sqrt{N} \qquad (6\text{-}14)$$

The percentage uncertainty V in the product kN is

$$V(kN) = [\sigma(kN)/kN] \times 100\% \qquad (6\text{-}15)$$
$$= 100\%/\sqrt{N} \qquad (6\text{-}16)$$

which is the same result as Equation 6-8. Thus, there is no statistical advantage gained or lost in multiplying the number of counts recorded by a constant. The percentage uncertainty still depends on the actual number of counts recorded.

    3. Products and Ratios

$$V(N_1 \overset{\times}{\div} N_2 \overset{\times}{\div} N_3 \overset{\times}{\div} \ldots) = \sqrt{1/N_1 + 1/N_2 + 1/N_3 + \cdots} \qquad (6\text{-}17)$$

    4. More Complicated Combinations
Many nuclear medicine procedures, e.g., thyroid uptakes, blood volume determinations, etc., use equations of the following general form

$$Y = k(N_1 - N_2)/(N_3 - N_4) \qquad (6\text{-}18)$$

Using the rules given above, one can show that

$$V_Y = \sqrt{(N_1 + N_2)/(N_1 - N_2)^2 + (N_3 + N_4)/(N_3 - N_4)^2} \times 100\% \qquad (6\text{-}19)$$
$$\sigma_Y = V_Y \times Y/100\% \qquad (6\text{-}20)$$

Example 6-3.
    A patient is injected with a radionuclide. At some later time a blood sample is withdrawn for counting in a well counter and $N_p = 1200$ counts are recorded. A blood sample withdrawn prior to injection gives a blood background of $N_{pb} = 400$ counts. A standard

prepared from the injection preparation records $N_s = 2000$ counts, and a "blank" sample records an instrument background of $N_b = 200$ counts. Calculate the ratio of net patient sample counts to net standard counts, and the uncertainty in this ratio.

Answer.

The ratio is
$$Y = (N_p - N_{pb})/(N_s - N_b)$$
$$= (1200 - 400)/(2000 - 200)$$
$$= 800/1800 = 0.44$$

The percentage uncertainty in the ratio is (Equation 6-19)

$$V_Y = \sqrt{(1200 + 400)/(800)^2 + (2000 + 200)/(1800)^2} \times 100\%$$
$$= 5.6\%$$

The uncertainty in Y is $5.6\% \times 0.44 \approx 0.02$; thus the ratio and its uncertainty are $Y = 0.44 \pm 0.02$.

D. APPLICATIONS OF STATISTICAL ANALYSIS

1. Effects of Averaging

If n counting measurements are used to compute an average result, the average $\overline{N}$ is a more reliable estimate of the true value than any one of the individual measurements. The uncertainty in $\overline{N}$, $\sigma_{\overline{N}}$, can be obtained by combining the rules for sums (Equation 6-13) and constant multipliers (Equation 6-14).

$$\sigma_{\overline{N}} = \sqrt{\overline{N}/n} \tag{6-21}$$

The uncertainty in $\overline{N}$ as an estimator of m therefore is smaller than the uncertainty in a single measurement by a factor $1/\sqrt{n}$.

2. Counting Rates

If N counts are recorded during a measuring time t, the average counting rate during that interval is $R = N/t$. Using Equation 6-14, the uncertainty in the counting rate R is

$$\sigma_R = (1/t)\sqrt{N} \tag{6-22}$$
$$= \sqrt{N/t^2} \tag{6-23}$$
$$= \sqrt{R/t} \tag{6-24}$$

The percentage uncertainty in R is

$$V_R = (\sigma_R/R) \times 100\% \qquad (6\text{-}25)$$
$$= 100\%/\sqrt{Rt} \qquad (6\text{-}26)$$

Example 6-4.
   In a 2 min counting measurement, 4900 counts are recorded. What is the average counting rate R (cpm) and its uncertainty?

Answer. $\qquad R = 4900/2 = 2450 \text{ cpm}$

$\qquad\qquad \sigma_R = \sqrt{2450/2} = 35 \text{ cpm}$

$\qquad\qquad V_R = 100\%/\sqrt{2450 \times 2} \approx 1.4\%$

Note from Equations 6-24 and 6-26 that *longer counting times produce smaller uncertainties in estimated counting rates.*

3. Significance of Differences Between Counting Measurements

Suppose two samples are counted and that counts N_1 and N_2 are recorded. The difference $N_1 - N_2$ may be due to an actual difference between sample activities or may be simply the result of random variations in counting rates. There is no way to state with absolute certainty that a given difference is or is not caused by random error; however, one can assess the "statistical significance" of the difference by comparing it to the expected random error. In general, differences of less than 2σ [i.e., $(N_1 - N_2) < 2(N_1 + N_2)^{1/2}$] are considered to be of marginal or no statistical significance because there is at least a 5 percent chance that such a difference is simply caused by random error. Differences greater than 3σ are considered significant (<1 percent chance caused by random error), while differences between 2σ and 3σ are in the questionable category, perhaps deserving repeat measurement and/or longer measuring times to determine their significance.
   If two counting rates R_1 and R_2 are determined from measurements using counting times t_1 and t_2, respectively, the uncertainty in their difference, $R_1 - R_2$ can be obtained by applying Equations 6-13 and 6-24.

$$\sigma(R_1 - R_2) = \sqrt{R_1/t_1 + R_2/t_2} \qquad (6\text{-}27)$$

Comparison of the observed difference to the expected random error difference can again be used to assess statistical significance, as described above.

4. Effects of Background

All nuclear counting instruments have background counting rates, consisting of electronic noise, detection of cosmic rays, natural radioactivity in the detector itself (e.g., ^{40}K), etc. If the background counting rate, measured with no sample present, is R_b and the gross counting rate with the sample is R_g, then the net sample counting rate is

$$R_s = R_g - R_b \qquad (6\text{-}28)$$

The uncertainty in R_s is (from Equation 6-27)

$$\sigma_{R_s} = \sqrt{R_g/t_g + R_b/t_b} \qquad (6\text{-}29)$$

The percentage uncertainty in R_s is

$$V_{R_s} = \frac{\sqrt{R_g/t_g + R_b/t_b}}{R_g - R_b} \times 100\% \qquad (6\text{-}30)$$

If the same counting time t is used for both sample and background counting,

$$\sigma_{R_s} = \frac{1}{\sqrt{t}} \sqrt{R_g + R_b} \qquad (6\text{-}31)$$

$$= \frac{1}{\sqrt{t}} \sqrt{R_s + 2R_b} \qquad (6\text{-}32)$$

Example 6-5

In 4 min counting measurements, gross sample counts are 6000 counts and background counts are 4000 counts. What is the net sample counting rate and its uncertainty?

$$Answer: R_g = 6000/4 = 1500 \text{ cpm}$$
$$R_b = 4000/4 = 1000 \text{ cpm}$$
$$R_s = 1500 - 1000 = 500 \text{ cpm}$$
$$\sigma_{R_s} = \frac{1}{\sqrt{4}} \sqrt{1500 + 1000}$$
$$= \tfrac{1}{2} \times \sqrt{2500}$$
$$= \tfrac{1}{2} \times (50)$$
$$= 25 \text{ cpm}$$

Therefore $R_s = 500 \pm 25$ cpm (± 5 percent). Compare this to the uncertainty in the gross counting rate R_g,

$$\sigma_{R_g} = \frac{1}{\sqrt{4}} \sqrt{1500} \approx 19 \text{ cpm } (\sim 1 \text{ percent})$$

and to the uncertainty in R_s that would be obtained if there were negligible background ($R_b \approx 0$),

$$\sigma_{R_s} = \frac{1}{\sqrt{4}} \sqrt{500} \approx 11 \text{ cpm } (\sim 2 \text{ percent})$$

Example 6-5 illustrates two important points:

1. *High background counting rates are undesirable because they increase uncertainties in net sample counting rates.*
2. *Small differences between relatively high counting rates can have relatively large uncertainties.*

5. Minimum Detectable Activity (MDA)

The minimum detectable activity (MDA) of a radionuclide for a particular counting system and counting time t is that activity that increases the counts recorded by an amount that is "statistically significant" in comparison to the random variation in background counts recorded during the same measuring time. In this instance, statistically significant means a counting rate increase of 3σ. The counting rate for the minimum detectable activity is therefore $3(R_b/t)^{1/2}$. (Equation 6-24)

Example 6-6.
A standard NaI(Tl) well counter has a background counting rate (full spectrum) of about 200 cpm. The sensitivity of the well counter for ^{131}I is about 10^6 cpm/μCi (Chapter 13, Table 13-2). What is the MDA for ^{131}I, using 4 min counting measurements?

Answer.
The MDA is that amount of ^{131}I giving $3(200/4)^{1/2} \approx 3 \times 7 = 21$ cpm. Thus

$$\text{MDA} = 21 \text{ cpm}/10^6 \text{ (cpm/}\mu\text{Ci)}$$
$$\approx 0.00002 \ \mu\text{Ci}$$

In SI units (1 μCi = 37 kBq), the MDA is 0.74 Bq, i.e., less than one dps.

6. Comparing Counting Systems

In Section B.1 it was noted that larger numbers of counts have smaller percentage uncertainties. Thus in general it is desirable from a statistical point of view to use a counting system with maximum sensitivity (large detector, wide pulse-height analyzer window, etc.) so that a maximum number of counts is obtained in a given measuring time; however, such systems are also more sensitive to background radiation and give higher background counting rates as well, which, as shown by Example 6-5, tends to increase statistical uncertainties. The trade-off between sensitivity and background may be analyzed as follows:

Suppose a counting system provides gross sample counts G_1, background counts B_1, and net sample counts $S_1 = G_1 - B_1$ and that a second system provides gross, background, and net counts G_2, B_2, and S_2 in the same counting time. One can compare the uncertainties in S_1 and S_2 to determine which system is statistically more reliable. The percentage uncertainty in S_1 is given by

$$V_1 = (\sqrt{G_1 + B_1}/S_1) \times 100\% \qquad (6\text{-}33)$$

$$= (\sqrt{S_1 + 2B_1}/S_1) \times 100\% \qquad (6\text{-}34)$$

Corresponding equations apply to the second system. The ratio of the percentage uncertainties for the net sample counts obtained with two systems is therefore

$$\frac{V_1}{V_2} = \frac{S_2 \sqrt{S_1 + 2B_1}}{S_1 \sqrt{S_2 + 2B_2}} \qquad (6\text{-}35)$$

If $V_1/V_2 < 1$, then $V_1 < V_2$, in which case system 1 is the statistically preferred system. Conversely, if $V_1/V_2 > 1$, system 2 is preferred.

If background counts are relatively small ($B_1 << S_1$, $B_2 << S_2$), Equation 6-35 can be approximated by

$$\frac{V_1}{V_2} \approx \frac{S_2 \sqrt{S_1}}{S_1 \sqrt{S_2}} \qquad (6\text{-}36)$$

$$\approx \sqrt{S_2/S_1} \qquad (6\text{-}37)$$

Thus when background levels are "small," only relative sensitivities are important. The system with the higher sensitivity gives the smaller uncertainty. On the other hand, if background counts are large ($B_1 >> S_1$, $B_2 >> S_2$), then

$$V_1/V_2 \approx (S_2/S_1) \sqrt{B_1/B_2} \tag{6-38}$$

Both sensitivity and background are important in this case. Note that Equations 6-35 through 6-38 also can be used with counting *rates* (cpm, cps) substituted for counts.

Example 6-7.
A sample is counted in a well counter using a "narrow" pulse-height analyzer window (N), and net sample and background counts are 500 counts and 200 counts, respectively. The sample is counted with the same system but using a "wide" window (W), and the net sample and background counts are 800 counts and 400 counts, respectively. Which window setting offers the statistical advantage?

Answer.
Background counts are neither "very small" nor "very large"; thus Equation 6-35 must be used:

$$V_N/V_W = (800 \times \sqrt{900})/(500 \times \sqrt{1600})$$
$$= (8 \times 3)/(5 \times 4)$$
$$= 6/5$$

Thus $V_N/V_W > 1$ and the statistical advantage belongs to the wider window setting, in spite of its higher background counting rate.

---

7. Estimating Required Counting Times

Suppose it is desired to determine net sample counting rate R_s to within a certain percentage uncertainty V. Suppose further that the approximate net sample and background counting rates are known to be R_s' and R_b', respectively (e.g., from quick preliminary measurements). If a counting time t is to be used for both the sample and background counting measurements, then the time required to achieve the desired level of statistical reliability is given by

$$t = [(R_s' + 2R_b')/R_s'^2] (100\%/V)^2 \tag{6-39}$$

Example 6-8.
Preliminary measurements in a sample counting procedure indicate gross and background counting rates of 900 cpm and 100 cpm, respectively. What counting time is required to determine net sample counting rate to within 5 percent?

Answer. $R_s' = 900 - 100 = 800$ cpm

$$t = [(800 + 2 \times 100)/800^2](100/5)^2$$
$$= (1000/800^2)(100/5)^2$$
$$= 0.625 \text{ min}$$

This time is used for both sample and background counting. Therefore the total counting time required is 1.25 min.

___

8. Optimal Division of Counting Times

In the preceding section it was assumed that equal counting times were used for the sample and background measurements. This is not necessary; in fact, statistically advantageous results may be obtained by using unequal times. The difference between two counting rates R_1 and R_2 is determined with the smallest statistical error if the total counting time $t = t_1 + t_2$ is divided according to

$$t_1/t_2 = \sqrt{R_1'/R_2'} \tag{6-40}$$

where R_1' and R_2' are counting rates estimated from preliminary measurements. Applying this to gross sample and background counting rate estimates, one obtains

$$t_g/t_b = \sqrt{R_g'/R_b'} \tag{6-41}$$

If $R_g' \approx R_b'$, approximately equal counting times are preferred; however, if the background counting rate is small ($R_b' \ll R_g'$), it is better to devote most of the available time to counting the sample.

___

Example 6-9.

In Example 6-8, what is the optimal division of a 1.25-min total counting time and the resulting uncertainty in the net sample counting rate?

Answer.

Applying Equation 6-41, with $R_g' = 900$ cpm and $R_b' = 100$ cpm,

$$t_g/t_b = \sqrt{900/100} = 3$$
$$t_g = 3t_b$$
$$t_g + t_b = 3t_b + t_b = 1.25 \text{ min}$$
$$t_b = 1.25 \text{ min}/4 \approx 0.3 \text{ min}$$
$$t_g \approx 1.25 - 0.3 = 0.95 \text{ min}$$

The percentage uncertainty in R_s given by Equation 6-39 is

$$V_{R_s} = \frac{\sqrt{R_g/t_g + R_b/t_b} \times 100\%}{R_g - R_b}$$

$$\approx \frac{\sqrt{900/0.95 + 100/0.3} \times 100\%}{800}$$

$$\approx 4.5\%$$

Thus a small statistical advantage (4.5 versus 5 percent) is gained by using an optimal division rather than equal counting times in this example.

9. Statistics of Ratemeters

The ratemeter is an analog device that indicates an average counting rate R during an averaging time that is proportional to the time constant τ (Chapter 5, Section D.2). The instantaneous ratemeter reading R fluctuates with a random error that is given by

$$\sigma_R = \sqrt{R/2\tau} \qquad (6\text{-}42)$$

and a percentage uncertainty

$$V_R = 100\%/\sqrt{2R\tau} \qquad (6\text{-}43)$$

From the standpoint of statistical variation, a ratemeter behaves as if it were using an averaging time 2τ.

Statistical fluctuations in ratemeter output are made smaller by using a longer time constant τ; however, this also smoothes out and distorts the actual changes in counting rate that occur during the study. The selection of a ratemeter time constant therefore is a trade-off between suppression of statistical fluctuations and accurate representation of the study. Figure 6-2 illustrates these tradeoffs for a simulated cardiac flow study. In general, the time constant must be shorter than the duration of any expected real change in counting rate in order to see that change at all, and it must be several times shorter ($\frac{1}{3}$–$\frac{1}{5}$) in order to see it represented accurately.

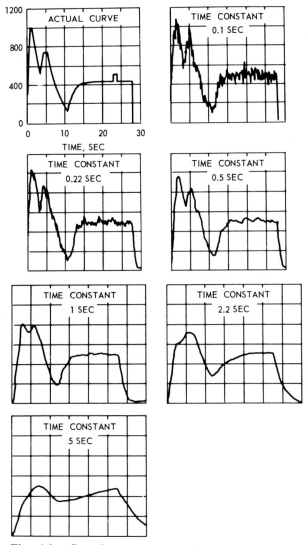

Fig. 6-2. Counting rate curves for a simulated cardiac study. Upper left, curve without statistical fluctuations. Other curves, ratemeter output curves with different time constants. [From Simmons GH: A Training Manual for Nuclear Medicine Technologists. Rockville, Md., Bureau of Radiological Health, Publ. No. BRH/DMRE 70-3, 1970, p. 136. Used by permission.]

E. STATISTICAL TESTS

In Section D.3 above, an example was given of a method for testing the statistical significance of the difference between two counting measurements. The test was based on the assumption of underlying Poisson distributions for the two individual measurements, with variances $\sigma^2 \approx N$. In this section we consider other tests for evaluating statistical parameters of *sets* of counting measurements. The discussion will focus on applications of these tests to nuclear counting data; however, as will be noted in the discussion, the tests also are applicable to other experimental data for which the underlying random variability is described by a Poisson or Gaussian distribution.

1. The Chi-Square Test

The χ^2 (*chi-square*) test is a means for testing whether random variations in a set of measurements are consistent with what would be expected for a Poisson distribution. This is a particularly useful test when a set of counting measurements are suspected to contain sources of random variation in addition to Poisson counting statistics, e.g., due to faulty instrumentation or other random variability between samples, animals, patients, measurement techniques, etc. The test is performed as follows:

1. Obtain a series of counting measurements (usually a total of 20 measurements is desirable).
2. Compute the mean,

$$\overline{N} = \sum_{i=1}^{n} \frac{N_i}{n}$$

and the quantity

$$\chi^2 = \sum_{i=1}^{n} \frac{(N_i - \overline{N})^2}{\overline{N}} \tag{6-44}$$

$$= (n - 1)\, SD^2/\overline{N} \tag{6-45}$$

where SD = standard deviation (Equation 6-9). Many pocket calculators have programs for calculating standard deviations; thus, Equation 6-45 may be the more convenient to use.

3. Refer to a χ^2 table (Table 6-2). In the row corresponding to the

number of measurements, n, go across to the tabulated value most closely corresponding to the calculated χ^2 value. (Note that some χ^2 tables use df = degrees of freedom instead of n. For these tables, use df = $n - 1$.)

4. Go up the selected column to find the probability value P.

P is the probability that random variations observed in a series of n measurements from a Poisson distribution would equal or exceed the calculated χ^2 value. Conversely, $1 - P$ is the probability that smaller variations would be observed. A P value of 0.5 (50 percent) would be "perfect." It indicates that the observed χ^2 value is in the middle of the range expected for a Poisson distribution. A low P value indicates that there is only a small probability that a Poisson distribution would give the χ^2 value as large as actually observed and suggests that additional sources of random error are present. In general, a range $0.02 < P < 0.98$ is considered an acceptable result. If $P < 0.01$, the variations are definitely too large. If $0.01 < P < 0.02$, the results are suspicious but the experiment is considered inconclusive and should be repeated.

A high P value (> 0.99) indicates that random variations are much smaller than expected and also is cause for concern. For example, it could indicate that periodic noise (e.g., 60 Hz line frequency) is being counted. Such signals are not subject to the same degree of random variation as are radiation counting measurements and therefore have very small χ^2 values. A result $0.98 < P < 0.99$ is again considered suspicious, but inconclusive, and thus deserving of repeat study.

Example 6-10.

Use the χ^2 test to determine the likelihood that the following set of 20 counting measurements were obtained from a Poisson distribution.

3875	3575
3949	4023
3621	3314
3817	3612
3790	3705
3902	3412
3851	3520
3798	3743
3833	3622
3864	3514

Answer.

Using a pocket calculator or by direct calculation, it can be shown that the mean and standard deviation of the counting measurements are

$$\overline{N} = 3717$$

$$SD = 187.4$$

Thus, from Equation 6-43,

$$\chi^2 = 19 \times (187.4)^2/3717$$

$$\approx 179.5$$

Using Table 6-2, the calculated value for χ^2 far exceeds the largest value for $n = 20$; (critical value $= 36.191$ for $P = 0.01$). Hence, we conclude that the probability is very small that the observed set of counting measurements were obtained from a Poisson distribution ($P << 0.01$). The observed standard deviation, $SD = 187.4$, also far exceeds what would be expected for a Poisson distribution, $\sqrt{N}= 61.0$. These results suggest the presence of additional sources of random variation beyond simple counting statistics in the data.

2. The *t*-Test

The *t*-test is used to determine the significance of the difference between the means of two sets of data. In essence, the test compares the difference in means relative to the observed random variations in each set. The test is applicable to any two Gaussian distributed sets of data; it is not necessary that they be Poisson-distributed.

Two different tests are used, depending on whether the two sets represent independent or paired data. *Independent* data are obtained from two *different* sample groups, e.g., two different groups of radioactive samples, two different groups of patients or animals, etc. *Paired* data are obtained from the *same* sample group but at different times or under different measurement conditions, e.g., the same samples counted on two different instruments or a group of patients or animals counted "before" and "after" a procedure. The test for paired data assumes that there is some degree of correlation between the two measurements of a pair, e.g., in an experiment comparing uptake of two different radiopharmaceuticals in animals, an animal with a "high" uptake for one radiopharmaceutical is likely also to have a "high" uptake for the other.

Table 6-2

Critical Values of χ^2

Number of Determinations, n	Probability, P						
	0.99	0.95	0.90	0.50	0.10	0.05	0.01
3	0.020	0.103	0.211	1.386	4.605	5.991	9.210
4	0.115	0.352	0.584	2.366	6.251	7.815	11.345
5	0.297	0.711	1.064	3.357	7.779	9.488	13.277
6	0.554	1.145	1.610	4.351	9.236	11.070	15.086
7	0.872	1.635	2.204	5.348	10.645	12.592	16.812
8	1.239	2.167	2.833	6.346	12.017	14.067	18.475
9	1.646	2.733	3.490	7.344	13.362	15.507	20.090
10	2.088	3.325	4.168	8.343	14.684	16.919	21.166
11	2.558	3.940	4.865	9.342	15.987	18.307	23.209
12	3.053	4.575	5.578	10.341	17.275	19.675	24.725
13	3.571	5.226	6.304	11.340	18.549	21.026	26.217
14	4.107	5.892	7.042	12.340	19.812	22.362	27.688
15	4.660	6.571	7.790	13.339	21.064	23.685	29.141
16	5.229	7.261	8.547	14.339	22.307	24.996	30.578
17	5.812	7.962	9.312	15.338	23.542	26.296	32.000
18	6.408	8.672	10.085	16.338	24.769	27.587	33.409
19	7.015	9.390	10.865	17.338	25.989	28.869	34.805
20	7.633	10.117	11.651	18.338	27.204	30.144	36.191
21	8.260	10.851	12.443	19.337	28.412	31.410	37.566
22	8.897	11.591	13.240	20.337	29.615	32.671	38.932
23	9.542	12.338	14.041	21.337	30.813	33.924	40.289
24	10.196	13.091	14.848	22.337	32.007	35.172	41.638
25	10.856	13.848	15.649	23.337	33.196	36.415	42.980
26	11.524	14.611	16.473	24.337	34.382	37.382	44.314
27	12.198	15.379	17.292	25.336	35.563	38.885	45.642
28	12.879	16.151	18.114	26.336	36.741	40.113	46.963
29	13.565	16.928	18.939	27.336	37.916	41.337	48.278
30	14.256	17.708	19.768	28.336	39.087	42.557	49.588

Adapted with permission from Simmons GH: A Training Manual for Nuclear Medicine Technologists. Rockville, Md., Bureau of Radiological Health, Publ. No. BRH/DMRE 70-3, 1970, p. 112.

To test the significance of the difference between the means of two sets of independent measurements, the following quantity is calculated

$$t = (X_1 - X_2)/\sqrt{(SD_1^2 + SD_2^2)/n} \qquad (6\text{-}46)$$

where X_1 and X_2 are the means of the two data sets, SD_1 and SD_2 are the standard deviations (calculated as in Equation 6-9), and $n = n_1 + n_2 - 2$, where n_1 = number of data values in set 1 and n_2 = number of data values in set 2. The calculated value of t then is compared to critical values of the t-distribution for the appropriate number of degrees of freedom, df = n.

Table 6-3 presents values of t that would be exceeded at various probability levels if the two sets of data actually were obtained from the *same* Guassian distribution. For example, for df = 10, a value of $t > 2.281$ would be obtained by chance with a probability of only 5% ($P = 0.05$). This probability is so small that if the critical value was exceeded the difference between the means usually would be considered to be "statistically significant", i.e., that the underlying distributions very likely are different.

Example 6-11.

Suppose the two columns of data in Example 6-10 actually represent counts measured on two different groups of animals, for the uptake of two different radiopharmaceuticals. Use the t-test to determine whether the means of the two sets of counts are significantly different.

Answer.

Using a pocket calculator or by direct calculation, the means and standard deviations of the two sets of data are found to be (1 = left column, 2 = right column)

$$\overline{X}_1 = 3830$$

$$SD_1 = 87.8$$

$$\overline{X}_2 = 3604$$

$$SD_2 = 195.1$$

Thus, from Equation 6-46,

$$t = (3830 - 3604)/(87.8^2 + 195.1^2)/18$$

$$\approx 2.99$$

From Table 6-3, the critical value of t for df = (10 + 10 - 2) = 18 an $P = 0.01$ is 2.878; thus, we can conclude that it is very unlikely that means of the two sets of data are the same ($P < 0.01$), and that they are in fact significantly different.

For paired comparisons, the same table of critical values is used but a different method is used for calculating t. In this case, the differences between pairs of measurements are determined, and t is calculated from

$$t = \sqrt{n - 2} \, |\overline{\Delta}|/SD \qquad (6\text{-}47)$$

Here, $|\overline{\Delta}|$ is the average magnitude (absolute value) and SD is the standard deviation of the differences (calculated as in Equation 6-9 with the N's replaced by Δs) and n is the number of paired measurements. The sign ($\pm$) of the difference Δ is significant and should be used in calculating $\overline{\Delta}$ and SD. The calculated value of t is compared to critical values in the t-distribution table using df $= (n - 1)$, and the probability values are interpreted in the same manner as for independent data.

Example 6-12.
  Suppose that the two columns of data in Example 6-10 represent counts measured on the same group of animals for the uptake of two different radiopharmaceuticals, i.e., opposing values in the two columns represent measurements on the same animal. Use the t-test to determine whether there is a significant difference in average uptake of the two radiopharmaceuticals in these animals.

Answer.
  The first step is to calculate the difference in counts for each pair of measurements. Subtracting the data value in the right-hand column from that in the left for each pair, one obtains for the differences,

$$3875 - 3575 = +300$$
$$3949 - 4023 = -80$$
$$\text{etc.}$$

The mean and standard deviation of the differences are found to be

$$\overline{\Delta} = +213.7$$
$$SD = 172.9$$

Using Equation 6-47

$$t = \sqrt{8} \times 213.7/172.9^2$$
$$\approx 3.50$$

From Table 6-3, the critical value of t for df $= n - 1 = 9$ and $P = 0.01$ is 3.250; thus, as in Example 6-11, we can conclude that the means of the two sets of data are significantly different.

Table 6-3
Critical Values of the t-Distribution

df	Level of Significance, P			
	0.1	*.05*	*.01*	*.001*
1	6.3138	12.7062	63.6567	636.6193
2	2.9200	4.3027	9.9248	31.5991
3	2.3534	3.1824	5.8409	12.9240
4	2.1318	2.7764	4.6041	8.6103
5	2.0150	2.5706	4.0322	6.8688
6	1.9432	2.4469	3.7074	4.9588
7	1.8946	2.3646	3.4995	5.4079
8	1.8595	2.3060	3.3554	5.0413
9	1.8331	2.2622	3.2498	4.7809
10	1.8125	2.2281	3.1693	4.5869
11	1.7959	2.2010	3.1058	4.4370
12	1.7823	2.1788	3.0545	4.3178
13	1.7709	2.1604	3.0123	4.2208
14	1.7613	2.1448	2.9768	4.1405
15	1.7531	2.1315	2.9467	4.0728
16	1.7459	2.1199	2.9208	4.0150
17	1.7396	2.1098	2.8982	3.9651
18	1.7341	2.1009	2.8784	3.9217
19	1.7291	2.0930	2.8609	3.8834
20	1.7247	2.0860	2.8453	3.8495
21	1.7207	2.0796	2.8314	3.8193
22	1.7171	2.0739	2.8188	3.7921
23	1.7139	2.0687	2.8073	3.7676
24	1.7109	2.0639	2.7969	3.7454
25	1.7081	2.0595	2.7874	3.7252
26	1.7056	2.0555	2.7787	3.7066
27	1.7033	2.0518	2.7707	3.6896
28	1.7011	2.0484	2.7633	3.6739
29	1.6991	2.0452	2.7564	3.6594
30	1.6973	2.0423	2.7500	3.6460
40	1.6839	2.0211	2.7045	3.5510
50	1.6759	2.0086	2.6778	3.4960
100	1.6602	1.9840	2.6259	3.3905
200	1.6525	1.9719	2.6006	3.3398
∞	1.6449	1.9600	2.5758	3.2905

Adapted with permission from Levin S: Statistical Methods, in Harbert J, Rocha AFG: Textbook of Nuclear Medicine, Vol 1 (2nd Ed.), Philadelphia, Lea and Febiger, 1984, Chap 4.

3. Treatment of "Outliers"

Occasionally, a set of data will contain what appears to be a spurious result, or "outlier," reflecting possible experimental or measurement error. Although generally it is inadvisable to discard data, statistical tests can be used to determine whether it is reasonable, from a *statistical* point of view, to do so. These tests involve calculating the standard deviation SD of the observed data set, and comparing this to the difference between the sample mean $\overline{X}$ and the suspected "outlier," X. The quantity calculated is

$$T = (X - \overline{X})SD \qquad (6\text{-}48)$$

which then is compared to a table of critical values (Table 6-4). The interpretation of the result is the same as for the *t*-test, i.e., the critical value is that value of T (also sometimes called the Thompson criterion) which would be exceeded by chance at a specified probability level if all the data values were obtained from the same Gaussian distribution. Rejection of data must be done with caution, e.g., in a series of 20 measurements, it is likely that at least one of the data values will exceed the critical value at the 5% confidence level.

Example 6-13.
  In the right-hand column of data in Example 6-10, the value 4023 appears to be an outlier, differing by several standard deviations from the mean of that column (see Example 6-11). Use the Thompson criterion to determine whether this data value may be discarded from the right-hand column of data.

Answer.
  From Example 6-11, the mean and standard deviation of the right-hand column of data are $\overline{X}_2 = 3604$, $SD_2 = 195.1$. Using Equation 6-48

$$T = (4023 - 3604)/195.1$$

$$= 419/195.1$$

$$= 2.15$$

According to Table 6-4, for 10 observations and $P = 0.05$, the critical value of T is 2.18. Since the observed value is smaller, we must conclude that there is a relatively high probability ($P > 0.05$) that the value could have been obtained by chance from the observed distribution, and therefore that it should *not* be discarded.

Table 6-4

Critical Values of the Thompson Criterion for Rejection
of a Single Outlier

Number of Observations, n	Level of Significance, P		
	0.05	*0.025*	*0.01*
3	1.15	1.15	1.15
4	1.46	1.48	1.49
5	1.67	1.71	1.75
6	1.82	1.89	1.94
7	1.94	2.02	2.10
8	2.03	2.13	2.22
9	2.11	2.21	2.32
10	2.18	2.29	2.41
11	2.23	2.36	2.48
12	2.29	2.41	2.55
13	2.33	2.46	2.61
14	2.37	2.51	2.66
15	2.41	2.55	2.71
16	2.44	2.59	2.75
17	2.47	2.62	2.79
18	2.50	2.65	2.82
19	2.53	2.68	2.85
20	2.56	2.71	2.88
21	2.58	2.73	2.91
22	2.60	2.76	2.94
23	2.62	2.78	2.96
24	2.64	2.80	2.99
25	2.66	2.82	3.01
30	2.75	2.91	
35	2.82	2.98	
40	2.87	3.04	
45	2.92	3.09	
50	2.96	3.13	
60	3.03	3.20	
70	3.09	3.26	
80	3.14	3.31	
90	3.18	3.35	
100	3.21	3.38	

Adapted with permission from Levin S: Statistical Methods, in Harbert J, Rocha AFG: Textbook of Nuclear Medicine, Vol 1 (2nd Ed.), Philadelphia, Lea and Febiger, 1984, Chap 4.

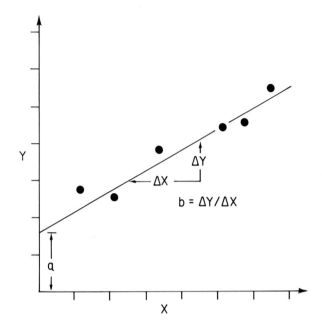

Fig. 6-3. Hypothetical example of data and linear regression curve. • = data values, —— = calculated regression
curve, $Y = a + bX$, $a = Y -$ axis intercept, $b =$ slope,
$\Delta Y/\Delta X$.

4. Linear Regression

Frequently, it is desired to know whether there exists a correlation
between a measured quantity and some other parameter, e.g., counts vs.
time, radionuclide uptake vs. organ weight, etc. The simplest such
relationship is described by an equation of the form

$$Y = a + bX \qquad (6\text{-}49)$$

Here, Y is the measured quantity and X is the parameter with which it is
suspected to be correlated. The graph of Y vs. X is a straight line, with
Y-axis intercept a and slope b (Figure 6-3).

To determine values for a and b from a set of data, and their
statistical significance, i.e., probability that there is indeed a correlation
between X and Y, the following quantities are calculated (1).

$$b = [n\Sigma X_i Y_i - \Sigma X_i \Sigma Y_i]/[n\Sigma X_i - (\Sigma X_i)^2] \qquad (6\text{-}50)$$

$$a = \overline{Y} - b\overline{X} \qquad (6\text{-}51)$$

$$(\text{SD}_{Y \cdot X})^2 = [(\text{SD}_Y)^2 - b^2(\text{SD}_X)^2] \qquad (6\text{-}52)$$

$$SD_b = SD_{Y \cdot X}/[SD_X \sqrt{n-1}] \qquad (6\text{-}53)$$

$$r = b\,(SD_X/SD_Y) \qquad (6\text{-}54)$$

Here n is the number of pairs of data values; X_i and Y_i are individual values of these pairs; $\overline{X}$ and $\overline{Y}$ are their means and SD_X and SD_Y their standard deviations calculated by the usual methods. The summations Σ in Equation 6-50 extend over all values of i $(1, 2, \ldots n)$. $SD_{Y \cdot X}$ is the "standard deviation of Y given X," i.e., the standard deviation of Y about the regression line; SD_b is the uncertainty (estimated standard deviation) in the calculated value of the slope b; and r is the correlation coefficient.

The correlation coefficient r has a value between ± 1, depending on whether the slope b is positive or negative. A value near zero suggests no correlation between X and Y, (i.e., $b \approx 0$) and a value near ± 1 suggests a strong correlation; however, the correlation coefficient is not considered to be a reliable indicator for the strength of the correlation because it depends on three different variables. In particular, the value of r can be increased by obtaining data over a wider range of values of the variable X, thus increasing SD_X in Equation 6-54.

A preferred method for evaluating the strength of the correlation and its statistical significance is to determine whether b is significantly different from zero. This can be done by calculating

$$t = b/SD_b \qquad (6\text{-}55)$$

and comparing this to critical values of the t-distribution (Table 6-3). The number of degrees of freedom is df $= (n - 2)$ where n is the number of (X, Y) data pairs. If the calculated value of t exceeds the tabulated critical value at a selected significance level, then one can conclude that the data support the hypothesis that Y is correlated with X.

REFERENCES

1. Crow EL, Davis FA, Maxfield MW: Statistics Manual. New York, Dover Publications, Inc., 1960, chap. 6.

   Additional discussion of nuclear counting statistics may be found in the following:
   Evans RD: The Atomic Nucleus. New York, McGraw-Hill, 1972, chap 26
   Martin P: Nuclear medicine statistics, in Rollo FD (ed): Nuclear Medicine Physics, Instrumentation, and Agents. St. Louis, C.V. Mosby Co., 1977, chap 13
   Quimby EH, Feitelberg S, Gross W: Radioactive Nuclides in Medicine and Biology (3rd ed.). Philadelphia, Lea & Febiger, 1970, chap 15

7

Production of Radionuclides

Most of the naturally occurring radionuclides are very long-lived (e.g., ^{40}K, $T_{1/2} \sim 10^9$ years) and/or represent very heavy elements (e.g., uranium and radium) that are unimportant in metabolic or physiological processes. Some of the first applications of radioactivity for medical tracer studies in the 1920s and 1930s made use of natural radionuclides; however, because of their generally unfavorable characteristics indicated above, they have found virtually no use in medical diagnosis since that time. The radionuclides used in modern nuclear medicine are all of the man-made or "artificial" variety. They are made by bombarding nuclei of stable atoms with subnuclear particles (neutrons, protons, etc.) so as to cause nuclear reactions to occur that convert a stable nucleus into an unstable (radioactive) one. This chapter describes the methods used to produce radionuclides for nuclear medicine.

A. REACTOR-PRODUCED RADIONUCLIDES

1. Reactor Principles

Nuclear reactors have for many years provided large quantities of radionuclides for nuclear medicine. Because of their long and continuing importance for this application, a brief description of their basic principles will be presented.

The "core" of a nuclear reactor contains a quantity of fissionable material, typically natural uranium (^{235}U and ^{238}U) enriched in ^{235}U

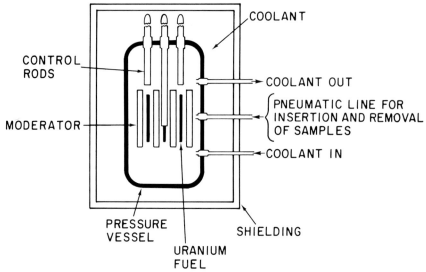

CONTROL RODS

COOLANT

MODERATOR

COOLANT OUT

PNEUMATIC LINE FOR INSERTION AND REMOVAL OF SAMPLES

COOLANT IN

PRESSURE VESSEL

URANIUM FUEL

SHIELDING

Fig. 7-1. Schematic representation of a nuclear reactor.

content. Uranium-235 undergoes spontaneous nuclear fission ($T_{1/2} \sim 7 \times 10^8$ years), splitting into two lighter *nuclear fragments* and emitting two or three *fission neutrons* in the process (Chapter 2, Section J). Spontaneous fission of ^{235}U is not a significant source of neutrons or energy of itself; however, the fission neutrons emitted stimulate additional fission events when they bombard ^{235}U and ^{238}U nuclei. The most important reaction is

$$^{235}U + n \rightarrow {}^{236}U^* \qquad (7-1)$$

The ^{236}U* nucleus is highly unstable and promptly undergoes nuclear fission, releasing additional fission neutrons. In the nuclear reactor, the objective is to have the fission neutrons emitted in each spontaneous or stimulated fission event stimulate, on the average, one additional fission event. This establishes a controlled, self-sustaining, *nuclear chain reaction*.

Figure 7-1 is a schematic representation of a nuclear reactor core. "Fuel" cells containing fissionable material—e.g., uranium—are surrounded by a *moderator* material. The purpose of the moderator is to slow down the rather energetic fission neutrons. Slow neutrons (also called *thermal neutrons*) are more efficient initiators of additional fission events. Commonly used moderators are "heavy water" (containing deuterium) and graphite. *Control rods* are positioned to either expose or shield the fuel cells from one another. The control rods contain materials that are strong neutron absorbers but that do not themselves undergo nuclear fission (e.g., cadmium or boron). The fuel cells and control rods are positioned carefully so as to establish the critical conditions for a controlled chain reaction. If the control rods were removed (or incorrectly positioned) conditions would exist wherein each fission event would stimulate more than one additional nuclear fission. This could lead to a "runaway" reaction and to a possible "meltdown" of the reactor core. (This sequence occurs in a very rapid time scale in nuclear explosives. Fortunately, the critical conditions of a nuclear explosion cannot be achieved in a nuclear reactor.) Insertion of additional control rods results in excess absorption of neutrons and terminates the chain reaction. This procedure is used to shut down the reactor.

Each nuclear fission event results in the release of a substantial amount of energy (200–300 MeV per fission fragment), most of which is dissipated ultimately as thermal energy. This energy can be used as a thermal power source in reactors. Situated around the reactor core are pneumatic lines for insertion of samples. These are used for the production of radionuclides.

2. Neutron Activation

Neutrons carry no net electrical charge. Thus they are neither attracted nor repelled by atomic nuclei. When neutrons (e.g., from a nuclear reactor core) strike a target, some of the neutrons are "captured" by nuclei of the target atoms. A target nucleus may be converted into a radioactive product nucleus as a result. Such an event is called *neutron activation*. Two types of reactions commonly occur.

In an *(n,γ) reaction* a target nucleus $_Z^A X$ captures a neutron and is converted into a product nucleus, $^{A+1}_Z X^*$, which is formed in an excited state. The product nucleus immediately undergoes deexcitation to its ground state by emitting a *prompt γ ray*. The reaction is represented schematically

$$_Z^A X(n, \gamma)^{A+1}_Z X \qquad (7\text{-}2)$$

The target and product nuclei of this reaction represent different isotopes of the same chemical element.

A second type of reaction is the *(n,p) reaction*. In this case, the target nucleus captures a neutron and promptly ejects a proton. This reaction is represented

$$_Z^A X(n,p)_{Z-1}^A Y \qquad (7\text{-}3)$$

Table 7-1

Some Reactor-produced Radionuclides Used in Nuclear
Medicine and Radiotracer Kinetics

Radionuclide	Decay Mode	Production Reaction	Natural Abundance of Target Isotope (%)	σ_c (b)*
^{14}C	β^-	$^{14}N(n,p)^{14}C$	99.6	1.81
^{24}Na	(β^-,γ)	$^{23}Na(n,\gamma)^{24}Na$	100	0.53
^{32}P	β^-	$^{31}P(n,\gamma)^{32}P$	100	0.19
		$^{32}S(n,p)^{32}P$	95.0	—
^{35}S	β^-	$^{35}Cl(n,p)^{35}S$	75.5	—
^{42}K	(β^-,γ)	$^{41}K(n,\gamma)^{42}K$	6.8	1.2
^{51}Cr	(EC,γ)	$^{50}Cr(n,\gamma)^{51}Cr$	4.3	17
^{59}Fe	(β^-,γ)	$^{58}Fe(n,\gamma)^{59}Fe$	0.3	1.1
^{75}Se	(EC,γ)	$^{74}Se(n,\gamma)^{75}Se$	0.9	30
^{125}I	(EC,γ)	$^{124}Xe(n,\gamma)^{125}Xe\overset{EC}{\rightarrow}{}^{125}I$	0.1	110
^{131}I	(β^-,γ)	$^{130}Te(n,\gamma)^{131}Te\overset{\beta^-}{\rightarrow}{}^{131}I$	34.5	0.24

*Thermal neutron capture cross-section, in barns, for (n,γ) reactions (see Section D.1).
Values from ref. 1.

Note that the target and product nuclei for an (n,p) reaction do not
represent the same chemical element.

In the above examples, the products ($^{A+1}_{Z}X$ or $_{Z-1}^{A}Y$) usually are
radioactive species. The quantity of radioactivity that is produced by
neutron activation depends on a number of factors, including the intensity
of the neutron flux, the neutron energies, etc. This is discussed in detail
in Section D of this chapter. Production methods for some reactor-
produced radionuclides for nuclear medicine are summarized in Table
7-1.

Reactor-produced radionuclides have the following general characteristics:

1. Because neutrons are added to the nucleus the products of neutron
    activation generally lie above the line of stability (Figure 1-7).
    Therefore they tend to decay by β^- emission.
2. The most common production mode is by the (n,γ) reaction, and the
    products of this reaction are not carrier-free because they are the
    same chemical element as the bombarded target material. It is
    possible to produce carrier-free products in a reactor by using (n,p)
    reaction (e.g., ^{32}P from ^{32}S) or by activating a short-lived intermediate
    product, e.g., ^{131}I from ^{131}Te using the reaction

$$^{130}Te(n,\gamma)^{131}Te\overset{\beta^-}{\rightarrow}{}^{131}I$$

3. Even in intense neutron fluxes, only a very small percentage of the target nuclei actually are activated, typically $1:10^6$–10^9 (Section D). Thus an (n,γ) product may have very low specific activity because of the overwhelming presence of a large amount of unactivated stable carrier (target material).

There are a few examples of the production of EC decay or β^+-emitting radionuclides with a nuclear reactor— e.g., ^{51}Cr by (n,γ) activation of ^{50}Cr. They may also be produced by using more complicated production techniques. An example is the production of ^{18}F (β^+, $T_{1/2} =$ 110 min). The target material is lithium carbonate, Li_2CO_3. The first step is the reaction

$$^6Li(n,\gamma)^7Li \tag{7-4}$$

Lithium-7 is very unstable and promptly disintegrates:

$$^7_3Li \rightarrow {}^4_2He + {}^3_1H + energy \tag{7-5}$$

Some of the energetic recoiling tritium nuclei ($^3_1$H) bombard stable ^{16}O nuclei, causing the reaction

$$^{16}_8O(^3_1H,n)^{18}_9F \tag{7-6}$$

Useful quantities of ^{18}F can be produced in this way. One problem is removal from the product (by chemical means) of the rather substantial quantity of radioactive tritium that is formed in the reaction. More satisfactory methods for producing ^{18}F involve the use of charged particle accelerators, as discussed in Section B.

Some of the fission fragments produced in the fission process are radioactive. This has been one source of ^{99}Mo, ^{131}I, and ^{133}Xe for nuclear medicine.

B. ACCELERATOR-PRODUCED RADIONUCLIDES

1. Charged-Particle Accelerators

Charged-particle accelerators are used to accelerate electrically charged subnuclear particles, such as protons, deuterons (^{2}H nuclei), tritons (^{3}H nuclei), and α particles ($^4_2$He nuclei), to very high energies. When directed onto a target material, these particles may cause nuclear reactions that result in the formation of radionuclides in a manner similar to neutron activation in a reactor. A major difference is that the particles, all of which are positively charged, must have very high energies, typically 10–20 MeV, to penetrate the repulsive coulomb forces surrounding the nucleus. Van de Graaff accelerators, linear accelerators, cyclotrons, and variations of cyclotrons have been used to accelerate charged particles. Some institutions have installed compact *medical cyclotrons* for on-site production of medical radionuclides. The principles of these machines will be described briefly.

2. Cyclotron Principles

A cyclotron consists of a pair of hollow, semicircular metal electrodes (called "dees" because of their shape), positioned between the poles of a large electromagnet (Figure 7-2). The dees are separated from one another by a narrow gap. Near the center of the dees is an ion source (typically an electrical arc device in a gas) that is used to generate the charged particles.

During operation, particles are generated in bursts by the ion source, and a high-frequency AC voltage generated by a high-frequency oscillator (typically 200 kV, 5 MHz) is applied across the dees. The particles are injected into the gap and immediately are accelerated toward one of the dees by the electrical field generated by the applied AC voltage. Inside the dee there is no electrical field, but because the particles are in a magnetic field they follow a curved circular path around to the opposite side of the dee. The AC voltage frequency is such that the particles arrive at the gap just as the voltage across the dees reaches its maximum value (200 kV) in the opposite direction. The particles are accelerated across the gap,

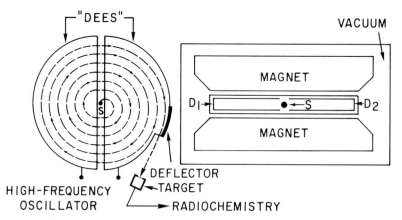

Fig. 7-2. Schematic representation of a cyclotron; top (left) and side (right) views. D_1 and D_2 are the "dees" to which the accelerating voltage is applied by a high-frequency oscillator. Target line may feed directly to a radiochemistry area.

gaining about 200 keV of energy in the process, and then continue on a circular path within the opposite dee.

Each time the particles cross the gap they gain energy, so the orbital radius continuously increases and the particles follow an outwardly spiraling path. The increasing speed of the particles exactly compensates for the increasing distance traveled per half orbit, and they continue to arrive back at the gap exactly in phase with the AC voltage. This condition applies so long as the charge-to-mass ratio of the accelerated particles remains constant. Because of their large relativistic mass increase, even at relatively low energies ($\leq$100 keV), it is not practical to accelerate electrons in a cyclotron. Protons can be accelerated to 20–30 MeV, and heavier particles to higher energies (in proportion to their rest mass), before relativistic mass changes become important.

Higher particle energies can be achieved in a variation of the cyclotron called the *synchrocyclotron*, in which the AC voltage frequency changes as the particles spiral outward and gain energy. These machines are used in high-energy nuclear physics research.

When the particles reach the maximum orbital radius allowed within the cyclotron dees, they may be directed onto a target placed directly in the orbiting beam path (internal beam irradiation), or, alternatively, the beam may be reflected by an electrostatic or electromagnetic device and directed onto an external target (external beam irradiation). The latter provides significantly less beam intensity (because of losses in the beam extraction process) but also allows greater flexibility in target design. Typical internal beam currents in medical cyclotrons are 100–500 μA, whereas external beam currents are 50–100 μA.

The energy of particles accelerated in a cyclotron is given by

$$E \text{ (MeV)} \approx 4.8 \times 10^{-3} (HRZ)^2/A \qquad (7\text{-}7)$$

Where H is the magnetic field strength in tesla, R is the radius of the particle orbit in cm, and Z and A are the atomic number (charge) and mass number of the accelerated particles, respectively. The energies that can be achieved are limited by the magnetic field strength and the dee size. In a typical medical cyclotron with magnetic field strength 1.5 tesla and a dee diameter 76 cm, protons ($Z = 1, A = 1$) and α particles ($Z = 2, A = 4$) can be accelerated to about 15 MeV, deuterons ($Z = 1, A = 2$) to about 8 MeV, and ${}^3_2$He particles to about 22 MeV.

3. Cyclotron-produced Radionuclides

Cyclotrons are used to produce a variety of radionuclides for nuclear medicine, some of which are listed in Table 7-2. General characteristics of cyclotron-produced radionuclides include the following:

Table 7-2
Some Cyclotron-produced Radionuclides Used in
Nuclear Medicine

Product	Decay Mode	Common Production Reaction	Natural Abundance of Target Isotope (%)
^{11}C	β^+	^{10}B(d,n)^{11}C	19.7
		^{11}B(p,n)^{11}C	80.3
^{13}N	β^+	^{12}C(d,n)^{13}N	98.9
^{15}O	β^+	^{14}N(d,n)^{15}O	99.6
^{18}F	β^+,EC	^{20}Ne(d,α)^{18}F	90.9
^{22}Na	β^+,EC	^{23}Na(p,2n)^{22}Na	100
^{43}K	(β^-,γ)	^{40}Ar(α,p)^{43}K	99.6
^{67}Ga	(EC,γ)	^{68}Zn(p,2n)^{67}Ga	18.6
^{111}In	(EC,γ)	^{109}Ag(α,2n)^{111}In	48.7
		^{111}Cd(p,n)^{111}In	12.8
^{123}I	(EC,γ)	^{122}Te(d,n)^{123}I	2.5
		^{124}Te(p,3n)^{123}I	4.6
^{201}Tl	(EC,γ)	^{201}Hg(d,2n)^{201}Tl	13.2

1. Positive charge is added to the nucleus in most activation processes. Therefore the products lie below the line of stability (Figure 1-7) and tend to decay by electron capture or β^+ emission.
2. Addition of positive charge to the nucleus changes its atomic number. Therefore cyclotron-activation products usually are carrier-free.
3. Cyclotrons generally produce smaller quantities of radioactivity than are obtained from nuclear reactors. In part this results from generally smaller "activation cross sections" for charged particle as compared to neutron irradiation (Section D) and in part from lower "beam intensities" obtained in cyclotrons as compared to nuclear reactors. Thus when obtained from commercial suppliers cyclotron products tend to be more expensive than reactor products.

Cyclotron products are attractive for nuclear medicine imaging studies because of the high photon/particle emission ratios that are obtained in β^+ and EC decay. Of special interest are the short-lived β^+ emitters ^{11}C ($T_{1/2}$ = 20 min), ^{13}N ($T_{1/2}$ = 10 min), and ^{15}O ($T_{1/2}$ = 2 min). These radionuclides represent elements that are important constituents of all biologic substances, and they can be used to label a wide variety of physiologically important tracers. In addition, the annihilation photons released following β^+ emission can be used for novel three-dimensional imaging techniques (Chapter 20, Section D). Because of their very short lifetimes, these radionuclides must be prepared on site, usually in a dedicated medical cyclotron. The high cost of owning and operating such machines has impeded their widespread use. Nevertheless, because of the importance of ^{11}C, ^{13}N, ^{15}O, and ^{18}F as medical radiotracers, greater use of medical cyclotrons is expected in the future.

C. PHOTONUCLEAR ACTIVATON

It is also possible to activate stable nuclei by bombarding them in very intense fields of very high energy photons ($\gtrsim$10 MeV). The typical reactions are (γ,n) and (γ,p), i.e., the high-energy photon ejects a neutron or proton from the nucleus. Intense fields of high-energy photons may be obtained from some medical linear accelerators used for radiation therapy. Medically interesting (γ,n) reactions that have been studied include the production of ^{11}C from ^{12}C, ^{13}N from ^{14}N, ^{15}O from ^{16}O, and ^{18}F from ^{19}F.[2] Note that since the (γ,n) reaction produces a neutron-deficient radionuclide, the products tend to be β^+ emitters; however, unlike the products of charged particle bombardment, they are not carrier-free. Another disadvantage of this mode of production is that the yields of radioactivity tend to be low. For these reasons, photonuclear activation techniques have not found widespread use in nuclear medicine.

D. EQUATIONS FOR RADIONUCLIDE PRODUCTION

1. Activation Cross-Sections

The amount of activity produced when a sample is irradiated in a particle (or photon) beam depends on the intensity of the particle beam, the number of target nuclei in the sample, and on the probability that a bombarding particle will interact with a target nucleus. The probability of interaction is determined by the *activation cross-section*. The activation cross-section is the effective "target area" presented by a target nucleus to a bombarding particle. It has dimensions of area and is symbolized by σ. The SI unit for σ is m^2. The traditional and more commonly used unit is the *barn* (1 b $= 10^{-28}$ m^2) or *millibarn* (1 mb $= 10^{-3}$ b $= 10^{-31}$ m^2). Activation cross-sections for a particular nucleus depend on the type of bombarding particle, the particular reaction involved, and the energy of the bombarding particles. Figure 7-3 shows the activation cross-sections for the production of ^{13}N from the ^{13}C(p,n)^{13}N reaction.

Because of their importance in radionuclide production by nuclear reactors, activation cross-sections for thermal neutrons have been measured in some detail. These are called *neutron-capture cross-sections*, symbolized by σ_c. Table 7-1 lists some values of σ_c of interest for radionuclide production in nuclear medicine.

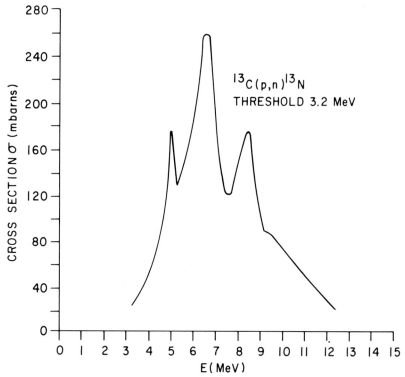

Fig. 7-3. Activation cross-section versus particle energy for the reaction
$^{13}C(p,n)^{13}N$. [From ref. 3: Dagley P, Haeberli W, Saladin J: Nucl Phys
24:353–371, 1961. With permission.]

2. Activation Rates

Suppose a sample containing n target nuclei per cm³, each having an
activation cross section σ, is irradiated in a beam having a *flux density* φ
(particles/cm²·sec) (Figure 7-4). It is assumed that the sample thickness Δx
(cm) is sufficiently thin that φ does not change much as the beam passes
through it. The total number of targets, per cm² of beam area, is $n\Delta x$.
They present a total area $n\sigma\Delta x$ per cm² of beam area. The reduction of
beam flux in passing through the target thickness Δx is therefore

$$\Delta\phi/\phi = n\sigma\Delta x \qquad (7\text{-}8)$$

The number of particles removed from the beam (i.e., the number of
nuclei activated) per cm² of beam area per second is

$$\Delta\phi = n\sigma\phi\Delta x \qquad (7\text{-}9)$$

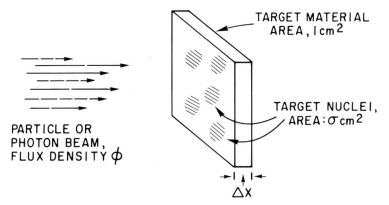

TARGET MATERIAL
AREA, I cm^2

TARGET NUCLEI,
AREA : σ cm^2

PARTICLE OR
PHOTON BEAM,
FLUX DENSITY ϕ

Δx

Fig. 7-4.   Activation targets in a particle or photon beam.

Each atom of target material has mass $AW/6.023 \times 10^{23}$) g, where AW is its atomic weight and 6.023×10^{23} is Avogadro's number. The total mass m of target material per cm^2 in the beam is therefore

$$m = n \times \Delta x \times AW/(6.023 \times 10^{23}) \qquad (7\text{-}10)$$

and the activation rate R per unit mass of target material is thus

$$R = \Delta\phi/m$$
$$= 6.023 \times 10^{23} \times \sigma \times \phi/AW \text{ (activations/g·sec)} \qquad (7\text{-}11)$$

Equation 7-11 can be used to calculate the rate at which target nuclei are activated in a particle or photon beam per gram of target material in the beam.

Example 7-1.
   What is the activation rate per gram of sodium for the reaction $^{23}Na(n,\gamma)^{24}Na$ in a reactor thermal neutron flux density of 10^{13} neutrons/cm^2·sec?

Answer.
   From Table 7-1, the thermal neutron capture cross section for ^{23}Na is $\sigma_c = 0.53$ b. The atomic weight of sodium is (approximately) 23. Therefore (Equation 7-11)

$$R = 6.023 \times 10^{23} \times 0.53 \times 10^{-24} \times 10^{13}/23$$
$$= 1.38 \times 10^{11} \text{ activations/g·sec}$$

Equation 7-11 and Example 7-1 describe situations in which the isotope represented by the target nucleus is 100 percent abundant in the irradiated sample (e.g., naturally occurring sodium is 100 percent ^{23}Na). When the target is not 100 percent abundant, then the activation rate *per gram of irradiated element* is decreased by the percentage abundance of the isotope of interest in the irradiated material.

Example 7-2.

Potassium-42 is produced by the reaction ^{41}K(n,γ)^{42}K. Naturally occurring potassium contains 6.8 percent ^{41}K, 93.2 percent ^{39}K. What is the activation rate of ^{42}K per gram of K in a reactor with thermal neutron flux density 10^{13} neutrons/cm$^2\cdot$sec?

Answer.

From Table 7-1, the neutron capture cross section of ^{41}K is 1.2 b. The atomic weight of ^{41}K is (approximately) 41. Thus (Equation 7-11)

$$R = 6.023 \times 10^{23} \times 1.2 \times 10^{-24} \times 10^{13}/41$$

$$= 1.76 \times 10^{11} \text{ activations/g}(^{41}\text{K})\cdot\text{sec}$$

The activation rate per gram of potassium is 6.8 percent of this, i.e.,

$$R = 0.068 \times 1.76 \times 10^{11}$$

$$= 1.20 \times 10^{10} \text{ activations/g(K)}\cdot\text{sec}$$

Activation rates are less than predicted by Equation 7-11 when the target thickness is such that there is significant attenuation of particle beam intensity as it passes through the target (i.e., some parts of the target are irradiated by a weaker flux density). Also, when "thick" targets are irradiated by charged-particle beams, the particles lose energy and activation cross-sections change as the beam penetrates the target. The equations for these conditions are beyond the scope of this book. They are discussed in the references listed at the end of the chapter.

3. Buildup and Decay of Activity

When a sample is irradiated in a particle or photon beam, the buildup and decay of product radioactivity is exactly analogous to a special case of parent-daughter radioactive decay discussed in Chapter 3, Section F.2. The irradiating beam acts as an inexhaustible, long-lived "parent," generating "daughter" nuclei at a constant rate. Thus as shown in Figure 3-6 the product activity starts from zero and increases with irradiation time, gradually approaching a "saturation level," at which its disintegration rate equals its production rate. The saturation level can be determined from Equation 7-11. The saturation *disintegration rate* per gram is just equal to R, the *activation rate* per gram, so the saturation specific activity A_s is

$$A_s \text{ (Ci/g)} = R/(3.7 \times 10^{10}) \qquad (7\text{-}12)$$

which when combined with Equation 7-11 and simplified yields

$$A_s \text{ (Ci/g)} = 1.63 \times \sigma \times F/AW \qquad (7\text{-}13)$$

where σ is the activation cross-section in barns, F is the particle or photon flux in units of $10^{11}/cm^2\cdot sec$, and AW is the atomic weight of the target material. The final equation for specific activity versus irradiation time is

$$A_t \text{ (Ci/g)} = A_s(1 - e^{-\lambda t}) \qquad (7\text{-}14)$$

where λ is the decay constant of the product (compare Equation 3-18). The specific activity of the target reaches 50 percent of the saturation level after irradiating for one daughter product half-life, 75 percent after two half-lives, and so on (Figure 3-6). No matter how long the irradiation, the sample specific activity cannot exceed the saturation level. Therefore it is unproductive to irradiate a target for longer than about 3–4 times the product half-life.

Example 7-3.

What is the saturation specific activity for the ^{42}K production problem described in Example 7-2? Compare this to the carrier-free specific activity of ^{42}K (the half-life of ^{42}K is 12.4 hours).

Answer.

Applying Equation 7-13 with $\sigma = 1.2$ b, $F = 10^2$, and AW ≈ 41,

$$A_s = 1.63 \times 1.2 \times 10^2/41$$

$$= 4.77 \text{ (Ci } ^{42}K/g \ ^{41}K)$$

If natural potassium is used, only 6.8 percent is ^{41}K. Therefore the saturation specific activity is

$$A_s = 4.77 \times 0.068$$

$$= 0.32 \text{ Ci } ^{42}K/g \text{ K}$$

The carrier-free specific activity of ^{42}K ($T_{1/2} \sim 0.5$ days) is (Equation 3-15)

$$\text{CFSA} \approx (1.3 \times 10^8)/(41 \times 0.5)$$

$$\approx 6.3 \times 10^6 \text{ Ci } ^{42}\text{K/g } ^{42}\text{K}$$

Example 7-3 illustrates the relatively low specific activity that usually is obtained by (n,γ) activation procedures in a nuclear reactor.

A parameter that is related directly to the saturation activity in an activation problem is the *production rate* $\dot{A}$. This is the rate at which radioactivity is produced during an irradiation, disregarding the simultaneous decay of radioactivity that occurs during the irradiation. It is the slope of the production curve at time $t = 0$ (before any of the generated activity has had opportunity to decay). The production rate can be shown by methods of differential calculus to be equal to

$$\dot{A} \text{ (Ci/g·hr)} = 0.693 \times A_s \text{ (Ci/g)}/T_{1/2}(\text{hr}) \qquad (7\text{-}15)$$

where $T_{1/2}$ is the half-life of the product.

Reactor production capabilities may be defined in terms of either saturation levels or production rates. If the irradiation time t is "short" in comparison to the product half-life, one can approximate the activity produced from the production rate according to

$$A_t \text{ (Ci/g)} \approx \dot{A} \times t \qquad (7\text{-}16)$$

$$\approx 0.693 \times A_s \times (t/T_{1/2}) \qquad (7\text{-}17)$$

where t and $T_{1/2}$ must be in the same units.

Example 7-4.

What is the production rate of ^{42}K for the problem described in Example 7-2, and what specific activity would be available after an irradiation period of 3 hours? (The half-life of ^{42}K is 12.4 hours.)

Answer.

From Example 7-3, $A_s = 0.32$ Ci ^{42}K/g K. Therefore (Equation 7-15)

$$A = (0.693 \times 0.32)/12.4$$

$$= 0.018 \text{ Ci } ^{42}\text{K/g K·hr}$$

After 3 hours, which is "short" in comparison to the half-life of ^{42}K, the specific activity of the target is (Equation 7-16)

$$A \ (\text{Ci/g}) \approx 0.018 \times 3$$

$$\approx 0.054 \ \text{Ci} \ {}^{42}\text{K/g K}$$

E. RADIONUCLIDE GENERATORS

A radionuclide generator consists of a parent-daughter radionuclide pair contained in an apparatus that permits separation and extraction of the daughter from the parent. The daughter product activity is replenished continuously by decay of the parent and may be extracted repeatedly.

Table 7-3 lists some radionuclide generators of interest to nuclear medicine. They are an important source of metastable radionuclides. The most important generator is the ${}^{99}\text{Mo}-{}^{99\text{m}}\text{Tc}$ system, because of the widespread use of ${}^{99\text{m}}\text{Tc}$ for radionuclide imaging. Technetium-99m emits γ rays (140 keV) that are very favorable for use with an Anger camera. It has a reasonable half-life (6 hours), delivers a relatively low radiation dose per emitted γ ray (Chapter 10), and can be used to label a wide variety of imaging agents.

A ${}^{99}\text{Mo}-{}^{99\text{m}}\text{Tc}$ generator is shown schematically in Figure 7-5. The ${}^{99}\text{Mo}$ activity in the form of molybdate ion, MoO_4 is bound to an alumina (Al_2O_3) column. The ${}^{99\text{m}}\text{Tc}$ activity, being chemically different, is not bound by the alumina and is eluted from the column with 5–25 ml of normal saline. Typically, 75–85 percent of the available ${}^{99\text{m}}\text{Tc}$ activity is extracted in a single elution. Technetium-99m activity builds up again after an elution, and maximum activity is available about 24 hours later (see Equation 3-20); however, usable quantities of ${}^{99\text{m}}\text{Tc}$ are available 3–6 hours later. Figure 7-6 shows the pattern of activity available in a ${}^{99\text{m}}\text{Tc}$ generator that is eluted at various intervals.

Commercially prepared generators are sterilized, well shielded, and largely automated in operation. Typically they are used for about one week and then discarded because of natural decay of the ${}^{99}\text{Mo}$ parent.

Table 7-3
Some Radionuclide Generators Used in Nuclear Medicine

Daughter†	Decay Mode	$T_{1/2}$	Parent	$T_{1/2}$
${}^{68}\text{Ga}$	β^+,EC	68 min	${}^{68}\text{Ge}$	275 days
${}^{82}\text{Rb}$	β^+,EC	1.3 min	${}^{82}\text{Sr}$	25 days
${}^{87\text{m}}\text{Sr}$	IT	2.8 hours	${}^{87}\text{Y}$	80 hours
${}^{99\text{m}}\text{Tc}$	IT	6 hours	${}^{99}\text{Mo}$	66 hours
${}^{113\text{m}}\text{In}$	IT	100 min	${}^{113}\text{Sn}$	120 days

†Generator product.

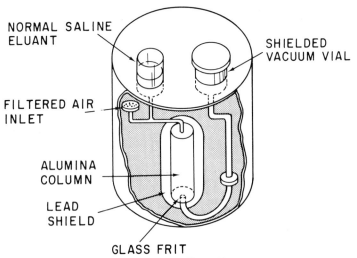

Fig. 7-5. Cross-sectional drawing of a ^{99}Mo-^{99m}Tc generator. (Courtesy of the Society of Nuclear Medicine and Thomas R. Gnau.)

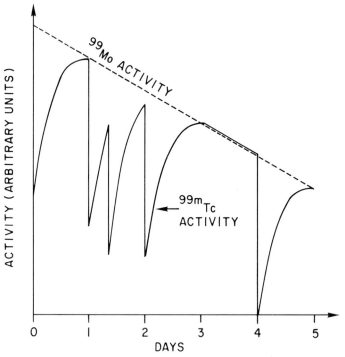

Fig. 7-6. Buildup and decay of ^{99m}Tc generator eluted on days 0, 1, 1.4, 2, and 4.

Molybdenum-99 activity is obtained by (n,γ) activation of stable molybdenum (23.8 percent ^{98}Mo) or by separation from reactor fission fragments. The latter, sometimes called "fission moly," has significantly higher specific activity. The volume of alumina required in a ^{99}Mo–^{99m}Tc generator is determined essentially by the amount of stable Mo-carrier that is present. Therefore "fission moly" generators require much smaller volumes of alumina per unit of ^{99}Mo activity. They can be eluted with very small volumes of normal saline ($\leq$5 ml), which is useful in some imaging techniques requiring bolus injections of very small volumes of high activity (~20mCi or 740 MBq) of ^{99m}Tc.

One problem with ^{99m}Tc generators is ^{99}Mo "breakthrough," i.e., partial elution of the ^{99}Mo parent along with ^{99m}Tc from the generator. From the standpoint of patient radiation safety, the amount of ^{99}Mo should be kept to a minimum. Maximum amounts, according to NRC regulations, are 1 μCi^{99}Mo/mCi^{99m}Tc(10^{-3}Bq^{99}Mo/Bq^{99m}Tc), not to exceed 5 μCi(185 kBq) of ^{99}Mo per administered dose. It is possible to assay ^{99}Mo activity in the presence of much larger ^{99m}Tc activity using NaI(Tl) counting systems (Chapter 13) by surrounding the sample with about 3 mm of lead, which is an efficient absorber of the 140 keV γ rays of ^{99m}Tc but which is relatively transparent to the 740–780 keV γ rays of ^{99}Mo (Chapter 9, Section B.1). Thus small quantities of ^{99}Mo can be detected in the presence of much larger amounts of ^{99m}Tc. Some dose calibrators are provided with a lead-lined container called a "moly shield" specifically for this purpose.

Other radioactive contaminants also are occasionally found in ^{99}Mo-^{99m}Tc generator eluate. The NRC-limit for other contaminants is 0.1 μCi/mCi^{99m}Tc(10^{-4}Bq/Bq^{99m}Tc). Methods for detecting other contaminants are discussed in reference 3.

A second major concern is breakthrough of aluminum ion, which interferes with labeling processes and also can cause clumping of red blood cells and possible microemboli. Current regulatory limits are 10 μg/ml for generators containing reactor-produced ^{99}Mo and 20 μg/ml for generators containing fission-produced ^{99}Mo. Chemical test kits are available from generator manufacturers to test for the presence of aluminum ion.

REFERENCES

1. Radiological Health Handbook. Rockville, Md., U.S. Dept. H.E.W., 1970, pp 231–380
2. Welch MJ: Production of radioisotopes for biomedical studies using photonuclear reactions, in: Proceedings of the International Conference on

Photonuclear Reactions and Applications, March 23–30, 1973, Asilomar, Pacific Grove, Calif. Livermore, Calif., Lawrence Livermore Laboratory, 1973
3. Briner W, Harris CG: Radionuclide contamination of eluates from fission-product molybdenum-technetium generators. J Nucl Med 15:466–467, 1974

Nuclear reactors and neutron activation equations are discussed in detail in the following:
Lapp RE, Andrews HL: Nuclear Radiation Physics (ed 4). Englewood Cliffs, N.J., Prentice-Hall, Inc., 1972, pp 341–386
Lenihan JMA: Nuclear activation analysis, in Hine GJ (ed): Instrumentation in Nuclear Medicine (vol 1). New York, Academic Press, 1967, pp 309–325

Medical cyclotrons are discussed in the following:
Hoop B Jr, Laughlin JS, Tilbury RS: Cyclotrons in Nuclear Medicine, in Hine GJ, Sorenson JA (eds): Instrumentation in Nuclear Medicine (vol 2). New York, Academic Press, 1974, pp 407–457

Generator systems and other aspects of radiopharmaceutical preparation and quality control are discussed in the following:
Castronovo FP: Principles, properties, and quality control of nuclear medicine agents, in Rollo FD (ed): Nuclear Medicine Physics, Instrumentation, and Agents. St. Louis, C.V. Mosby Co., 1977, chap 16

8

Passage of Charged
Particles Through Matter

High-energy charged particles, such as α particles or β particles, lose energy and slow down as they pass through matter as a result of collisions with atoms and molecules. Energy is transferred to the absorbing matter in the process, with the principle result being ionization and excitation of atoms and molecules. Most of this energy ultimately is degraded into heat (atomic and molecular vibrations); however, the ionization effect has other important consequences. Ionization is the underlying mechanism for most radiation detectors (Chapter 4) and also is responsible for most radiobiologic effects (Chapter 10). For this reason, high-energy charged particles are called *ionizing radiations*.

Electrons are the most important type of charged particle encountered in nuclear medicine. High-energy electrons are emitted in several important modes of radioactive decay, including β^- and β^+ decay and internal conversion, and in the Auger effect (Chapter 2). In addition, high-energy electrons are generated when γ rays and x rays interact with matter and are responsible for the ultimate deposition of energy from these radiations in an absorbing medium (Chapter 9).

This chapter will emphasize the interactions of electrons with matter. Except for differences in sign, the forces experienced by positive and negative electrons (e.g., β^+ and β^- particles) are identical. There are minor differences between the interactions of these two types of particles, but they are not of importance to nuclear medicine and will not be discussed here. In this chapter, the term "electrons" will be meant to include both the positive and negative types. The annihilation effect, which occurs when a positive electron has lost all of its kinetic energy and stopped, is discussed in Chapter 2, Section G.

A. INTERACTIONS OF CHARGED PARTICLES WITH MATTER

1. Interaction Mechanisms

The "collisions" that occur between a charged particle and atoms or molecules involve electrical forces of attraction or repulsion, rather than actual mechanical contact. For example, a charged particle passing near an atom exerts electrical forces on the orbital electrons of that atom. In a close encounter, the strength of the forces may be sufficient to cause an orbital electron to be separated from the atom, thus causing *ionization* (Figure 8-1A). An ionization interaction looks like a collision between the

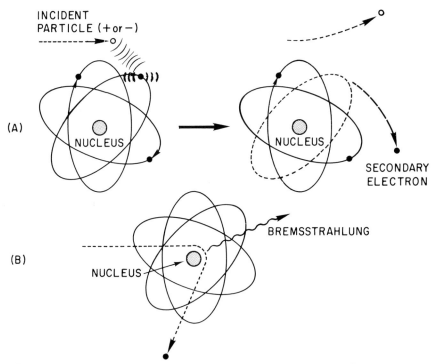

Fig. 8-1. Interactions of charged particles with atoms. (A) Interaction with an orbital electron resulting in ionization. Less close encounters may result in atomic excitation without ionization. (B) Interaction with a nucleus, resulting in bremsstrahlung production. [Repulsion by orbital electron (A) and attraction toward nucleus (B) indicates incident particles are negatively charged in examples shown.]

charged particle and an orbital electron. The charged particle loses energy in the collision. Part of this energy is used to overcome the binding energy of the electron to the atom, and the remainder is given to the ejected *secondary electron* as kinetic energy. Ionization involving an inner shell electron eventually leads to the emission of characteristic x rays or Auger electrons; however, these effects generally are very small, since most ionization interactions involve outer shell electrons. The ejected electron may be sufficiently energetic to cause *secondary ionizations* on its own. Such an electron is called a *delta* (δ) *ray*.

A less close encounter between a charged particle and an atom may result in an orbital electron being raised to an *excited state,* thus causing atomic or molecular *excitation.* These interactions generally result in smaller energy losses than occur in ionization events. The energy transferred to an atom in an excitation interaction is dissipated in molecular vibrations, atomic emission of infrared, visible, or UV radiation, etc.

A third type of interaction occurs when the charged particle actually penetrates the orbital electron cloud of an atom and collides with its nucleus. For a heavy charged particle of sufficiently high energy, e.g., and α particle or a proton, this may result in nuclear reactions of the types used for the production of radionuclides (Chapter 7, Section B); however, for both heavy charged particles and electrons, a more likely result is that that particle will simply be deflected by the strong electrical forces exerted on it by the nucleus (Figure 8-1B). The particle is rapidly decelerated and loses energy in the "collision." The energy appears as a photon of electromagnetic radiation, called *bremsstrahlung* (German, "braking radiation").

The energy of bremsstrahlung photons can range anywhere from nearly zero (events in which the particle is only slightly deflected) up to a maximum equal to the full energy of the incident particle (events in which the particle is virtually stopped in the collision). Figure 8-2 shows the energy spectrum for bremsstrahlung photons generated in aluminum by β particles from a $^{90}Sr-^{90}Y$ source mixture (E_β^{max} = 2.27 MeV) and illustrates that most of the photons are in the lower energy range.

2. Collisional Versus Radiation Losses

Energy losses incurred by a charged particle in ionization and excitation events are called *collisional losses,* while those incurred in nuclear encounters, resulting in bremsstrahlung production, are called *radiation losses.* In the nuclear medicine energy range, collisional losses are by far the dominating factor (see Figure 8-5). Radiation losses increase with increasing particle energy and with increasing atomic number of the absorbing medium. An approximation for percentage radiation losses for β particles having maximum energy E_β^{max} (MeV) is

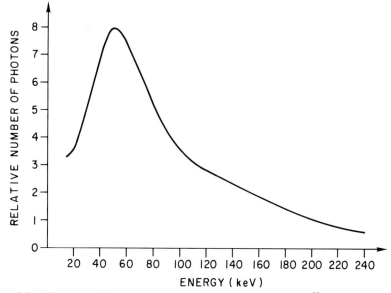

Fig. 8-2.   Bremsstrahlung spectrum for β particles emitted by ^{90}(Sr + Y) mixture ($E_β^{max}$ = 2.27 MeV) in aluminum. [Adapted with permission from Mladjenovic M: Radioisotope and Radiation Physics. New York, Academic Press, 1973, p. 121.]

$$\text{percentage radiation losses} \approx (ZE_β^{max}/3000) \times 100\% \qquad (8\text{-}1)$$

where Z is the atomic number of the absorber. This approximation is accurate to within about 30 percent. For a mixture of elements an "effective" atomic number for bremsstrahlung production should be used:

$$Z_{eff} = \Sigma f_i Z_i^2 / \Sigma f_i Z_i \qquad (8\text{-}2)$$

where $f_1, f_2, \ldots$ are the fractions by weight of the elements $Z_1, Z_2, \ldots$ in the mixture.

Example 8-1.
Calculate the percentage radiation losses for ^{32}P β particles in water and in lead.

Answer.
$E_β^{max}$ = 1.7 MeV for ^{32}P (Appendix B). Water is comprised of 2/18 parts hydrogen (Z = 1, AW~1) and 16/18 parts oxygen (Z = 8, AW~16); thus its effective atomic number for bremsstrahlung production is (equation 8-2)

$$Z_{eff} = [(1/9)(1)^2 + (8/9)(8)^2]/[(1/9)(1) + (8/9)(8)]$$
$$= 7.9$$

The percentage radiation losses in water are therefore (Equation 8-1) $(7.9 \times 1.7/3000) \times 100\% \sim 0.4\%$, and in lead $(Z = 82)$ they are $(82 \times 1.7/3000) \times 100\% \approx 4.6\%$. The remaining 99.6% and 95.4%, respectively, are dissipated as collisional losses.

Example 8-1 demonstrates that high-energy electrons in the nuclear medicine energy range dissipate most of their energy in collisional losses. Bremsstrahlung production accounts for only a small fraction of their energy. Nevertheless, bremsstrahlung can be important in some situations, such as the shielding of relatively large quantities of an energetic β-particle emitter (e.g., tens of mCi of ^{32}P). The β particles themselves are easily stopped by only a few millimeters of plastic, glass, or lead (Section B.2); however, the bremsstrahlung photons they generate are much more penetrating and may require additional shielding around the primary β-particle shielding. It is helpful in such situations to use a low-Z material, such as plastic, for the primary β-particle shielding, and then to surround this with a higher-Z material, such as lead, for bremsstrahlung shielding (Figure 8-3). This arrangement minimizes bremsstrahlung production by the β particles in the shielding material.

Bremsstrahlung production and radiation losses for α particles and other heavy charged particles are very small because the amount of bremsstrahlung production is inversely proportional to the mass of the incident charged particle. Alpha particles, protons, etc. are several

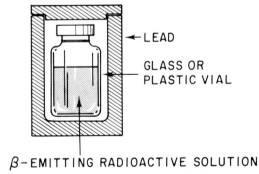

β−EMITTING RADIOACTIVE SOLUTION

Fig. 8-3. Preferred arrangement for shielding energetic β-emitting radioactive solution. Glass or plastic walls of vial stop the β particles with minimum bremsstrahlung production, and lead container absorbs the few bremsstrahlung photons produced.

thousand times heavier than electrons and therefore dissipate only a few hundredths of a percent or less of their energy as radiation losses. These particles, even at energies up to 100 MeV, dissipate nearly all of their energy as collisional losses.

3. Charged-Particle Tracks

A charged particle passing through matter leaves a track of secondary electrons and ionized atoms in its path. In soft tissue and materials of similar density, the tracks are typically about 100 μm wide, with occasionally longer side tracks generated by energetic δ rays. The tracks are studied in nuclear physics using film emulsions, cloud chambers,† and other devices.

When a heavy particle, such as an α particle, collides with an orbital electron, its direction is virtually unchanged and it loses only a small fraction of its energy (rather like a bowling ball colliding with a small lead shot). The maximum fractional energy loss by a heavy particle of mass M colliding with a light particle of mass m is approximately $(4m/M)$, or about 0.05 percent $[4 \times (\frac{1}{4})/1840]$ for an α particle colliding with an electron. Heavy particles also undergo relatively few bremsstrahlung-producing collisions with nuclei. As a result, their tracks tend to be straight lines, and they experience an almost continuous slowing down in which they lose small amounts of energy in a large number of individual collisions.

By contrast, electrons can undergo large-angle deflections in collisions with orbital electrons and can lose a large fraction of their energy in these collisions. These events are more like collisions between billiard balls of equal mass. Electrons also undergo occasional collisions with nuclei in which they are deflected through large angles and bremsstrahlung photons are emitted. For these reasons, electron tracks are tortuous and their exact shape and length is unpredictable.

An additional difference between electrons and heavy particles is that for a given amount of kinetic energy, an electron travels at a much faster speed. For example, a 4 MeV α particle travels at about 10 percent of the speed of light, whereas a 1 MeV electron travels at 90 percent of the speed of light. As a result, an electron spends a much briefer time in the vicinity of an atom than an α particle of similar energy and is therefore less likely to interact with the atom. Also, an electron carries only one unit of

---

† A cloud chamber consists of a cylinder with a piston at one end and viewing windows at the other end and around the sides. The cylinder contains a water–alcohol vapor mixture under pressure. When the piston is rapidly withdrawn to suddenly decrease the pressure and temperature of the vapor, droplets of condensed liquid are formed around ionized nuclei. Ionization tracks existing in the chamber at the time thus can be visualized and photographed through the viewing windows.

α – PARTICLE TRACK

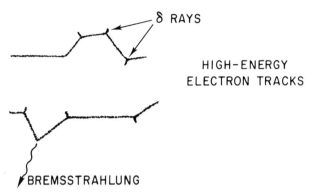

δ RAYS

HIGH-ENERGY
ELECTRON TRACKS

BREMSSTRAHLUNG

Fig. 8-4.   Representation of α-particle and electron tracks in an absorber. Alpha particles leave short, straight, densely ionized tracks, whereas electron paths are tortuous and much longer; δ rays are energetic secondary electrons.

electrical change, versus two for α particles, and thus exerts weaker forces on orbital electrons. For these reasons, electrons experience less frequent interactions and lose their energy more slowly than α particles; they are much less densely ionizing, and they travel farther before they are stopped than α particles or other heavy charged particles of similar energy.

To illustrate these differences Figure 8-4 shows (in greatly enlarged detail) some possible tracks for β particles and for α particles in water. The actual track lengths are on the order of microns for α particles and fractions of a centimeter for β particles. This is discussed further in Section B.

4. Deposition of Energy
Along a Charged-Particle Track

The rate at which a charged particle loses energy determines the distance it will travel and the density of ionization along its track. Energy loss rates and ionization densities depend on the type of particle and its energy and on the composition and density of the absorbing medium. Density affects energy loss rates because it determines the density of atoms along the particle path. In the nuclear medicine energy range ($\lesssim 10$ MeV), energy loss rates for charged particles increase linearly with the density of the absorbing medium. (At higher energies, density effects are more complicated, as discussed in the references listed at the end of the chapter.)

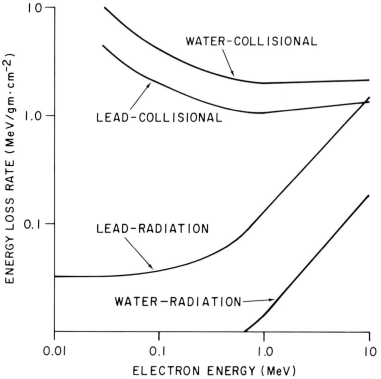

Fig. 8-5.   Collisional (ionization, excitation) and radiation (bremsstrahlung) energy losses versus electron energy in lead and in water. [Adapted with permission from Johns HE, Cunningham JR: The Physics of Radiology (ed 3). 1971, p 47. Courtesy of Charles C Thomas, Publisher, Springfield, Illinois.]

Figure 8-5 shows collisional and radiation energy loss rates for electrons in the energy range 0.01–10 MeV in water and in lead. Energy loss rates $\Delta E/\Delta x$ are expressed in MeV/g·cm^{-2} to normalize for density effects:

$$\Delta E/\Delta x(\text{MeV/g} \cdot \text{cm}^{-2}) = \frac{\Delta E/\Delta x(\text{MeV/cm})}{\rho(\text{g/cm}^3)} \qquad (8\text{-}3)$$

Thus for a given density ρ the energy loss rate in MeV/cm is given by

$$\Delta E/\Delta x(\text{MeV/cm} = \Delta E/\Delta x(\text{MeV/g·cm}^{-2}) \times \rho \; (\text{g/cm}^3) \qquad (8\text{-}4)$$

Collisional loss rates $\Delta E/\Delta x_{\text{coll}}$ decrease with increasing electron energy, reflecting the velocity effect mentioned in Section A.3. Also,

$\Delta E/\Delta x_{coll}$ decreases with increasing atomic number of the absorbing medium because in atoms of higher atomic number, inner shell electrons are "screened" from the incident electron by layers of outer shell electrons, making interactions with inner shell electrons less likely in these atoms. Gram for gram, lighter elements are better absorbers of electron energy than are heavier elements.

Radiation loss rate $\Delta E/\Delta x_{rad}$ increase with increasing electron energy and increasing atomic number of the absorber, as discussed in Section A.2.

The total energy loss rate of a charged particle, $\Delta E/\Delta x_{total}$, expressed in MeV/cm, is also called the *linear stopping power, S_l*. A closely related parameter is the LET, or *linear energy transfer, L,* which refers to energy lost that is deposited "locally" along the track. L differs from S_l in that it does not include radiation losses. These result in the production of bremsstrahlung photons, which may deposit their energy at some distance from the particle track. For both electrons and α particles in the nuclear medicine energy range, however, radiation losses are small, and the two quantities S_l and L are practically identical.

The average value of the linear energy transfer measured along a charged particle track, $\overline{L}$, is an important parameter in health physics (Chapter 23, Section A). $\overline{L}$ is expressed usually in units of keV/μm. For electrons in the energy range 10 keV–10 MeV traveling through soft tissue, L has values in the range 0.2–2 keV/μm. Lower-energy electrons, e.g., β particles emitted by ^{3}H, $\overline{E}_\beta = 5.6$ keV, have somewhat higher values of $\overline{L}$. Alpha particles have values of $\overline{L} \approx 100$ keV/μm.

Specific ionization, SI, refers to the total number of ionizations (primary and secondary) per unit track length along a charged particle track. The ratio of linear energy transfer divided by specific ionization is W, the *average energy expended per ionization event:*

$$W = L/SI \qquad (8\text{-}5)$$

This quantity has been measured and found to have a relatively narrow range of values in a variety of gases (25–45 eV/ionization) independent of the type or energy of the incident particle. The value for air is 33.7 eV/ionization. W is not the same as the *ionization potential I,* which is the average energy *required* to cause an ionization in a material (averaged over all the electron shells). Ionization potentials for gases are in the range 10–15 eV. The difference between W and I is energy dissipated by a charged particle in excitation events. Apparently, over half of the energy of a charged particle is expended in this way. Similar ratios between W and I are found in semiconductor solids, except that in these materials the values of W and I are both about a factor of 10 smaller than for gases (Table 4-1).

Because W does not change appreciably with particle type or energy, specific ionization is proportional to linear energy transfer L along a charged particle track. Figure 8-6 shows specific ionization in air for electrons as a function of their energy. The curve indicates that specific ionization increases with decreasing energy down to an energy of about 100 eV. This behavior reflects the fact that energy loss rates and L increase as the electron slows down. Below about 100 eV, the electron energy is inadequate to cause ionizations efficiently, and specific ionization decreases rapidly to zero.

Specific ionizations for α particles are typically 100 times greater than for electrons of the same energy because of their greater charge and much lower velocities, leading to greater rates of energy loss, as discussed in Section A.3.

The fact that specific ionization increases as a particle slows down leads to a marked increase in ionization density near the end of its track. This effect is especially pronounced for heavy particles. Figure 8-7 shows a graph of ionization density versus distance traveled for α particles in air. The peak near the end of the α particle range is called the *Bragg ionization peak*. A similar increase in ionization density is seen at the end of an electron track; however, the peak occurs when the electron energy has been reduced to less than about 1 keV, and it accounts for only a small fraction of its total energy.

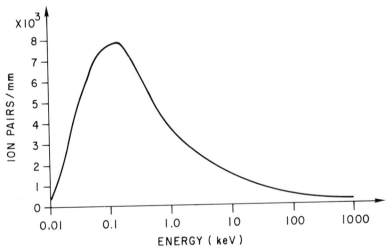

Fig. 8-6.   Specific ionization (SI) for electrons versus energy in water. [Adapted with permission from Mladjenovic M: Radioisotope and Radiation Physics. New York, Academic Press, 1973, p. 145.]

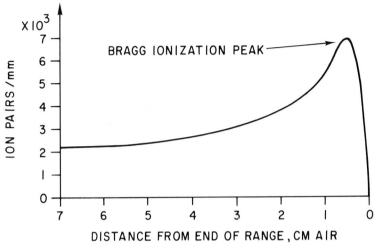

Fig. 8-7. Specific ionization (SI) versus distance traveled for α particles in air. [Adapted with permission from Mladjenovic M: Radioisotope and Radiation Physics. New York, Academic Press, 1973, p 111.]

5. The Cerenkov Effect

An additional charged-particle interaction deserving brief mention is the *Cerenkov* (pronounced cher-EN-kof) *effect*. This effect occurs when a charged particle travels in a medium at a speed greater than the speed of light in that medium. The restriction that a particle cannot travel faster than the speed of light applies to the speed of light in a vacuum, $c \cong 3 \times 10^8$ m/sec; however, a 1 MeV β particle emitted in water solution travels with a velocity $v \approx 0.8c$, whereas the speed of light in water (refractive index $n = 1.33$) is $c' = c/n \approx 0.75c$. Under these conditions, the particle creates an electromagnetic "shock wave" in much the same way that an airplane traveling faster than the speed of sound creates an acoustic shock wave. The electromagnetic shock wave appears as a burst of visible radiation, typically bluish in color, called *Cerenkov radiation*. The Cerenkov effect can occur for electrons with energies of a few hundred keV; however, for heavy particles such as α particles and protons, energies of several thousands of MeV are required to meet the velocity requirements.

The Cerenkov effect accounts for a very small fraction (<<1 percent) of electron energies in the nuclear medicine energy range, but it is detectable in water solutions containing an energetic β-particle emitter (e.g., ^{32}P) using liquid scintillation counting apparatus. The Cerenkov effects also is responsible for the bluish glow that is seen around the core of an operating nuclear reactor.

B. CHARGED-PARTICLE RANGES

1. Alpha Particles

An α particle loses energy in a more or less continuous slowing down process as it travels through matter. The particle is deflected only slightly in its collisions with atoms and orbital electrons. As a result, the distance traveled, or *range*, of an α particle depends only on its initial energy and on its average energy loss rate in the medium. For α particles of the same energy, the range is quite consistent from one particle to the next. A transmission curve, showing percent transmission for α particles versus thickness of absorber, remains essentially flat at 100 percent until the maximum range is reached; then it falls rapidly to zero (Figure 8-8). The *mean range* is defined as the thickness resulting in 50 percent transmission. There is only a small amount of range fluctuation, or *range straggling*, about the mean value. Typically, range straggling amounts to only about 1 percent of the mean range.

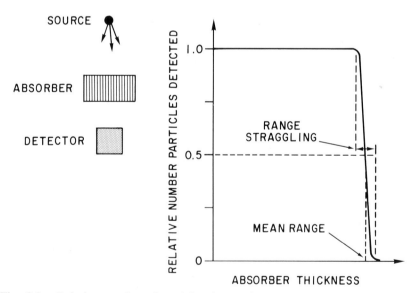

Fig. 8-8.   Relative number of particles detected versus absorber thickness in a transmission experiment with α particles. Range straggling is exaggerated for purposes of illustration.

For α particles emitted in radioactive decay ($E = 4 - 8$ MeV), an approximation for the mean range in air is

$$R(cm) = 0.325E^{3/2}(MeV) \tag{8-6}$$

Example 8-2.
Calculate the mean range in air of α particles emitted by ^{241}Am($E_\alpha = 5.49$ MeV).

Answer.

$$R(cm) = 0.325(5.49)^{3/2}$$
$$= 0.325(\sqrt{5.49})^3$$
$$\approx 4.2 \text{ cm}$$

Example 8-2 illustrates that α particles have very short ranges. They produce densely ionized tracks over this short range.

Example 8-3.
Estimate the average value of specific ionization in air for α particles emitted by ^{241}Am.

Answer.
$W = 33.7$ eV/ionization in air. Therefore the number N of ionizations caused by an α particle of energy 5.49 MeV is

$$N = 5.49 \times 10^6 \text{ eV}/33.7 \text{ eV/ionization}$$
$$\approx 1.63 \times 10^5 \text{ ionizations}$$

Over a distance of travel of 4.2 cm, the average specific ionizations $\overline{SI}$ is therefore

$$\overline{SI} \approx 1.63 \times 10^5 \text{ ionizations}/4.2 \text{ cm}$$
$$\approx 3.9 \times 10^4 \text{ ionizations/cm}$$

Compare the result in Example 8-3 with the values shown in Figures 8-6 and 8-7. Only near the very end of their ranges ($E \lesssim 1$ keV) do electrons have specific ionizations comparable to the *average* values for α particles.

Alpha particle ranges in materials other than air can be estimated using the equation

$$R_x = R_A(\rho_A\sqrt{A_x}/\rho_x\sqrt{A_A}) \tag{8-7}$$

where R_A is the range of the α particle in air, ρ_A ($= 0.001293$ g/cm^3) and A_A (≈ 14) are the density and (average) mass number of air, and ρ_X and A_X are the same quantities for the material of interest. This estimation is accurate to within about 15 percent.

Example 8-4.

What is the approximate mean range of α particles emitted by ^{241}Am in soft tissue?

Answer.

The elemental compositions of air and soft tissue are similar; thus $A_A \approx A_X$ may be assumed. From Example 8-2, $R_A = 4.2$ cm. Therefore the approximate range in soft tissue is

$$R \approx 4.2 \text{ cm} \times 0.001293$$

$$\approx 0.0054 \text{ cm}$$

$$\approx 54 \text{ } \mu m$$

Examples 8-2 and 8-4 illustrate that α particles have very short ranges in air as well as in soft tissue and other solid materials. The very short ranges of α particles means that they constitute an almost negligible hazard as an external radiation source. Only a few centimeters of air, a sheet of paper, or a rubber glove provide adequate shielding protection. Even those particles that do reach the skin deliver a radiation dose only to the most superficial layers of skin. Alpha-particle emitters become a radiation hazard only when ingested; then, because of their densely ionizing nature, they become very potent radiation hazards (Chapter 23, Section A).

2. Beta Particles

In contrast to α particles, which have precise and predictable ranges, electrons have ranges that are quite variable from one electron to the next, even for electrons of exactly the same energy in a specific absorbing material. This is because of the possibility of scattering events and nuclear, bremsstrahlung-producing collisions that can deflect an electron through large angles or stop it completely in a single interaction.

A transmission experiment with β particles results in a curve of the type illustrated in Figure 8-9. Transmission begins to decrease immedi-

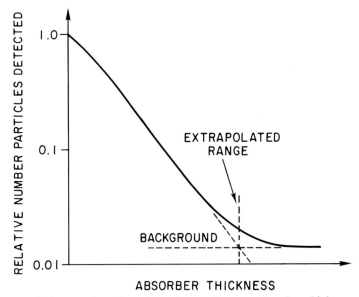

Fig. 8-9. Relative number of particles detected versus absorber thickness in an electron absorption experiment. (Compare with Figure 8-8.)

ately when absorber is added because even thin absorbers can remove a few electrons by the processes mentioned above. When the transmission curve is plotted on semilog graph paper, it follows at first a more or less straight-line decline until it gradually merges with a long, relatively flat tail. The tail of the curve does not reflect β particle transmission, but rather represents the detection of relatively penetrating bremsstrahlung photons generated by the β particles in the absorber and possibly in the source and source holder. Extraneous instrument and radiation background also may contribute to the tail of the curve.

The thickness of absorber corresponding to the intersection between the extrapolation of the linearly descending portion and the tail of the curve is called the *extrapolated range R_e* of the electrons. This is slightly less (perhaps by a few percent) than the maximum range R_m, which is the actual maximum thickness of absorber penetrated by the maximum energy β particles (Figure 8-9); however, because the difference is small and because R is very difficult to measure, R_e is usually specified as the β-particle range.

The extrapolated range for a monoenergetic beam of electrons of energy E is the same as that for a beam of β particles of maximum energy $E_\beta^{max} = E$. In both cases, range is determined by the maximum energy of electrons in the beam. The shapes of the transmission curves for monoenergetic electrons and for β particles are somewhat different, however. Specifically, the curve for β particles declines more rapidly for very thin absorbers because of rapid elimination of low-energy electrons in the β-particle energy spectrum (Figure 2-2).

Electron ranges are found to be inversely proportional to the density ρ of the absorbing material. To normalize for density effects, electron ranges usually are expressed in g/cm² of absorber. This is the weight of a 1 cm² section cut from a thickness of an absorber equal to the range of electrons in it. It is related to the range in centimeters according to

$$R_e(\text{g/cm}^2) = R_e(\text{cm}) \times \rho(\text{g/cm}^3) \qquad (8\text{-}8)$$

$$R_e(\text{cm}) = R_e(\text{g/cm}^2)/\rho(\text{g/cm}^3) \qquad (8\text{-}9)$$

It is also found that electron ranges in different elements, when expressed in g/cm², are practically identical. There are small differences in electron energy loss rates in different elements, as discussed in Section A.4, but they have only a small effect on total ranges. Figure 8-10 shows a curve for extrapolated ranges, in g/cm² of absorber, versus electron energy (or maximum β-particle energy, E_β^{max}) that is reasonably accurate for all absorbers.

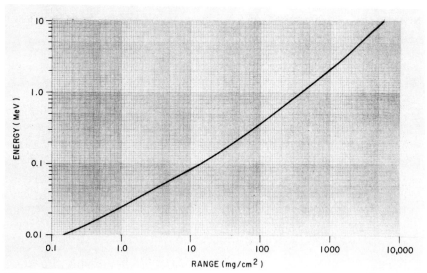

Fig. 8-10. Extrapolated range versus electron energy. Curve applies to all absorbers. Range in cm is obtained by dividing range in g/cm² by absorber density in g/cm³. [Adapted with permission from Radiological Health Handbook. Rockville, Md., U.S. Dept. H.E.W., 1970, p. 123.]

Table 8-1
Maximum Beta-Particle Ranges for Some Commonly
Used β Emitters

		Ranges (cm) in		
Radionuclide	E_β^{max} (MeV)	Air	Water	Aluminum
^{3}H	0.0186	4.6	0.00059	0.00022
^{14}C†	0.156	22.4	0.029	0.011
^{32}P	1.70	610	0.79	0.29

†Ranges for ^{35}S (E_β^{max} = 0.167 MeV) are nearly the same as those for ^{14}C.

Example 8-5.
Using Figure 8-10, determine the range of 1 MeV electrons in air
(ρ = 0.001293 g/cm^3), water (ρ = 1 g/cm^3), and lead (ρ = 11.3
g/cm^3).

Answer.
The range of a 1 MeV electron is 0.4 g/cm^2 (400 mg/cm^2). Thus

$$R_e = (0.4 \text{ g/cm}^2)/0.001293 \approx 309 \text{ cm in air}$$

$$R_e = 0.4/1 = 0.4 \text{ cm in water (or soft tissue)}$$

$$R_e = 0.4/11.3 = 0.035 \text{ cm in lead}$$

Example 8-5 illustrates that electron ranges can be several meters in
air but that they are only a few millimeters or fractions of a millimeter in
solid materials or liquids. Some ranges for β particles emitted by
radionuclides of medical interest are summarized in Table 8-1.

REFERENCES
Discussion of charged particle interactions and their passage through matters
is found in the following:
Johns HE, Cunningham JR: The Physics of Radiology (ed 4). Springfield, Ill.,
Charles C Thomas, 1983, Chap 6
Lapp RE, Andrews HL: Nuclear Radiation Physics (ed 4). Englewood Cliffs,
N.J., Prentice-Hall, Inc., 1972, pp 196–203, 261–279
Mladjenovic M: Radioisotope and Radiation Physics. New York, Academic
Press, 1973, Chap 4–6

Useful tabulations of charged particle ranges and other absorption data are
found in the following:
Radiological Health Handbook, Rockville, Md., U.S. Dept. H.E.W., 1970, pp
122–126

9

Passage of High-Energy Photons Through Matter

High-energy photons (γ rays, x rays, annihilation radiation, and bremsstrahlung) transfer their energy to matter in complex interactions with atoms, nuclei, and electrons. For practical purposes, however, these interactions can be viewed as simple "collisions" between a photon and a target atom, nucleus, or electron. These interactions do not cause ionization directly, as do the charged-particle interactions described in Chapter 8; however, some of the photon interactions result in the ejection of orbital electrons from atoms or in the creation of positive-negative electron pairs. These electrons in turn cause ionization effects, which are the basis for mechanisms by which high-energy photons are detected and by which they cause radiobiologic effects. For these reasons, high-energy photons are classified as *secondary ionizing* radiation.

There are nine possible interactions between photons and matter, of which only five are of significance to nuclear medicine. These five interactions, and mathematical aspects of the passage of photon beams through matter, will be discussed in this chapter.

A. INTERACTION MECHANISMS

1. The Photoelectric Effect

The *photoelectric effect* is an atomic absorption process in which an atom absorbs totally the energy of an incident photon. The photon disappears and the energy absorbed is used to eject an orbital electron from the atom. The ejected electron is called a *photoelectron*. It receives

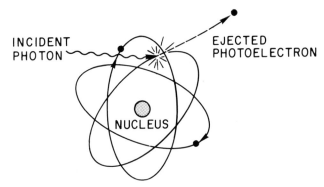

Fig. 9-1. Schematic representation of the photoelectric
effect. The incident photon transfers its energy to a photoelectron and disappears.

kinetic energy E_{pe} equal to the difference between the incident photon
energy E_0 and the binding energy of the electron shell from which it was
ejected. For example, if a K shell electron is ejected, the kinetic energy of
the photoelectron is

$$E_{pe} = E_0 - K_B \qquad (9\text{-}1)$$

where K_B is the K shell binding energy for the atom from which it is
ejected (Chapter 1, Section C.2). The photoelectric effect looks like a
"collision" between a photon and an orbital electron in which the
electron is ejected from the atom and the photon disappears (Figure 9-1).

Photoelectrons cannot be ejected from an electron shell unless the
absorbed photon energy exceeds the binding energy of that shell. (Values
of K shell binding energies for the elements are listed in Appendix A.) If
sufficient photon energy is available, the photoelectron is most likely to be
ejected from the innermost possible shell. For example, ejection of a K
shell electron is four to seven times more likely than ejection of an L shell
electron when the energy requirement of the K shell is met, depending on
the absorber element.

The photoelectric effect creates a vacancy in an orbital electron shell,
which in turn leads to the emission of characteristic x rays (or Auger
electrons). In low-Z elements, binding energies and characteristic x-ray
energies are only a few keV or less. Thus binding energy is a small factor
in photoelectric interactions in body tissues. In heavier elements, however, such as iodine, or lead, binding energies are in the 20–100 keV
range, and they may account for a significant fraction of the absorbed
photon energy.

Table 9-1
Ranges of Photoelectrons in Soft Tissue

E (keV)	Range (mm)	E (keV)	Range (mm)
34	0.023	270	0.64
40	0.034	400	1.24
68	0.070	590	2.8
86	0.108	1240	4.4
146	0.180		

From Mladjenovic M: Radioisotope and Radiation Physics. New York, Academic Press, 1973, chap 7. Used by permission.

The kinetic energy imparted to the photoelectron is deposited near the site of the photoelectric interaction by the ionization and excitation interactions of high-energy electrons described in Chapter 8, Section A. Table 9-1 lists some ranges of photoelectrons in soft tissue as a function of their energy.

2. Compton Scattering

Compton scattering is a collision between a photon and a loosely bound outer shell orbital electron of an atom. In Compton scattering, because the incident photon energy greatly exceeds the binding energy of the electron to the atom, the interaction looks like a collision between the photon and a "free" electron (Figure 9-2).

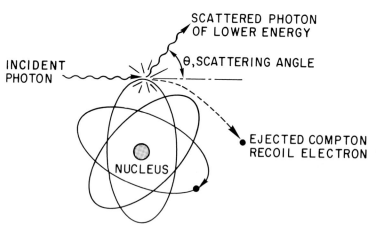

Fig. 9-2.   Schematic representation of Compton scattering. The incident photon transfers part of its energy to a Compton recoil electron and is scattered in another direction of travel (θ, scattering angle).

The photon does not disappear in Compton scattering. Instead, it is deflected through a scattering angle θ. Part of its energy is transferred to the *recoil electron;* thus the photon loses energy in the process. The energy of the scattered photon is related to the scattering angle θ by considerations of energy and momentum conservation according to

$$E_{sc} = E_0/[1 + (E_0/0.511)(1 - \cos\theta)] \qquad (9\text{-}2)$$

where E_0 and E_{sc} are the incident and scattered photon energies in MeV, respectively. The energy of the recoil electron, E_{re}, is thus

$$E_{re} = E_0 - E_{sc} \qquad (9\text{-}3)$$

The energy transferred does not depend on the density, atomic number, or any other property of the absorbing material. Compton scattering is strictly a photon–electron interaction.

The amount of energy transferred to the recoil electron in Compton scattering ranges from nearly zero for $\theta \approx 0°$ ("grazing" collisions) up to some maximum value E_{re}^{max} that occurs in 180° *backscattering* events. The minimum energy for scattered photons, E_{sc}^{min}, also occurs for 180° backscattering events. The minimum energy of Compton-scattered photons can be calculated from Equation 9-2 with $\theta = 180°$ ($\cos 180° = -1$):

$$E_{sc}^{min} = E_0/[1 + 2E_0/0.511] \qquad (9\text{-}4)$$

Thus

$$E_{re}^{max} = E_0 - E_{sc}^{min} \qquad (9\text{-}5)$$

$$= E_0 \left[1 - \frac{1}{(1 + 2E_0/0.511)} \right] \qquad (9\text{-}6)$$

$$= E_0^2/(E_0 + 0.2555) \qquad (9\text{-}7)$$

The energy of backscattered photons, E_{sc}^{min}, and the maximum energy transferred to the recoil electron, E_{re}^{max}, have characteristic values that depend on E_0, the energy of the incident photon. These energies are of interest in pulse-height spectrometry because they result in characteristic structures in pulse-height spectra (Chapter 11, Section B.1).

Table 9-2 lists some values of E_{sc}^{min} and E_{re}^{max} for some γ- and x-ray emissions from radionuclides of interest in nuclear medicine. Note that for relatively low photon energies (e.g., ^{125}I), the recoil electron receives

Table 9-2
Scattered Photon and Recoil Electron Energies for 180°
Compton Scattering Interactions

Radionuclide	Photon Energy (keV)	E_{sc}^{min} (keV)	E_{re}^{max} (keV)
^{125}I	27.5	24.8	3.3
^{133}Xe	81	62	19
^{99m}Tc	140	91	49
^{131}I	364	150	214
β^+ (annihilation)	511	170	341
^{60}Co	1330	214	1116
—	∞	256	—

only a small fraction of the incident photon energy, even in 180° scattering events. Thus photon energy changes very little in Compton scattering at low photon energies. This has important implications in the elimination of Compton-scattered photons by energy discrimination techniques (Chapter 11, Section B.3). At higher energies the energy distribution changes. E_{sc}^{min} approaches a maximum value of 256 keV. The remaining energy, which now accounts for most of the incident photon energy, is transferred to the recoil electron in 180° scattering events.

Note also that the energy of Compton-scattered photons is never zero—i.e., a photon cannot transfer all of its energy to an electron in a Compton-scattering event.

The angular distribution of Compton-scattered photons also depends on the incident photon energy. Figure 9-3 shows that at relatively low energies (10–100 keV) Compton scattering tends to be in either the forward or backward direction, with a minimum at right angles (90-deg) to the direction of the incident photons. At higher energies ($\gtrsim 0.5$ MeV) Compton scattering is increasingly toward the forward direction.

3. Pair Production

Pair production occurs when a photon interacts with the electric field of a charged particle. Usually the interaction is with an atomic nucleus, but occasionally it is with an electron. In pair production, the photon disappears and its energy is used to create a positive–negative electron pair (Figure 9-4). Because each electron has a rest mass equivalent to 0.511 MeV, a minimum photon energy of 2×0.511 MeV = 1.022 MeV must be available for pair production to occur. The difference between the incident photon energy E_0 and the 1.022 MeV of energy required to create the electron pair is imparted as kinetic energy to the two electrons, E_{e+} and E_{e-}:

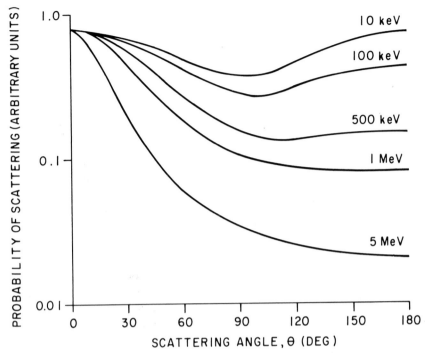

Fig. 9-3.   Relative probability of Compton scattering versus scattering angle θ for different incident photon energies.

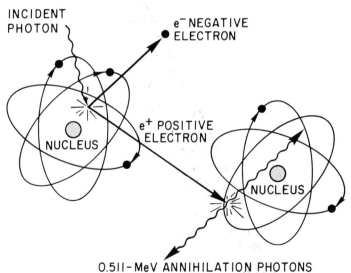

Fig. 9-4.   Schematic representation of pair production. Energy of incident photon is converted into electrons (total 1.022 MeV mass-energy equivalent) plus their kinetic energy. Positive electron position eventually undergoes mutual annihilation with a negative electron, producing two 0.511 MeV annihilation photons.

183

$$E_{e+} + E_{e-} = E_0 - 1.022 \text{ MeV} \tag{9-8}$$

The energy sharing is more or less random from one interaction to the next, usually within the 20–80 percent sharing range.

The two electrons dissipate their kinetic energy primarily in ionization and excitation interactions. When the positive electron has lost its kinetic energy and stopped, it undergoes mutual annihilation with a negative electron, and a pair of 0.511 MeV *annihilation photons* are emitted in opposite directions from the site of the annihilation event (Chapter 2, Section G). Annihilation photons usually travel for some distance before interacting again. Thus usually only the kinetic energy of the two electrons (Equation 9-8) is deposited at the site of the interaction in pair production.

4. Coherent (Rayleigh) Scattering

Coherent or *Rayleigh scattering* is a type of scattering interaction that occurs between a photon and an atom as a whole. Because of the great mass of an atom (for example, in comparison to the recoil electron in the Compton scattering process), very little recoil energy is absorbed by the atom. The photon is therefore deflected with essentially no loss of energy.

Coherent scattering is important only at relatively low energies (≤ 50 keV). It can be of significance in some precise photon transmission measurements—e.g., in x-ray CT scanning—because it is a mechanism by which photons are removed from a photon beam. Coherent scattering is also an important interaction in x-ray crystallography; however, because it is not an effective mechanism for transferring photon energy to matter, it is of little practical importance in nuclear medicine.

5. Photonuclear Reactions

Photonuclear reactions were discussed as methods for generating radionuclides in Chapter 7, Section C. These reactions require a minimum photon energy of about 2 MeV, and they are not significant in most elements until photon energies exceed about 10 MeV. Also, even at these energies, the probability of photonuclear reactions is much smaller than that of Compton scattering or pair production. Therefore photonuclear reactions are of no practical importance in terms of photon beam attenuation or the transfer of photon energy to matter.

6. Deposition of Photon Energy in Matter

The most important interactions in the transfer of photon energy to matter are the photoelectric effect, Compton scattering, and pair production. The transfer of energy occurs typically in a series of these interac-

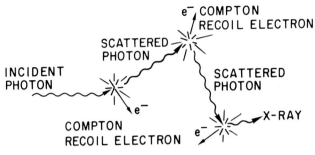

Fig. 9-5. Multiple interactions of a photon passing through matter. Energy is transferred to electrons in a sequence of photon-energy degrading interactions.

tions in which energy is transferred to electrons, and, usually, secondary photons, of progressively less energy (Figure 9-5). The products of each interaction are secondary photons and high-energy electrons (Table 9-3). The high-energy electrons ultimately are responsible for the deposition of energy in matter. Ionization and excitation by these electrons are the mechanisms underlying all of the photon detectors described in Chapter 4. The electrons also are responsible for radiobiologic effects caused by γ-ray, x-ray, or bremsstrahlung radiation. Because of this, the average LET of photons for radiobiologic purposes is the same as for electrons of similar energy, i.e., 0.2–2 keV/μm (Chapter 23, Section A).

B. ATTENUATION OF PHOTON BEAMS

1. Attenuation Coefficients

When a photon passes through a thickness of absorber material, the probability that it will experience an interaction depends on its energy and on the composition and thickness of the absorber. The dependence on

Table 9-3
Products of the Three Major Photon Interaction
Processes

Interaction	Secondary Photon(s)	High-Energy Secondary Electron(s)
Photoelectric	Characteristic x rays	Photoelectrons
		Auger electrons
Compton	Scattered photon	Recoil electron
Pair production	Annihilation photons	Positive-negative electron pair

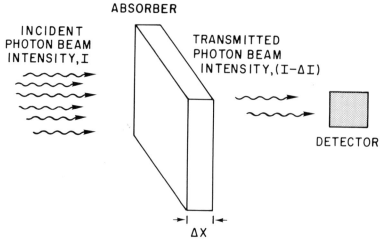

Fig. 9-6.   Photon beam transmission measurement.

thickness is relatively simple; the thicker the absorber, the greater the probability of an interaction. The dependence on absorber composition and photon energy, however, is more complicated.

Consider the photon transmission measurement diagrammed in Figure 9-6. A beam of photons of intensity I (photons/cm^2·sec) is directed onto an absorber of thickness Δx. Because of composition and photon energy effects, it will be assumed for the moment that the absorber is comprised of a single element of atomic number Z and that the beam is monoenergetic with energy E. A photon detector records transmitted beam intensity. It is assumed that only those photons passing through the absorber without interaction are recorded. (The validity of this assumption will be discussed further in Sections B.2 and B.3.)

For a "thin" absorber, such that beam intensity is reduced by only a small amount, i.e., less than about 10 percent, it is found that the fractional decrease in beam intensity ($\Delta I/I$) is related to absorber thickness Δx according to

$$\Delta I/I \approx -\mu_l \Delta x \qquad (9\text{-}9)$$

the minus sign indicating beam intensity decreases with increasing absorber thickness. The quantity μ_l is called the *linear attenuation coefficient* of the absorber. It has dimensions (thickness)$^{-1}$ and usually is expressed in cm^{-1}. This quantity reflects the "absorptivity" of the absorbing material.

The quantity μ_l is found to increase linearly with absorber density ρ. Density effects are factored out by dividing μ_l by density ρ:

$$\mu_m = \mu_l/\rho \tag{9-10}$$

The quantity μ_m has dimensions cm^2/g and is called the *mass attenuation coefficient* of the absorber. It depends on the absorber atomic number Z and photon energy E. This sometimes is emphasized by writing it $\mu_m(Z,E)$.

It is possible to measure μ_m or μ_l in different absorber materials by transmission measurements with monoenergetic photon beams. Most tables, however, are based on theoretical calculations from atomic and nuclear physics. An extensive tabulation of values of μ_m versus photon energy for different absorber materials is found in reference 1. Some values of interest to nuclear medicine, taken from these tables, are presented in Appendix D. Usually, values of μ_m rather than μ_l are tabulated because they do not depend on the physical state (density) of the absorber. Given a value of μ_m from the tables, μ_l for an absorber can be obtained from

$$\mu_l(cm^{-1}) = \mu_m(cm^2/g) \times \rho(g/cm^3) \tag{9-11}$$

The mass attenuation coefficient for a *mixture of elements* can be obtained from the values for its component elements according to

$$\mu_m(mix) = \mu_{m1}f_1 + \mu_{m2}f_2 + \cdots \tag{9-12}$$

where $\mu_{m1}, \mu_{m2}, \ldots$ are the mass attenuation coefficients for elements 1, 2, ... and $f_1, f_2, \ldots$ are the fractions by weight of these elements in the mixture. For example, the mass attenuation coefficient for water (2/18 H, 16/18 O, by weight) is given by

$$\mu_m(H_2O) = (2/18)\mu_m(H) + (16/18)\mu_m(O) \tag{9-13}$$

The mass attenuation coefficient μ_m can be broken down into components according to

$$\mu_m = \tau + \sigma + \kappa \tag{9-14}$$

where τ is that part of μ_m due to the photoelectric effect, σ is the part due to Compton scattering, and κ is the part due to pair production. Thus, for example, τ would be the mass attenuation coefficient of an absorber in the absence of Compton scattering and pair production. Note that μ_m involves both absorption and scattering processes. Thus μ_m is properly called an *attenuation* coefficient rather than an *absorption* coefficient.

The relative magnitudes of τ, σ, and κ vary with atomic number Z and

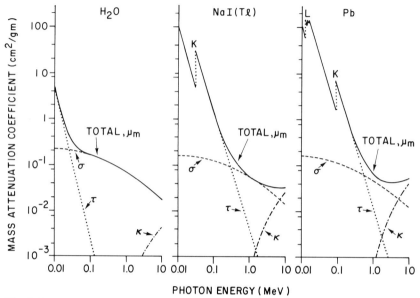

Fig. 9-7. Photoelectric (τ), Compton (σ), pair-production (κ), and total (μ_m) mass attenuation coefficients (cm²/g) for H₂O, NaI(Tl), and Pb from 0.01 to 10 MeV. K and L are absorption edges. The curves for μ_l are obtained by multiplying by the appropriate density values.

photon energy E. Figure 9-7 shows graphs of μ_m and its components, τ, σ, and κ versus photon energy from 0.01 to 10 MeV in water, NaI(Tl), and lead. The following points are illustrated by these graphs:

1. The photoelectric component τ decreases rapidly with increasing photon energy and increases rapidly with increasing atomic number of the absorber ($\tau \sim Z^3/E^3$). The photoelectric effect is thus the dominating effect in heavy elements at low photon energies. The photoelectric component also increases abruptly at energies corresponding to orbital electron binding energies of the absorber elements. At the K shell binding energies of iodine ($K_B = 33.2$ keV) and lead ($K_B = 88.0$ keV), the increase is a factor of 5–6. These abrupt increases are called *K absorption edges*. They result from the fact that photoelectric absorption involving K shell electrons cannot occur until the photon energy exceeds the K shell binding energy. L absorption edges also are seen at $E \sim 13$–16 keV in the graph for lead. L absorption edges in water and iodine and the K absorption edge for water also exist, but they occur at energies less than those shown in the graphs.

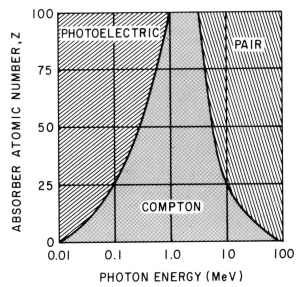

Fig. 9-8.   Predominating (most probable) interaction versus
photon energy for absorbers of different atomic numbers.

2. The Compton scatter component σ decreases slowly with increasing
    photon energy E and with increasing absorber atomic number Z. The
    changes are so small that for practical purposes σ usually is consid-
    ered to be invariant with Z and E. Compton scattering is the
    dominating interaction for intermediate values of Z and E.
3. The pair-production component κ is zero for photon energies less
    than the threshhold energy for this interaction at 1.02 MeV; then it
    increases logarithmically with increasing photon energy and with
    increasing atomic number of the absorber (κ $\sim Z \log E$). Pair
    production is the dominating effect at higher photon energies in
    absorbers of high atomic number.

    Figure 9-8 shows the dominating (most probable) interaction versus
photon energy E and absorber atomic number Z. Note that Compton
scattering is the dominating interaction for $Z \lesssim 20$ (body tissues) over
most of the nuclear medicine energy range.

2. Thick Absorbers, Narrow-Beam Geometry

The transmission of a photon beam through a "thick" absorber—that
is, one in which the probability of photon interaction is not small
($\gtrsim 10\%$)—depends on the geometric arrangement of the photon source,
absorber, and detector. Specifically, transmission depends on whether or

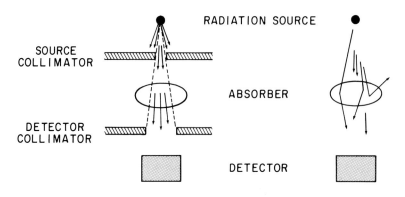

Fig. 9-9. Narrow-beam and broad-beam geometries for photon-beam attenuation measurements. Narrow-beam geometry is designed to minimize the number of scattered photons recorded.

not scattered photons are recorded as part of the transmitted beam. An arrangement that is designed to minimize the recording of scattered photons is called *narrow-beam geometry*. Conversely, an arrangement in which many scattered photons are recorded is called *broad-beam geometry*. (They also are called *good geometry* and *poor geometry,* respectively.) Figure 9-9 shows examples of these geometries.

Conditions of narrow-beam geometry usually require that the beam be collimated with a narrow aperture at the source so that only a narrow beam of photons is directed onto the absorber. This minimizes the probability that photons will strike neighboring objects (e.g., the walls of the room) and scatter toward the detector. Matching collimation on the detector helps to prevent photons that are multiple scattered in the absorber from being recorded. In addition, it is desirable to place the absorber about halfway between the source and the detector.

Under conditions of narrow-beam geometry the transmission of a monoenergetic photon beam through an absorber is described by an exponential equation,

$$I(x) = I(0)e^{-\mu x} \tag{9-15}$$

where $I(x)$ is the beam intensity transmitted through a thickness x of absorber, $I(0)$ is the intensity recorded with no absorber present, and μ_l is the linear attenuation coefficient of the absorber at the photon energy of interest. In contrast to charged particles, photons do not have a definite maximum range. There is always some finite probability that a photon will penetrate even the thickest absorber [i.e., I(x) in Equation 9-15 never reaches zero].

Equation 9-15 is exactly analogous to Equation 3-5 for the decay of radioactivity, with the attenuation coefficient μ_l replacing the decay constant λ and absorber thickness x replacing decay time t. Analogous to the concept of half-life in radioactive decay, the thickness of an absorber that decreases recorded beam intensity by one half is called the *half-value thickness* (HVT) or *half-value layer* (HVL). It is related to the linear attenuation coefficient according to

$$\text{HVT} = 0.693/\mu_l \qquad (9\text{-}16)$$

$$\mu_l = 0.693/\text{HVT} \qquad (9\text{-}17)$$

(Compare these equations with Equations 3-6 and 3-7.)

Some radiation shielding problems require the use of relatively thick absorbers; for this purpose it is sometimes useful to know the *tenth-value thickness* (TVT)—that is, the thickness of absorber that decreases transmitted beam intensity by a factor of 10. This quantity is given by

$$\text{TVT} = 2.30/\mu_l \qquad (9\text{-}18)$$

$$= 3.32 \times \text{HVT} \qquad (9\text{-}19)$$

Some half-value thicknesses for water and tenth-value thicknesses for lead are listed in Table 9-4.

The quantity

$$X_m = 1/\mu_l \qquad (9\text{-}20)$$

is called the *mean free path* for photons in an absorber. It is the *average distance* traveled by a photon in the absorber before experiencing an interaction. Mean free path is related to half-value thickness according to

Table 9-4
Half-Value Thicknesses in Water and Tenth-Value
Thicknesses in Lead (Narrow-Beam Conditions)

Radionuclide	Photon Energy (keV)	HVT in Water (cm)	TVT in Lead (mm)
^{125}I	27.5	1.7	0.06
^{133}Xe	81	4.3	1.0
^{99m}Tc	140	4.6	0.9
^{131}I	364	6.3	7.7
β^+ (annihilation)	511	7.1	13.5
^{60}Co	1330	11.2	36.2

Table 9-5
Comparison of Photon Mean Free Paths (MFP) and
α-Particle and Electron Ranges

Photon or Particle Energy (MeV)	Photon MFP (cm H_2O)	Electron Range (cm H_2O)	α-Particle Range (cm Air)
0.01	0.20	0.00016	—
0.1	5.95	0.014	0.1
1	14.14	0.40	0.5
10	45.05	5.20	10.3

$$X_m = 1.44 \times \text{HVT} \qquad (9\text{-}21)$$

(Compare this to equation 3-10; note analogy to average lifetime, τ.)

Table 9-5 compares mean free paths for photons in water against ranges for electrons in water and α particles in air as a function of their energy. Although the concepts of photon mean free path and charged particle ranges are different, the comparison gives an indication of relative penetration by these two types of radiations. Over the energy range 0.01–10 MeV, photons are much more penetrating than electrons or α particles. For this reason they are sometimes called *penetrating radiation*.

The quantity $e^{-\mu x}$ (or $I(x)/I(0)$ in equation 9-15), the fraction of beam intensity transmitted by an absorber, is called its *transmission factor*. The transmission factor can be determined using the methods described for determining decay factors in Chapter 3, Section C. For example, the graph shown in Figure 3-3 can be used with "decay factor" replaced by "transmission factor" and "number of half-lives" replaced by "number of half-value thickness."

Example 9-1.

Determine the transmission factor for 140 keV photons in 10 cm of soft tissue (water) by direct calculation.

Answer.

From Table 9-4, HVT = 4.6 cm in water at 140 keV. Thus $\mu_l = 0.693/4.6 = 0.151$ cm^{-1}, and the transmission factor is

$$I(10)/I(0) = \exp(-0.151 \times 10) = e^{-1.51}$$

(recall that $\exp(x) = e^x$). Using a pocket calculator or from Appendix C,

$$e^{-1.51} = 0.22$$

Thus the transmission of 140 keV photons through 10 cm of water is 22.2 percent.

Example 9-2.
Determine the transmission factor for 511 keV photons in 1 cm of lead using graphical methods.

Answer.
From Table 9-4, the TVT of 511 keV photons in lead is 13.5 mm. From Equation 9-19, HVT = TVT/3.32 = 1.35 cm/3.32 = 0.4 cm. Thus 1 cm = 2.5 HVTs. From Figure 3-3, the transmission (decay) factor for 2.5 HVTs ($T_{1/2}$'s) is approximately 0.18 (18 percent transmission).

It must be remembered that the answers obtained in Examples 9-1 and 9-2 apply only to narrow-beam conditions. Broad-beam conditions are discussed in the following section.

3. Thick Absorbers, Broad-Beam Geometry

Practical problems of photon beam attenuation in nuclear medicine usually involve broad-beam conditions. Examples are the shielding of radioactive materials in lead containers and the penetration of body tissues by photons emitted from radioactive tracers localized in internal organs. In both of these examples, a considerable amount of scattering occurs in the absorber material surrounding or overlying the radiation source.

The factor by which transmission is increased in broad-beam conditions, relative to narrow-beam conditions, is called the *buildup factor B*. Thus the transmission factor T for broad-beam conditions is given by

$$T = Be^{-\mu_l x} \tag{9-22}$$

where μ_l and x are the linear attenuation coefficient and thickness, respectively, of the absorber.

Buildup factors for various source-absorber-detector geometries have been calculated. Some values for water and lead for a source embedded in or surrounded by scattering and absorbing material are listed in Table 9-6. Note that B depends on photon energy and on the product $\mu_l x$ for the absorber.

Example 9-3.
In Example 9-2, the transmission factor for 511 keV photons in 1 cm of lead was found to be 18 percent, for narrow-beam conditions. Estimate the actual transmission for broad-beam conditions

(e.g., a vial of β^+-emitting radioactive solution in a lead container of 1 cm wall thickness).

Answer.

For 511 keV photons, HVT = 0.4 cm (Example 9-2). Thus $\mu_l =$ 0.693/(0.4 cm)$\approx$ 1.73 cm^{-1}, and, for $x = 1$ cm, $\mu_l x \approx 1.73$. Taking values for 0.5 MeV ($\approx$511 keV) from Table 9-6 and using linear interpolation between values for $\mu_x = 1$ ($B = 1.24$) and $\mu_x = (B = 1.42)$, one obtains

$$B = 1.24 + (0.73)(1.42 - 1.24)$$

$$= 1.37$$

Thus the actual transmission factor is

$$T \approx 1.37 \times 0.18$$

$$\approx 0.25$$

or 25 percent. For $B = 1.37$, the transmission in broad-beam conditions is 37 percent greater than calculated for narrow-beam conditions.

Example 9-3 illustrates that scatter effects can be significant in broad-beam conditions. The thickness of lead shielding required to

Table 9-6
Buildup Factors in Water and in Lead[†]

Material	Photon Energy (MeV)	$\mu_l x$						
		1	*2*	*4*	*7*	*10*	*15*	*20*
Water	0.255	3.09	7.14	23.0	72.9	166	456	982
	0.5	2.52	5.14	14.3	38.8	77.6	178	334
	1.0	2.13	3.71	7.68	16.2	27.1	50.4	82.2
	2.0	1.83	2.77	4.88	8.46	12.4	19.5	27.7
	4.0	1.58	2.17	3.34	5.13	6.94	9.97	12.9
	10.0	1.33	1.63	2.19	2.97	3.72	4.90	5.98
Lead	0.5	1.24	1.42	1.69	2.00	2.27	2.65	2.73
	1.0	1.37	1.69	2.26	3.02	3.74	4.81	5.86
	2.0	1.39	1.76	2.51	3.66	4.84	6.87	9.00
	4.0	1.27	1.56	2.25	3.61	5.44	9.80	16.3
	10.0	1.11	1.23	1.58	2.52	4.34	12.5	39.2

[†]Data taken from ref. 2.

achieve a given level of protection is greater than that calculated using narrow-beam equations.

Example 9-4.
Estimate the thickness of lead shielding required to achieve an actual transmission of 18 percent in the problem described in Example 9-3.

Answer.
Since $B = 1.37$, it is necessary to further reduce transmission by approximately $1/1.37 \approx 0.73$ to correct for scattered radiation. According to Figure 3-3, this would require approximately 0.45 HVTs, or about 0.18 cm (1 HVT = 0.4 cm). This is only an estimate, since the HVT used applies to narrow-beam conditions. A more exact answer could be obtained by successive approximations.

Broad-beam conditions also arise in problems of internal radiation dosimetry—e.g., when it is desired to calculate the radiation dose to an organ delivered by a radioactive concentration in another organ. This problem is discussed further in Chapter 10, Section B.4.

4. Polyenergetic Sources

Many radionuclides emit photons of more than one energy. The photon transmission curve for such an emitter consists of a sum of exponentials, one component for each of the photon energies emitted. The transmission curve has an appearance similar to the decay curve for a mixed radionuclide sample shown in Figure 3-4. The transmission curve drops steeply at first as the lower-energy ("softer") components of the beam are removed. Then it gradually flattens out, reflecting greater penetration by the higher-energy ("harder") components of the beam. The average energy of photons in the beam increases with increasing absorber thickness. This effect is called *beam hardening*.

It is possible to detect small amounts of a high-energy photon emitter in the presence of large amounts of a low-energy photon emitter by making use of the beam-hardening effect. For example, a 3 mm thickness of lead is several TVTs for the 140 keV γ rays of ^{99m}Tc, but it is only about one HVT for the 700–800 keV γ rays of ^{99}Mo. Thus a 3 mm thick lead shield placed around a vial containing ^{99m}Tc solution permits detection of small amounts of ^{99}Mo contamination with minimal interference from the ^{99m}Tc γ rays (Chapter 7, Section E.).

REFERENCES

1. Hubbell JH: Photon cross-sections, attenuation coefficients, and energy absorption coefficients from 10 keV to 100 GeV. Natl Stand Ref Data Ser Natl Bur Stand 29, 1969
2. Radiological Health Handbook. Rockville, Md., U.S. Dept. H.E.W., 1971, pp 145–146

Additional discussion of photon interactions and photon-beam transmission is found in the following:

Lapp RE, Andrews HL: Nuclear Radiation Physics (ed 4). Englewood Cliffs, N.J., Prentice-Hall, Inc., 1972, pp 233–247

Mladjenovic M: Radioisotope and Radiation Physics. New York, Academic Press, 1973, chap 7

Applications of quantitative photon-beam transmission measurements in nuclear medicine are discussed in the following:

Sorenson JA, Cameron JR: Transmission scanning techniques, in Hine GJ, Sorenson JA (eds): Instrumentation in Nuclear Medicine (vol 2). New York, Academic Press, 1974, pp 350–384

10
Internal Radiation Dosimetry

Absorption of energy from ionizing radiation can cause damage to living tissues. This is used to advantage in radionuclide therapy, but it is a limitation for diagnostic applications because of the potential hazard for the patient. In either case, it is necessary to analyze the energy distribution in body tissues quantitatively in order to ensure an accurate therapeutic prescription or to assess potential risks to the patient. The study of radiation effects on living organisms is the subject of *radiation biology* (or radiobiology) and is discussed in several excellent texts, some of which are listed at the end of this chapter.

One of the most important factors to be evaluated in the assessment of radiation effects on an organ is the amount of radiation energy deposited in that organ. Calculation of radiation energy deposited by internal radionuclides is the subject of *internal radiation dosimetry*. There are two general methods by which these calculations may be performed: the *classical method* and the *absorbed fraction method*. Although the classical method is somewhat simpler, and the results by the two methods are not greatly different, the absorbed fraction method is more versatile and gives more accurate results. Therefore it has gained acceptance as the standard method for performing internal dosimetry calculations. The procedures to be followed in using this method will be summarized in this chapter. Descriptions of the classical method are found in references listed at the end of this chapter. Dosimetry calculations for external radiation sources as well as some health physics aspects of radiation dosimetry are discussed in Chapter 23. Some radiation dose estimates for nuclear medicine procedures are summarized in Appendix E.

A. RADIATION DOSE: QUANTITIES AND UNITS

Radiation dose D refers to the quantity of radiation energy deposited in an absorber per gram of absorber material. This quantity applies to any kind of absorber material, including body tissues. The basic unit of radiation dose is the *rad*,†

$$1 \text{ rad} = 100 \text{ ergs energy deposited/g absorber} \qquad (10\text{-}1)$$

The SI unit for absorbed dose is the *gray*, abbreviated Gy:

$$1 \text{ Gy} = 1 \text{ joule energy deposited/kg absorber} \qquad (10\text{-}2)$$

Since 1 joule = 10^7 ergs, 1 Gy is equivalent to 100 rads or, alternatively, 1 rad = 10^{-2} Gy. As with units of activity, the transition from traditional to SI units is in progress, but traditional units continue to dominate day-to-day practice in the U.S. In this chapter, radiation doses are presented in rads, with values in grays also indicated in selected examples.

It is sometimes of interest to know the total amount of energy deposited in a volume of tissue, such as an entire organ. This quantity is called *integral dose*. It is the product of absorbed dose in rads times tissue mass in grams for the tissue volume of interest, and has units g·rad is equivalent to 100 ergs of radiation energy deposited in the tissue volume.

B. CALCULATION OF RADIATION DOSE (ABSORBED FRACTION METHOD)

1. Basic Procedure and Some Practical Problems

The absorbed fraction dosimetry method allows one to calculate the radiation dose delivered to a *target organ* from radioactivity contained in one or more *source organs* in the body (Figure 10-1). The source and target may be the same organ, and, in fact, frequently the most important contributor to radiation dose is radioactivity contained within the target organ itself. Generally, organs other than the target organ are considered to be source organs if they contain concentrations of radioactivity that exceed the average concentration in the body.

The general procedure for calculating the radiation dose to a target organ from radioactivity in a source organ is a three-step process:

---

† Rad is an acronym for *r*adiation *a*bsorbed *d*ose.

SOURCE
ORGANS

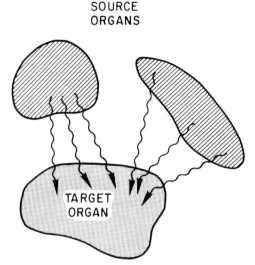

Fig. 10-1.   Absorbed dose delivered to a target organ from
one or more source organs containing radioactivity is calculated by the absorbed fraction dosimetry method.

1. The amount of activity and time spent by the radioactivity in the
    source organ is determined. Obviously, the greater the activity and
    the longer the time that it is present, the greater is the radiation dose
    delivered by it.
2. The total amount of radiation energy emitted by the radioactivity in
    the source organ is calculated. This depends primarily on the energy
    of the radionuclide emissions and their frequency of emission (num-
    ber per disintegration).
3. The fraction of energy emitted by the source organ that is absorbed
    by the target organ is determined. This depends on the type and
    energy of the emissions (absorption characteristics in body tissues)
    and on the anatomic relationships between source and target organs
    (size, shape, and distance between them).

    Each of these steps involves certain difficulties. Step 2 involves
physical characteristics of the radionuclide, which generally are known
accurately. Step 3 involves patient anatomy, which can be quite different
from one patient to the next. Step 1 is perhaps the most troublesome.
Such data on radiopharmaceutical distribution as are available usually are
obtained from studies on a relatively small number of human subjects or
animals. There are variations in metabolism and distribution of
radionuclides among human subjects, especially in different disease

states. Also, the distribution of radioactivity within an organ may be inhomogeneous, leading to further uncertainties in the dose specification for that organ.

Because of these complications and variables, radiation dose calculations are made for anatomic models that incorporate "average" anatomic sizes and shapes. The radiation doses that are calculated are *average* values $\overline{D}$ for the organs in this anatomic model. An exception is made when one is specifically interested in a *surface dose* to an organ from activity contained within that organ—e.g., the dose to the bladder wall due to bladder contents. This is considered to have a value one-half the average dose to the organ.

It must be remembered that in spite of the refined mathematical models used in the absorbed fraction model the results obtained are only *estimates* of *average* values and should be used for *guideline* purposes only in evaluating the potential radiation effects on a patient.

2. Cumulated Activity, $\tilde{A}$

The radiation dose delivered to a target organ depends on the amount of activity present in the source organ and on the length of time for which the activity is present. These two factors together determine the *cumulated activity* $\tilde{A}$ in the source organ. This quantity is the product of activity and time and has units of $\mu Ci \cdot hr$.

Cumulated activity is essentially a measure of the total number of radioactive disintegrations occurring during the time that radioactivity is present in the source organ (1 $\mu Ci = 3.7 \times 10^4$ dis/sec; 1 hr = 3600 sec; therefore 1 $\mu Ci \cdot hr = 3.7 \times 10^4 \times 3600 = 1.332 \times 10^8$ dis). The corresponding SI unit for cumulated activity is the bequerel $\cdot$ sec; 1 Bq$\cdot$sec $\sim 7.51 \times 10^{-9}$ mCi$\cdot$hr, or 1 mCi$\cdot$hr $= 1.332 \times 10^8$ Bq$\cdot$sec. The radiation dose delivered by activity in a source organ is proportional to its cumulated activity.

The amount of activity contained in a source organ generally changes with time, owing to physical decay of the radionuclide and biologic uptake and excretion processes. If the time–activity curve is known, the cumulated activity is obtained by measuring the area under this curve (Figure 10-2). Mathematically, if the time–activity curve is described by a function $A(t)$, then

$$\tilde{A} = \int_0^\infty A(t) \, dt \qquad (10\text{-}3)$$

where it is assumed that activity is administered to the patient at time $t = 0$ and is measured to complete disappearance from the organ ($t = \infty$).

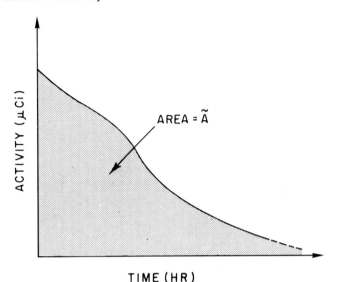

TIME (HR)

Fig. 10-2. Hypothetical time–activity curve for radioactivity in a source organ. Cumulated activity $\tilde{A}$ in μCi·hr is the area under the curve (equivalent to the integral in Equation 10-3).

Time–activity curves can be quite complex, and thus Equation 10-3 may be difficult to analyze. Frequently, however, certain assumptions can be made to simplify this calculation.

Situation 1: Uptake by the organ is "instantaneous" (i.e., very rapid with respect to the half-life of the radionuclide), and there is no biologic excretion. The time–activity curve is then described by ordinary radioactive decay (Equations 3-6 and 3-8):

$$A(t) = A_0 e^{-0.693t/T_p} \tag{10-4}$$

where T_p is the physical half-life of the radionuclide and A_0 is the activity initially present in the organ. Thus

$$\tilde{A} = A_0 \int_0^\infty e^{-0.693t/T_p} \, dt \tag{10-5}$$

$$= T_p A_0/0.693 \tag{10-6}$$

$$= 1.44 T_p A_0 \tag{10-7}$$

The quantity $1.44T_p$ is the average lifetime of the radionuclide (Chapter 3, Section B.3). Thus the cumulated activity in a source organ,

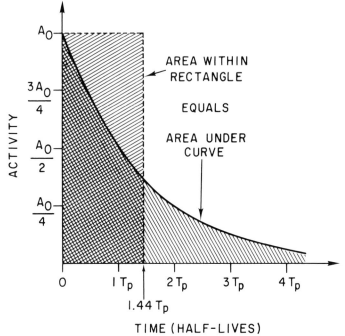

Fig. 10-3. Illustration of relationship between $\bar{A}$ and average lifetime ($1.44T_p$) of a radionuclide for simple exponential decay.

when eliminated by physical decay only, is the same as if activity were present at a constant level A_0 for a time equal to the average lifetime of the radionuclide (Figure 10-3).

Example 10-1.
What is the cumulated activity in the liver for an injection of 3 mCi of a ^{99m}Tc-labeled sulfur colloid, assuming that 60 percent of the injected colloid is trapped by the liver and retained there indefinitely?

Answer.

$$\bar{A} = 1.44 \times 3.0 \text{ mCi} \times 0.60 \times 6.0 \text{ hr}$$

$$= 15.6 \text{ mCi·hr}$$

$$= 15,600 \text{ μCi·hr}$$

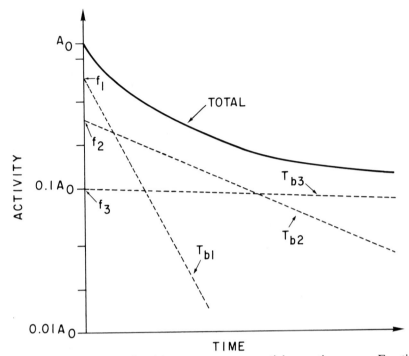

Fig. 10-4. Illustration of multicomponent exponential excretion curve. Fraction f_1 is excreted with biologic half-life T_{b1}, f_2 with half-life T_{b2}, f_3 with half-life T_{b3}, etc.

Situation 2:   Uptake is instantaneous, and clearance is by biologic excretion only (no physical decay, or half-life very long in comparison to biologic excretion).   In this situation, biologic excretion must be carefully analyzed. Frequently, it can be described by a set of exponential excretion components, with a fraction f_1 of the initial activity A_0 being excreted with a (biologic) half-life T_{b1}, a fraction f_2 with half-life T_{b2}, and so on (Figure 10-4). The cumulative activity then is given by

$$\bar{A} = A_0 \int_0^\infty f_1 e^{-0.693t/T_{b1}} \, dt + A_0 \int_0^\infty f_2 e^{-0.693t/T_{b2}} \, dt + \ldots \qquad (10\text{-}8)$$

$$= 1.44 T_{b1} f_1 A_0 + 1.44_{b2} f_2 A_0 + \ldots \qquad (10\text{-}9)$$

Example 10-2.
Suppose that 3 mCi of ^{99m}Tc-labeled microspheres are injected into a patient, with essentially instantaneous uptake of activity by the lungs. What is the cumulated activity in the lungs if 60 percent of

the activity is excreted from the lungs with a biologic half-life of 15 min and 40 percent with a biologic half-life of 30 min?

Answer.

Because ^{99m}Tc physical decay is much slower than the biologic excretion processes, we may assume that no physical decay occurs during the time that activity is present in the lungs. Thus (Equation 10-9)

$\tilde{A}$ = (1.44 × ¼ hr × 0.60 × 3.0 mCi) + (1.44 × ½ hr × 0.40 × 3.0 mCi)

= (0.65 + 0.86) mCi·hr

= 1.51 mCi·hr

= 1510 μCi·hr

Situation 3: Uptake is instantaneous, but clearance is by both physical decay and biologic excretion. In this case, if biologic excretion is described by a single-component exponential curve with biologic half-life T_b and the physical half-life is T_p, then the total clearance is described by a single-component exponential curve with an *effective half-life* T_e given by

$$1/T_e = 1/T_p + 1/T_b \tag{10-10}$$

or

$$T_e = T_p T_b/(T_p + T_b) \tag{10-11}$$

Cumulated activity is given by

$$\tilde{A} = 1.44 T_e A_o \tag{10-12}$$

If there is more than one component to the biologic excretion curve, then each component (in Equation 10-9) has an effective half-life given by Equation 10-11 for that component.

Note that if physical decay is very slow in comparison to biologic excretion ($T_p >> T_b$), then $T_e \approx T_b$, whereas if biologic excretion is slow in comparison to physical decay ($T_b >> T_p$), then $T_e \approx T_p$. Note also that the effective half-life always is shorter than either the physical or the biologic half-life.

Example 10-3.

Suppose in Example 10-2 that because of a metabolic defect 60 percent of the activity is excreted from the lungs with a half-life of 2 hr and 40 percent with a half-life of 3 hr. What is the cumulated activity in the lungs for a 3 mCi injection for this patient?

Answer.
The effective half-lives for the two components of biologic excretion are (Equation 10-11)

$$T_{e1} = 6 \times 2/(6 + 2) = 1.5 \text{ hr}$$
$$T_{e2} = 6 \times 3/(6 + 3) = 2 \text{ hr}$$

Thus applying Equation 10-9, with T_e replacing T_b

$$\tilde{A} = (1.44 \times 1.5 \text{ hr} \times 0.60 \times 3.0 \text{ mCi}) + (1.44 \times 2 \text{ hr} \times 0.40 \times 3.0 \text{ mCi})$$

$$= (3.89 + 3.46) \text{ mCi·hr}$$

$$= 7.35 \text{ mCi·hr}$$

$$= 7350 \text{ } \mu\text{Ci·hr}$$

Situation 4: Uptake is not instantaneous. The equations developed thus far will overestimate radiation doses when uptake by the source organ is not rapid in comparison to physical decay, i.e., if a significant amount of physical decay occurs during the uptake process. This situation arises with radionuclides that have a slow pattern of uptake in comparison to their physical half-life. Frequently, uptake can be described by an exponential equation of the form

$$A(t) = A_0(1 - e^{-0.693t/T_u}) \tag{10-13}$$

where T_u is the biologic uptake half-time. In this case, cumulated activity is given by

$$\tilde{A} = 1.44A_0T_e(T_{ue}/T_u) \tag{10-14}$$

where T_e is the effective excretion half-life (Equation 10-11) and T_{ue} is the effective uptake half-time

$$T_{ue} = T_uT_p/(T_u + T_p) \tag{10-15}$$

Example 10-4.
A radioactive gas having a half-life of 20 sec is injected in an intravenous solution. It appears in the lungs with an uptake half-time of 30 sec and is excreted (by exhalation) with a biologic half-life of 10 sec. What is the cumulated activity in the lungs for a 10 mCi injection?

Answer.

The effective uptake half-time is (Equation 10-15)

$$T_{ue} = 20 \times 30/(20 + 30) = 12 \text{ sec}$$

and the effective excretion half-life is

$$T_e = 20 \times 10/(20 + 10) = 6.7 \text{ sec}$$

Thus (Equation 10-14)

$$\tilde{A} = 1.44 \times 10 \text{ mCi} \times 6.7 \text{ sec} \times (12 \text{ sec}/30 \text{ sec})$$

$$= 38.6 \text{ mCi·sec}$$

$$= 38,600 \text{ } \mu\text{Ci·sec}$$

$$= 10.7 \text{ } \mu\text{Ci·hr}$$

---

3. Equilibrium Absorbed Dose Constant, Δ

Given $\tilde{A}$ for the source organ, the next step is to calculate the radiation energy emitted by this activity. Energy emitted per unit of cumulated activity is given by the *equilibrium absorbed dose constant* Δ. The factor Δ must be calculated for each type of emission for the radionuclide. It is given by†

$$\Delta_i = 2.13 N_i E_i \text{ g·rad}/\mu\text{Ci·hr} \qquad (10\text{-}16)$$

where E_i is the average energy (in MeV) of the ith emission and N_i is the relative frequency of that emission (number emitted per disintegration).

Example 10-5.

A certain radionuclide decays by emitting β particles in 100 percent of its disintegrations with $\overline{E}_\beta = 0.3$ MeV. This is followed in 80 percent of its disintegrations by emission of a 0.2 MeV γ ray and in 20 percent by emission of a 0.195 MeV conversion electron and a 0.005 MeV characteristic x ray. What are the equilibrium absorbed dose constants for the emissions of this radionuclide?

---

† Essentially the energy emitted per nuclear disintegration: 1 MeV/dis = 2.13 g·rad/μCi·hr.

Answer.

$$\Delta_\beta = 2.13 \times 1.0 \times 0.30 = 0.639 \text{ g·rad/}\mu\text{Ci·hr}$$

$$\Delta_\gamma = 2.13 \times 0.80 \times 0.20 = 0.341 \text{ g·rad/}\mu\text{Ci·hr}$$

$$\Delta_e = 2.13 \times 0.20 \times 0.195 = 0.083 \text{ g·rad/}\mu\text{Ci·hr}$$

$$\Delta_x = 2.13 \times 0.2 \times 0.005 = 0.0021 \text{ g·rad/}\mu\text{Ci·hr}$$

The product of cumulated activity $\bar{A}$ and equilibrium absorbed dose constant Δ_i is the radiation energy emitted by the ith emission, in g·rad, during the time that radioactivity is present in a source organ.

Example 10-6.

Assume that the radionuclide in Example 10-5 is used for the problem described in Example 10-4. What is the total amount of energy emitted from radioactivity contained in the lungs in Example 10-4?

Answer.

The total energy emitted per μCi·hr is the sum of the equilibrium absorbed dose constants for the β, γ, conversion electron, and x-ray emissions:

$$\Delta = \Delta_\beta + \Delta_\gamma + \Delta_e + \Delta_x$$

$$= 1.07 \text{ g·rad/}\mu\text{Ci·hr}$$

The cumulated activity is 10.7 μCi·hr. Thus the total energy emitted is

$$\bar{A} \times \Delta = 11.4 \text{ g·rad}$$

$$= 1140 \text{ ergs (1 g·rad} = 100 \text{ ergs)}$$

Values of Δ are presented in Appendix B for some of the radionuclides of interest in nuclear medicine.

4. Absorbed Fraction, ϕ

The final step is to determine the fraction of the energy emitted by the source organ that is absorbed by the target organ. This is given by the *absorbed fraction* ϕ. The absorbed fraction depends on the amount of radiation energy reaching the target organ (tissue and distance attenuation between source and target organs) and on the volume and composition (e.g., lung, bone, etc.) of the target organ. The value of ϕ depends on the type and energy of the emission and on the anatomic relationship of the source–target pair. Thus a value of ϕ must be determined for each type of emission from the radionuclide and for each source–target pair in a dosimetry calculation. The notation $\phi_i(r_k \leftarrow r_h)$ is used to indicate absorbed fraction for energy delivered from a source organ (or region), r_h, to a target organ, r_k, for the ith emission of the radionuclide.

The total energy absorbed by a target organ is thus given by

$$\text{Total energy absorbed (g·rad)} = \bar{A} \sum_i \phi_i(r_k \leftarrow r_h) \Delta_i \qquad (10\text{-}17)$$

The summation Σ_i includes values of ϕ_i and Δ_i for all the emissions of the radionuclide and values of $\phi_i(r_k \leftarrow r_h)$ for the appropriate source–target pair. $\bar{A}$ is the cumulated activity in the source organ h. The energy absorbed by the target organ divided by the target organ mass m_t gives the *average absorbed dose* $\overline{D}$ in rads to the target organ from activity in the source organ,

$$\overline{D}(r_k \leftarrow r_h) = (\bar{A}/m_t) \sum_i \phi_i(r_k \leftarrow r_h) \Delta_i \qquad (10\text{-}18)$$

The total dose to the target organ is then obtained by summing the doses from all of the source organs in the body.

Values of ϕ have been calculated for humanoid models incorporating organs and anatomic structures of "average" size and shape (Figure 10-5) and published by the Medical Internal Radiation Dosimetry (MIRD) committee of the Society of Nuclear Medicine.[1] Organ masses used for these calculations are given in Table 10-1.

The calculations of ϕ values are complex and the tables are quite lengthy for "penetrating" radiations (photons with energy $\gtrsim 10$ keV) because of the energy dependence of photon attenuation and absorption; however, the situation is simpler for nonpenetrating radiations (photons with energy $\lesssim 10$ keV and electrons), for which it can be assumed that the emitted energy is "locally absorbed," i.e., within the source organ itself. For these emissions, $\phi = 1$ when the target and the source are the same organ, $\phi = 0$ otherwise. In dosimetry calculations, it is useful to sum the equilibrium absorbed dose constants for the nonpenetrating radiations and treat them as a single parameter, Δ_{np}, because the absorbed fractions for all of these emissions are equal (unity when the source and target are the same organ, zero otherwise).

Example 10-7.

Compute the absorbed dose delivered to the lung by nonpenetrating radiations in the problem described by Examples 10-4 and 10-5.

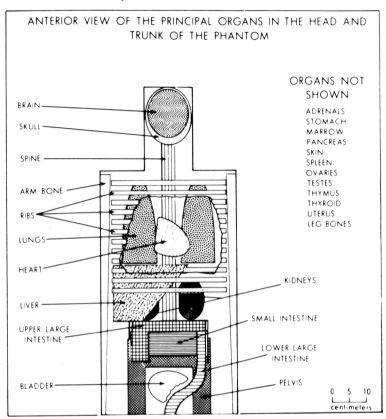

ANTERIOR VIEW OF THE PRINCIPAL ORGANS IN THE HEAD AND
TRUNK OF THE PHANTOM

ORGANS NOT
SHOWN

ADRENALS
STOMACH
MARROW
PANCREAS
SKIN
SPLEEN
OVARIES
TESTES
THYMUS
THYROID
UTERUS
LEG BONES

BRAIN
SKULL
SPINE
ARM BONE
RIBS
LUNGS
HEART
LIVER
UPPER LARGE
INTESTINE
BLADDER

KIDNEYS
SMALL INTESTINE
LOWER LARGE
INTESTINE
PELVIS

0   5   10
centimeters

Fig. 10-5.   Representation of an "average man" used for MIRD dose calculations and tables. [From ref. 1: Snyder WS, Ford MR, Warner GG, et al: Estimates of absorbed fractions for monoenergetic photon sources uniformly distributed in various organs of a heterogenous phanton. J Nucl Med, 1969, p. 9. With permission of The Society of Nuclear Medicine]

Answer.

The nonpenetrating radiations are the β particles (Δ_β = 0.639 g·rad/μCi·hr), conversion electrons (Δ_e = 0.083·rad/μCi·hr), and 5 keV characteristic x rays (Δ_x = 0.0021g·rad/μCi·hr). Thus Δ_{np} = 0.724g·rad/μCi·hr. Cumulated activity is $\tilde{A}$ = 10.7 μCi·hr. Lung mass is 1000 g (Table 10-1). Thus the average radiation dose delivered by these emissions to the lungs is

$$\overline{D} = (10.7 \ \mu Ci \cdot hr) \times (0.724 g \cdot rad/\mu Ci \cdot hr) \times (\phi = 1)/1000 \ g$$

$$= 0.0077 \ rad$$

$$= 7.7 \ mrad$$

In SI units (1 rad = 10^{-2} Gy) the dose is $\overline{D}$ = 7.7 × 10^{-5} Gy.

Table 10-1

Organ Masses Used for MIRD Calculations and Tables

Body organs	Abbreviation	Mass (g)
Adrenals	AD	15.5
Bladder		
Wall	BLADW	45.13
Contents	BLADC	200
Gastrointestinal tract		
Stomach		
Wall	STW	150
Contents	STC	246.9
Small intestine and contents	SI	1,044
		wall plus contents
Upper large intestine		
Wall	ULIW	209.2
Contents	ULIC	200
Lower large intestine		
Wall	LLIW	160.1
Contents	LLIC	136.8
Kidneys (both)	KI	284.2
Liver	LI	1,809
Lungs (both, including blood)	LU	999.2
Other tissue	OT	48,480
		(2,800 g suggested for muscle; 12,500 g for separable adipose tissue)
Ovaries (both)	OV	8.268
Pancreas	PA	60.27
Salivary glands	SALG	Not represented
Skeleton	SKEL	10,470
Cortical bone	CORTB	4,000
Trabecular bone	TRAB	1,000
Red marrow	RM	1,500
Yellow marrow	YM	1,500
Cartilage	CART	1,100
Other constituents	—	1,370
Spleen	SP	173.6
Testes	TE	37.08
Thyroid	THY	19.63
Uterus	UT	65.4
Total body	TB	69,880

From ref. 2: Snyder WS, Ford MR, Warner GG, et al: "S" Absorbed Dose per Unit Cumulated Activity for Selected Radionuclides and Organs. MIRD Pamphlet No 11, New York, Society of Nuclear Medicine, 1975. p. 60 with permission.

5. Specific Absorbed Fraction, Φ, and the Dose Reciprocity Theorem

The *specific absorbed fraction* is given by

$$\Phi = \phi/m_t \qquad (10\text{-}19)$$

It is the fraction of radiation emitted by the source organ that is absorbed *per gram* of target organ mass. The absorbed dose equation can be written using specific absorbed fractions as

$$\overline{D}(r_k \leftarrow r_h) = \tilde{A}\sum_i \Phi_i(r_k \leftarrow r_h)\Delta_i \qquad (10\text{-}20)$$

The *dose reciprocity theorem* says that for a given organ pair the specific absorbed fraction is the same, regardless of which organ is the source and which is the target:

$$\Phi(r_k \leftarrow r_h) = \Phi(r_h \leftarrow r_k) \qquad (10\text{-}21)$$

This simply says that the energy absorbed per gram is the same for radiation traveling from r_h to r_k as it is for radiation traveling from r_k to r_h, a fact that seems intuitively obvious.

The dose reciprocity theorem is useful when tables for ϕ are not available for all source–target organ pairs. If $\phi(r_k \leftarrow r_h)$ is known, then $\phi(r_h \leftarrow r_k)$ can be obtained from the dose reciprocity theorem:

$$\phi(r_h \leftarrow r_k)/m_h = \phi(r_k \leftarrow r_h)/m_k \qquad (10\text{-}22)$$

$$\phi(r_h \leftarrow r_k)/ = (m_h/m_k)\phi(r_k \leftarrow r_h) \qquad (10\text{-}23)$$

6. Mean Dose per Cumulated Activity, S

Radiation dose calculations for penetrating radiations can be quite tedious, especially when there are multiple emissions to consider. The problem has been simplified by the introduction of S, the mean dose per unit cumulated activity:

$$S(r_k \leftarrow r_h) = (1/m_k) \sum_i \Delta_i \phi_i(r_k \leftarrow r_h) \qquad (10\text{-}24)$$

$$= \sum_i \Delta_i \Phi_i(r_k \leftarrow r_h) \qquad (10\text{-}25)$$

The quantity S has units rad/μCi·hr. It has been calculated for different source–target organ pairs for a number of radionuclides of interest in nuclear medicine[3] (Tables 10-2 and 10-3). Given the appropriate value of

Table 10-2

S, Absorbed Dose per Unit Cumulative (rad/μCi · hr) for ^{99m}Tc

Target Organs	Adrenals	Bladder Contents	Intestinal Tract Stomach Contents	SI Contents	ULI Contents	LLI Contents	Kidneys	Liver	Lungs	Other Tissue (Muscle)
Adrenals	3.1E-03	1.5E-07	2.7E-06	1.0E-06	9.1E-07	3.6E-07	1.1E-05	4.5E-06	2.7E-06	1.4E-06
Bladder wall	1.3E-07	1.6E-04	2.7E-07	2.6E-06	2.2E-06	6.9E-06	2.8E-07	1.6E-07	3.6E-08	1.8E-06
Bone (total)	2.0E-06	9.2E-07	9.0E-07	1.3E-06	1.1E-06	1.6E-06	1.4E-06	1.1E-06	1.5E-06	9.8E-07
GI (stom. wall)	2.9E-06	2.7E-07	1.3E-04	3.7E-06	3.8E-06	1.8E-06	3.6E-06	1.9E-06	1.8E-06	1.3E-06
GI (SI)	8.3E-07	3.0E-06	2.7E-06	7.8E-05	1.7E-05	9.4E-06	2.9E-06	1.6E-06	1.9E-07	1.5E-06
GI (ULI wall)	9.3E-07	2.2E-06	3.5E-06	2.4E-05	1.3E-04	4.2E-06	2.9E-06	2.5E-06	2.2E-07	1.6E-06
GI (LLI wall)	2.2E-07	7.4E-06	1.2E-06	7.3E-06	3.2E-06	1.9E-04	7.2E-07	2.3E-07	7.1E-08	1.7E-06
Kidneys	1.1E-05	2.6E-07	3.5E-06	3.2E-06	2.8E-06	8.6E-07	1.9E-04	3.9E-06	8.4E-07	1.3E-06
Liver	4.9E-06	1.7E-07	2.0E-06	1.8E-06	2.6E-06	2.5E-07	3.9E-06	4.6E-05	2.5E-06	1.1E-06
Lungs	2.4E-06	2.4E-08	1.7E-06	2.2E-07	2.6E-07	7.9E-08	8.5E-07	2.5E-06	5.2E-05	1.3E-06
Marrow (red)	3.6E-06	2.2E-06	1.6E-06	4.3E-06	3.7E-06	5.1E-06	3.8E-06	1.6E-06	1.9E-06	2.0E-06
Other tissue (muscle)	1.4E-06	1.8E-06	1.4E-06	1.5E-06	1.5E-06	1.7E-06	1.3E-06	1.1E-06	1.3E-06	2.7E-06
Ovaries	6.1E-07	7.3E-06	5.0E-07	1.1E-05	1.2E-05	1.8E-05	1.1E-06	4.5E-07	9.4E-08	2.0E-06
Pancreas	9.0E-06	2.3E-07	1.8E-05	2.1E-06	2.3E-06	7.4E-07	6.6E-06	4.2E-06	2.6E-06	1.8E-06
Skin	5.1E-07	5.5E-07	4.4E-07	4.1E-07	4.1E-07	4.8E-07	5.3E-07	4.9E-07	5.3E-07	7.2E-07
Spleen	6.3E-06	6.6E-07	1.0E-05	1.5E-06	1.4E-06	8.0E-07	8.6E-06	9.2E-07	2.3E-06	1.4E-06
Testes	3.2E-08	4.7E-06	5.1E-08	3.1E-07	2.7E-07	1.8E-06	8.8E-08	6.2E-08	7.9E-09	1.1E-06
Thyroid	1.3E-07	2.1E-09	8.7E-08	1.5E-08	1.6E-08	5.4E-09	4.8E-08	1.5E-07	9.2E-07	1.3E-06
Uterus (nongravid)	1.1E-06	1.6E-05	7.7E-05	9.6E-06	5.4E-06	7.1E-06	9.4E-07	3.9E-07	8.2E-08	2.3E-06
Total body	2.2E-06	1.9E-06	1.9E-06	2.4E-06	2.2E-06	2.3E-06	2.2E-06	2.2E-06	2.0E-06	1.9E-06

Source Organs

Source Organs

Target Organs	Ovaries	Pancreas	Red Marrow	Cort. Bone	Trab. Bone	Skin	Spleen	Testes	Thyroid	Total Body
			Skeleton							
Adrenals	3.3E-07	9.1E-06	2.3E-06	1.1E-06	1.1E-06	6.8E-07	6.3E-06	3.2E-08	1.3E-07	2.3E-06
Bladder wall	7.2E-06	1.4E-07	9.9E-07	5.1E-07	5.1E-07	4.9E-07	1.2E-07	4.8E-06	2.1E-09	2.3E-06
Bone (total)	1.5E-06	1.5E-06	4.0E-06	1.2E-05	1.0E-05	9.9E-07	1.1E-06	9.2E-07	1.0E-06	2.5E-06
GI (stom. wall)	8.1E-07	1.8E-05	9.5E-07	5.5E-07	5.5E-07	5.4E-07	1.0E-05	3.2E-08	4.5E-08	2.2E-06
GI (SI)	1.2E-05	1.8E-06	2.6E-06	7.3E-07	7.3E-07	4.5E-07	1.4E-06	3.6E-07	9.3E-09	2.5E-06
GI (ULI wall)	1.1E-05	2.1E-06	2.1E-06	6.9E-07	6.9E-07	4.6E-07	1.4E-06	3.1E-07	1.1E-08	2.4E-06
GI (LLI wall)	1.5E-05	5.7E-07	2.9E-06	1.0E-06	1.0E-07	4.8E-07	6.1E-07	2.7E-06	4.3E-09	2.3E-06
Kidneys	9.2E-07	6.6E-06	2.2E-06	8.2E-07	8.2E-07	5.7E-07	9.1E-06	4.0E-08	3.4E-08	2.2E-06
Liver	5.4E-07	4.4E-06	9.2E-07	6.6E-07	6.6E-07	5.3E-07	9.8E-07	3.1E-08	9.3E-08	2.2E-06
Lungs	6.0E-08	2.5E-06	1.2E-06	9.4E-07	9.4E-07	5.8E-07	2.3E-06	6.6E-09	9.4E-07	2.0E-06
Marrow (red)	5.5E-06	2.8E-06	3.1E-05	4.1E-06	9.1E-06	9.5E-07	1.7E-06	7.3E-07	1.1E-06	2.9E-06
Other tissue (muscle)	2.0E-06	1.8E-06	1.2E-06	9.8E-07	9.8E-07	7.2E-07	1.4E-06	1.1E-06	1.3E-06	1.9E-06
Ovaries	4.2E-03	4.1E-07	3.2E-06	7.1E-07	7.1E-07	3.8E-07	4.0E-07	0.0	4.9E-09	2.4E-06
Pancreas	5.0E-07	5.8E-04	1.7E-06	8.5E-07	8.5E-07	3.3E-07	1.9E-05	5.5E-08	7.2E-08	2.4E-06
Skin	4.1E-07	4.0E-07	5.9E-07	6.5E-07	6.5E-07	1.6E-05	4.7E-07	1.4E-06	7.3E-07	1.3E-06
Spleen	4.9E-07	1.9E-05	9.2E-07	5.8E-07	5.8E-07	5.4E-07	3.3E-04	1.7E-08	1.1E-07	2.2E-06
Testes	0.0	5.5E-08	4.5E-07	6.4E-07	6.4E-07	9.1E-07	4.8E-08	1.4E-03	5.0E-10	1.7E-06
Thyroid	4.9E-09	1.2E-07	6.8E-07	7.9E-07	7.9E-07	6.9E-07	8.7E-08	5.0E-10	2.3E-03	1.5E-06
Uterus (nongravid)	2.1E-05	5.3E-07	2.2E-06	5.7E-07	5.7E-07	4.0E-07	4.0E-07	0.0	4.6E-09	2.6E-06
Total body	2.6E-06	2.6E-06	2.2E-06	2.0E-06	2.0E-06	1.3E-06	2.2E-06	1.9E-06	1.8E-06	2.0E-06

Adapted from ref. 2: Snyder WS, Ford MR, Warner GG, et al: "S," Absorbed Dose per Unit Cumulated Activity for Selected Radionuclides and Organs. MIRD Pamphlet No 11, New York, Society of Nuclear Medicine, 1975. With permission.
†The notation "E-03" means "× 10⁻³", etc.

Table 10-3

S, Absorbed Dose per Unit Cumulative Activity (rad/μCi · hr) for ^{131}I

				Source Organs						
				Intestinal Tract						Other Tissue
Target Organs	Adrenals	Bladder Contents	Stomach Contents	SI Contents	ULI Contents	LLI Contents	Kidneys	Liver	Lungs	(Muscle)
Adrenals	3.1E-02	6.1E-07	6.3E-06	3.9E-06	2.7E-06	1.4E-06	3.2E-05	1.4E-05	6.9E-06	4.2E-06
Bladder wall	3.3E-07	1.2E-03	1.0E-06	8.5E-06	5.6E-06	1.7E-05	1.0E-06	7.4E-07	1.8E-07	5.0E-06
Bone (total)	4.1E-06	1.8E-06	1.8E-06	2.5E-06	2.2E-06	3.2E-06	3.0E-06	2.3E-06	3.0E-06	3.0E-06
GI (Stom. wall)	8.2E-06	8.8E-07	9.7E-04	9.9E-06	1.0E-05	5.0E-06	9.4E-06	5.4E-06	5.2E-06	3.9E-06
GI (SI)	2.6E-06	7.6E-06	7.3E-06	6.0E-04	4.6E-05	2.6E-05	7.8E-06	4.6E-06	6.9E-07	4.4E-06
GI (ULI wall)	2.8E-06	6.6E-06	9.5E-06	6.5E-05	1.1E-03	1.2E-05	8.1E-06	7.0E-06	9.1E-07	4.6E-06
GI (LLI wall)	8.4E-07	2.0E-05	3.6E-06	1.9E-05	8.4E-06	1.7E-03	2.4E-06	8.1E-07	2.6E-07	4.8E-06
Kidneys	3.2E-05	9.6E-07	9.5E-06	8.7E-06	7.7E-06	2.5E-06	1.5E-03	1.1E-05	2.7E-06	4.0E-06
Liver	1.4E-05	7.2E-07	5.6E-06	5.1E-06	7.1E-06	9.0E-07	1.1E-05	3.0E-04	6.8E-06	3.1E-06
Lungs	6.7E-06	1.1E-07	5.0E-06	8.5E-07	8.9E-07	2.8E-07	2.5E-06	6.8E-06	4.5E-04	3.7E-06
Marrow (red)	7.5E-06	4.1E-06	3.2E-06	7.9E-06	6.9E-06	9.7E-06	7.6E-06	3.3E-06	3.8E-06	4.1E-06
Other tissue (muscle)	4.2E-06	5.0E-06	3.9E-06	4.4E-06	4.1E-06	4.8E-06	4.0E-06	3.1E-06	3.7E-06	1.9E-05
Ovaries	1.6E-06	1.9E-05	1.4E-06	2.7E-05	3.4E-05	5.0E-05	3.4E-06	9.6E-07	4.0E-07	5.6E-06
Pancreas	2.4E-05	7.9E-07	5.0E-05	5.8E-06	5.8E-06	2.0E-06	1.8E-05	1.2E-05	7.5E-06	5.0E-06
Skin	1.8E-06	1.7E-06	1.5E-06	1.4E-06	1.4E-06	1.6E-06	1.8E-06	1.6E-06	1.8E-06	2.4E-06
Spleen	1.8E-05	5.6E-07	2.7E-05	4.4E-06	3.7E-06	2.5E-06	2.4E-05	2.7E-06	6.2E-06	4.1E-06
Testes	1.7E-07	1.4E-05	1.3E-07	1.0E-06	1.2E-06	5.7E-06	3.9E-07	3.0E-07	5.7E-08	3.4E-06
Thyroid	5.2E-07	2.1E-08	3.9E-07	9.5E-08	1.0E-07	4.1E-08	2.4E-07	5.7E-07	3.0E-06	3.8E-06
Uterus (nongravid)	3.4E-06	4.3E-05	2.4E-06	2.5E-05	1.3E-05	1.7E-05	2.6E-06	1.2E-06	2.7E-07	5.9E-06
Total body	1.1E-05	5.9E-06	6.7E-06	1.0E-05	8.2E-06	8.8E-06	1.1E-05	1.1E-05	9.9E-06	9.8E-06

Source Organs

Target Organs	Ovaries	Pancreas	Skeleton Red Marrow	Cort. Bone	Trab. Bone	Skin	Spleen	Testes	Thyroid	Total Body
Adrenals	1.4E-06	2.3E-05	6.1E-06	4.3E-06	4.3E-06	2.1E-06	1.8E-05	1.7E-07	5.2E-07	1.2E-05
Bladder wall	1.9E-05	5.0E-07	2.1E-06	1.6E-06	1.6E-06	1.7E-06	4.5E-07	1.4E-05	2.1E-08	1.1E-05
Bone (total)	2.9E-06	2.8E-06	2.5E-05	9.2E-05	6.5E-05	2.4E-06	2.3E-06	2.0E-06	2.2E-06	1.0E-05
GI (Stom. wall)	2.3E-06	5.0E-05	2.9E-06	1.6E-06	1.6E-06	1.7E-06	2.7E-05	2.5E-07	2.6E-07	1.1E-05
GI (SI)	3.3E-05	5.1E-06	7.4E-06	2.2E-06	2.2E-06	1.5E-06	3.9E-06	1.4E-06	3.4E-08	1.1E-05
GI (ULI wall)	3.1E-05	6.1E-06	5.8E-06	2.0E-06	2.0E-06	1.5E-06	3.7E-06	9.7E-07	3.5E-08	1.1E-05
GI (LLI wall)	4.0E-05	1.5E-06	8.4E-06	2.8E-06	2.8E-06	1.6E-06	1.9E-06	7.8E-06	3.4E-08	1.1E-05
Kidneys	3.0E-06	1.8E-05	6.5E-06	2.6E-06	2.6E-06	2.0E-06	2.4E-05	2.4E-07	1.4E-07	1.1E-05
Liver	1.7E-06	1.2E-05	2.8E-06	1.9E-06	1.9E-06	1.8E-06	3.0E-06	1.4E-07	4.0E-07	1.1E-05
Lungs	2.7E-07	6.8E-06	3.4E-06	2.8E-06	2.8E-06	1.9E-06	6.2E-06	4.0E-08	2.9E-06	1.0E-05
Marrow (red)	9.8E-06	5.4E-06	2.3E-04	1.0E-05	1.0E-04	2.3E-06	3.5E-06	1.6E-06	2.4E-06	1.1E-05
Other tissue (muscle)	5.6E-06	5.0E-06	3.6E-06	3.0E-06	3.0E-06	2.4E-06	4.1E-06	3.4E-06	3.8E-06	9.8E-06
Ovaries	3.9E-02	1.1E-06	8.4E-06	2.6E-06	2.6E-06	1.1E-06	2.4E-06	0.0	4.1E-08	1.1E-05
Pancreas	1.5E-06	4.7E-03	4.6E-06	2.8E-06	2.8E-06	1.6E-06	5.4E-05	1.6E-07	2.4E-07	1.1E-05
Skin	1.4E-06	1.4E-06	2.0E-06	2.3E-06	2.3E-06	1.6E-04	1.6E-06	4.3E-06	2.4E-06	8.3E-06
Spleen	1.8E-06	5.4E-05	2.4E-06	2.2E-06	2.2E-06	1.8E-06	2.6E-03	2.3E-07	3.6E-07	1.1E-05
Testes	0.0	2.0E-07	1.1E-06	1.7E-06	1.7E-06	2.6E-06	2.4E-07	1.3E-02	7.2E-09	1.0E-05
Thyroid	4.1E-08	4.7E-07	2.3E-06	2.8E-06	2.8E-06	2.3E-06	3.8E-07	7.2E-09	2.2E-02	9.7E-06
Uterus (nongravid)	5.4E-05	1.8E-06	5.8E-06	1.7E-06	1.7E-06	1.4E-06	1.2E-06	0.0	3.8E-08	1.1E-05
Total body	1.2E-05	1.1E-05	1.0E-05	9.9E-06	9.9E-06	8.3E-06	1.1E-05	9.8E-06	9.5E-06	9.9E-06

Adapted from ref. 2: Snyder WS, Ford MR, Warner GG, et al: "S," Absorbed Dose per Unit Cumulated Activity for Selected Radionuclides and Organs. MIRD Pamphlet No 11, New York, Society of Nuclear Medicine, 1975.

†The notation "E-03" means "$\times 10^{-3}$," etc.

S and a value for cumulated activity $\tilde{A}$, the average dose to an organ is given by

$$\overline{D}(r_k \leftarrow r_h) = \tilde{A} \ (r_k \leftarrow r_h) \tag{10-26}$$

Example 10-8.
Calculate the radiation dose to the liver for an injection of 3 mCi of ^{99m}Tc sulfur colloid. Assume that 60 percent of the activity is trapped by the liver, 30 percent by the spleen, and 10 percent by red bone marrow, with instantaneous uptake and no biologic excretion.

Answer.
The cumulated activities for the three source organs are (Equation 10-7)

$$A_{LI} = 1.44 \times 6.0 \ hr \times 0.60 \times 3.0 \ mCi = 15,600 \ \mu Ci \cdot hr$$

$$A_{SP} = 1.44 \times 6.0 \ hr \times 0.30 \times 3.0 \ mCi = 7780 \ \mu Ci \cdot hr$$

$$A_{RM} = 1.44 \times 6.0 \ hr \times 0.10 \times 3.0 \ mCi = 2590 \ \mu Ci \cdot hr$$

The values for S are (Table 10-2)

$$S(LI \leftarrow LI) = 4.6 \times 10^{-5} \ rad/\mu Ci \cdot hr$$

$$S(LI \leftarrow SP) = 9.8 \times 10^{-7} \ rad/\mu Ci \cdot hr$$

$$S(LI \leftarrow RM) = 9.2 \times 10^{-7} \ rad/\mu Ci \cdot hr$$

Therefore the absorbed doses are

$$\overline{D}(LI \leftarrow LI) = 15,600 \ \mu Ci \cdot hr \times 4.6 \times 10^{-5} \ rad/\mu Ci \cdot hr = 0.718 \ rad$$

$$\overline{D}(LI \leftarrow SP) = 7,780 \ \mu Ci \cdot hr \times 9.8 \times 10^{-7} \ rad/\mu Ci \cdot hr = 0.0076 \ rad$$

$$\overline{D}(LI \leftarrow RM) = 2,590 \ \mu Ci \cdot hr \times 9.2 \times 10^{-7} \ rad/\mu Ci \cdot hr = 0.0024 \ rad$$

The total dose (average) to the liver is therefore

$$\overline{D} = 0.718 + 0.0076 + 0.0024 \ rad = 0.728 \ rad$$

In SI units (1 rad $= 10^{-2}$ Gy) the total dose to the liver is $\overline{D} = 7.28 \times 10^{-3}$ Gy.

Example 10-8 demonstrates that most of the dose delivered to an organ that concentrates the radionuclide arises from the radioactivity in the target organ itself [D(LI←LI)].

Example 10-9.

A patient is to be treated with ^{131}I for hyperthyroidism. It is determined by prior studies with a tracer dose of ^{131}I that the patient's thyroidal iodine uptake is 60 percent, and the biologic half-life of iodine in the thyroid gland is 2 days. Assuming instantaneous uptake ($T_u << T_p$ = 8 days), what is the dose to the thyroid from radioactivity contained in the thyroid for this patient, per mCi^{131}I?

Answer.

The effective half-life of ^{131}I in the thyroid for this patient is (Equation 10-11)

$$T_e = 8 \times 2/(8 + 2) = 16/10 \text{ days}$$

$$= 38.4 \text{ hr}$$

Therefore the cumulated activity per mCi administered is (Equation 10-12)

$$\tilde{A} = 1.44 \times 38.4 \text{ hr} \times 0.60 \times 1000 \text{ }\mu\text{Ci}$$

$$= 33,200 \text{ }\mu\text{Ci}\cdot\text{hr/mCi administered}$$

The dose per μCi·hr is (Table 10-3)

$$S(THY \leftarrow THY) = 2.2 \times 10^{-2} \text{ rad/}\mu\text{Ci}\cdot\text{hr}$$

Thus the average absorbed dose for the thyroid is

$$\overline{D}(THY \leftarrow THY) = 33,200 \times 2.2 \times 10^{-2}$$

$$= 730 \text{ rads/mCi administered}$$

In SI units (1 rad = 10^{-2} Gy, 1 mCi = 3.7×10^4 Bq) the average dose for the thyroid is $\overline{D}(THY \leftarrow THY)$ = 1.97×10^{-7} Gy/Bq administered.

One could include the radiation dose to the thyroid from activity in other organs in Example 10-9; however, inspection of Table 10-3 reveals that in comparison to the thyroid as the source organ, other organs have much smaller values of S. This, plus the fact that other organs concentrate much less of the activity than the thyroid, eliminates the need to consider them as source organs in this calculation.

REFERENCES

Society of Nuclear Medicine (MIRD) publications presenting the basic data required for absorbed fraction dosimetry are the following:

1. Snyder WS, Ford MR, Warner GG, et al: Estimates of absorbed fractions for monoenergetic photon sources uniformly distributed in various organs of a heterogeneous phantom. J Nucl Med [Suppl 3, Pamphlet No. 5], 1969, p 9
2. Snyder WS, Ford MR, Warner GG, et al: "S," Absorbed Dose per Unit Cumulated Activity for Selected Radionuclides and Organs. MIRD Pamphlet No 11, New York, Society of Nuclear Medicine, 1975

Descriptions of the classical internal dosimetry method are found in the following:

Greenfield MA, Lane RG: Radioisotope dosimetry, in Blahd WH (ed): Nuclear Medicine (ed 2). New York, McGraw-Hill, 1971, chap 5 [also gives comparisons of radiation doses calculated by the absorbed fraction and classical methods]

Quimby EH, Feitelberg S, Gross W: Radioactive Nuclides in Medicine and Biology. Philadelphia, Lea & Febiger, 1970, chap 9

Recommended basic textbooks on radiation biology are the following:

Hall EJ: Radiobiology for the Radiologist (ed 2): New York, Harper & Row, 1978

Altman KF, Gerber GB, Okada S: Radiation Biochemistry: Cells (vol 1); Tissues and Body Fluids (vol 2). New York, Academic Press, 1970

11

Pulse-Height Spectrometry

Most of the radiation measurement systems used in nuclear medicine use pulse-height analysis (Chapter 5, Section C) to sort out the different radiation energies striking the detector. This is called *pulse-height*—or *energy—spectrometry*. It is used to discriminate against background radiation sources, scattered radiation, etc., and to identify the emission energies of unknown radionuclides. In this chapter we discuss the basic principles of pulse-height spectrometry and some of its characteristics as applied to different types of detectors.

A. BASIC PRINCIPLES

Pulse-height spectrometry is used to examine the amplitudes of signals (electrical current or light) from a radiation detector in order to determine the energies of radiations striking the detector, or to select for counting only those energies within a desired energy range. This can be accomplished only with those detectors that provide output signals with amplitudes proportional to radiation energy detected, e.g., proportional counters, scintillation detectors, and semiconductor detectors (Chapter 4). A pulse-height, or energy, *spectrometer* consists of such a radiation detector and its high voltage supply, preamplifier, amplifier, and pulse-height analyzer (see Figure 5-1). A pulse-height *spectrum* is a display showing number of events detected ("counts") versus the amplitude of those events. This is provided most conveniently by a multichannel analyzer (see Figure 5-9), but it also can be obtained with a single-channel

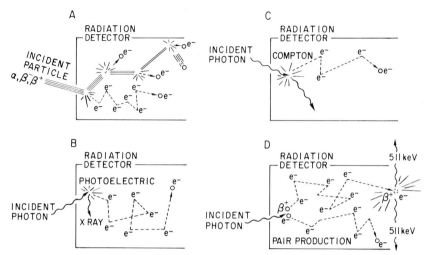

Fig. 11-1. Deposition of radiation energy in a radiation detector. (A) Energy transfer from an incident charged particle to electrons in multiple ionization events. Open circles, electrons generated in primary ionization events; other electrons are released in secondary ionization events. (B–D) Energy transfer from incident photon to electrons in (B) photoelectric, (C) Compton, and (D) pair-production interactions.

analyzer. For example, a 100-channel spectrum of a 0–10 V range of amplifier output signals could be recorded by using a 0.1 V window width and counting one channel at a time at 0.1 V increments from 0 to 10 V.

The spectrum recorded from a radiation source depends not only on the energy of the emissions from the source but also on the type of radiation detector used. It also depends on the mechanisms by which the radiation energy is deposited in the detector. It is important to remember that the amplitude of the signal from a proportional, scintillation, or semiconductor detector depends on the amount of radiation energy *deposited in the detector*, which may be *less* than the full energy of the detected particle of photon.

In the case of particle types of radiation (β particles, α particles, etc.), energy is transferred to the detector by collisions with atomic electrons in *primary ionization events*. These electrons may be given sufficient energy to cause *secondary ionizations* in collisions with other atomic electrons (Figure 11-1A). About 80 percent of the total ionization from particle-type radiation is the result of secondary ionization. The total amount of ionization produced (primary plus secondary) determines the amplitude of signal out of the detector (electrical current or light). Whether or not the full energy of the incident particle is deposited in the detector depends primarily on the range of the particle in the detector material. Particle ranges are very short in solids and liquids: thus the energy transfer is complete in most solid and liquid detectors (e.g., liquid scintillation detectors, Chapter 14, Section B), and the amplitude of signal from the detector is thus proportional to particle energy. In gas-filled detectors (e.g., proportional counters), however, or in very thin solid detectors (e.g., some semiconductor detectors) that do not have sufficient thickness to stop the particle, the energy transfer may be incomplete. In this case, the amplitude of the signal from the detector will not reflect the total energy of the incident particle.

In the case of photons (γ rays, x rays, bremsstrahlung), energy is transferred to the detector primarily in photoelectric, Compton, or pair-production interactions. A part of the incident photon energy is transferred as kinetic energy to photoelectrons, Compton electrons, or positive-negative electron pairs, respectively, which in turn transfer their kinetic energy to the detector in secondary ionization events (Figure 11-1B–D). Whether or not the amplitude of the signal out of the detector reflects the full energy of the incident photon depends on the fate of the remaining energy, which is converted into one or more *secondary photons* (characteristic x ray, Compton-scattered photon, or annihilation photons). A secondary photon may deposit its energy in the detector by additional interactions;† however, if it *escapes* from the detector, then the energy deposited in the detector and the amplitude of the signal from the detector do not reflect the full energy of the incident photon. The amplitude of the signal from the detector reflects only *the amount of energy deposited in it* by the radiation event.

B. SPECTROMETRY WITH NaI(Tl)

Because of its favorable performance/cost ratio, NaI(Tl) is the most commonly used detector in nuclear medicine. The basic principles of pulse-height spectrometry will be illustrated for this detector. Since NaI(Tl) is used almost exclusively for detecting photons (γ rays or x rays, primarily), only photon spectrometry will be considered here.

1. The Ideal Pulse-Height Spectrum

Suppose that a monoenergetic γ-ray source is placed in front of a radiation detector. Assume, further, that the energy of the γ rays, E_γ, is less than 1.02 MeV, so that pair-production interactions do not occur. The

---

† Note that multiple events involving a single radiation event occur so rapidly in the detector that they appear to be a single event.

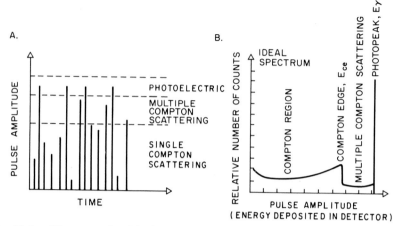

Fig. 11-2.   Elements of an ideal γ-ray pulse-height spectrum. (A) Pulses from the detector representing different types of γ-ray interactions in the detector. (B) Distribution (relative number) of pulses versus amplitude (or energy deposited in the detector). Only the photopeak represents deposition of the full energy of the γ ray in the detector.

principle γ-ray interactions with the detector will be by photoelectric absorption and Compton scattering. Most of the photoelectric interactions result in full deposition of the γ-ray energy in the detector (the characteristic x ray usually is also absorbed in the detector). Pulse amplitudes from these events are proportional to E_γ (Figure 11-2A). With an *ideal* radiation detector, this would produce a single narrow line in the pulse-height spectrum, called the *photopeak*, at a location corresponding to the γ-ray energy E_γ (Figure 11-2B).

In Compton scattering, only a part of the γ-ray energy is transferred to the detector, via the Compton recoil electron. If the scattered γ ray also is absorbed in the detector, the event produces a pulse in the photopeak. If the scattered γ ray escapes, the energy deposited in the detector is less than E_γ. The energy deposited in the detector in a single Compton scattering event ranges from near zero (small-angle scattering event) up to a maximum value E_{ce}, corresponding to the energy of the recoil electron for 180° Compton scattering events

$$E_{ce} = E_\gamma^2/(E_\gamma + 0.2555) \qquad (11\text{-}1)$$

where E_γ is in MeV. This equation is derived from Equation 9-7. The ideal spectrum therefore includes a distribution of pulse amplitudes ranging from nearly zero amplitude up to some maximum amplitude corresponding to the energy given by Equation 11-1 (Figure 11-2). This part of the spectrum is called the *Compton region*. The sharp edge in the spectrum at E_{ce} is called the *Compton edge*.

Another possibility is that a Compton-scattered γ ray may experience additional Compton-scattering interactions in the detector. Multiple Compton scattering events produce the distribution of pulses with amplitudes between the Compton edge and the photopeak.

2. The Actual Spectrum

In practice, the actual spectrum obtained with a NaI(Tl) spectrometer is quite different from the ideal one shown in Figure 11-2B. For example, Figure 11-3 shows a spectrum obtained from a ^{137}Cs radiation source, which emits 662 keV γ rays and ~30 keV barium x rays. The spectrum was recorded with a multichannel analyzer, 0.01 V per channel, with amplifier gain adjusted so that 662 keV of energy corresponds to 6.62 V of pulse amplitude. Thus the horizontal axis has been translated from pulse amplitude (0 –10 V) into energy (0 –1000 keV).

The first feature noted is that the spectrum is "smeared out." The

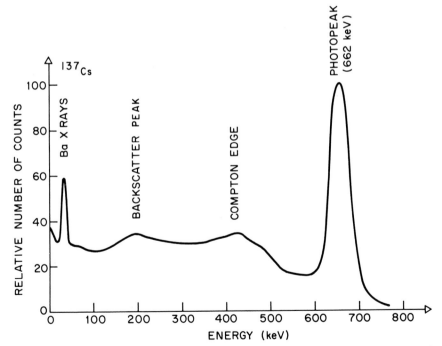

Fig. 11-3.   Actual pulse-height spectrum recorded with a NaI(Tl) detector and ^{137}Cs (662 keV γ rays, ~30 keV Ba x rays). Compare to Figure 11-2B.

photopeak is not a sharp line, as shown in Figure 11-2B, but a somewhat broadened peak, and the Compton edge is rounded. This is caused by the imperfect energy resolution of the NaI(Tl) detector, discussed in Section B.6.

Another structure that may appear in the spectrum is a *backscatter peak*. This is caused by detection of γ rays that have been scattered toward the detector after undergoing a 180° scattering outside the detector. Certain detector configurations enhance the intensity of the backscatter peak. For example, in the well counter (Chapter 13, Section A), a γ ray may pass through the detector without interaction, then scatter back into the detector from the shielding material surrounding it and be detected.

Note that the energy of the backscatter peak, E_b, is the energy of the *scattered γ ray* after 180° scattering, whereas the energy of the Compton edge, E_{ce}, is the energy given to the *recoil electron* in a 180° scattering event. Therefore

$$E_b + E_{ce} = E_\gamma \qquad (11\text{-}2)$$

Equation 11-2 is helpful for identifying backscatter peaks.

Another structure that may appear is an *iodine escape peak*. This results from photoelectric absorption interactions with iodine atoms in the NaI(Tl) crystal, followed by escape from the detector of the characteristic iodine K-x ray, which has energy of approximately 30 keV. The iodine escape peak occurs at an energy $E_\gamma - 30$ keV; that is, 30 keV below the photopeak. Iodine escape peaks may be prominent with low-energy γ-ray emitters, e.g., ^{197}Hg (Figure 11-4). Low-energy γ rays are detected by absorption primarily in a thin layer close to the entrance surface of the NaI(Tl) crystal where there is a reasonable probability that the iodine x ray will escape from the detector. With increasing γ-ray energy, the interactions tend to occur deeper within the detector, and there is less likelihood of x-ray escape. Also, the relative difference between the photopeak and escape peak energies becomes smaller, and it becomes more difficult to distinguish between them.

Lead x-ray peaks are seen frequently in systems employing lead shielding and collimation. This peak is caused by photoelectric interactions of the incident γ rays with lead atoms followed by emission of characteristic 80–90 keV lead x rays, which are then detected by the detector.

If the γ-ray energy exceeds 1.02 MeV, pair production interactions can occur. The kinetic energy given to the positive-negative electron pair is $E_\gamma - 1.02$ MeV (Chapter 9, Section A.3). When the positron comes to rest, it combines with an electron to create a pair of 511 keV annihilation

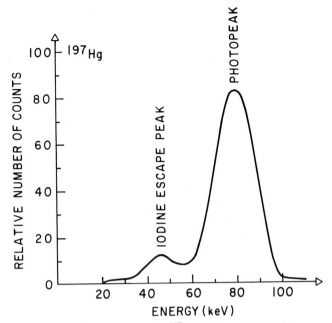

Fig. 11-4. Pulse-height spectrum for ^{197}Hg (E_γ = 77.3 keV) recorded with NaI(Tl). Iodine escape peak (45–50 keV) is due to escape of characteristic iodine x ray (~30 keV) following photoelectric absorption event in detector.

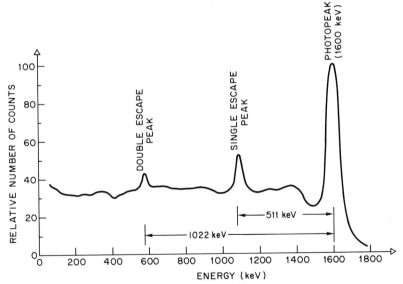

Fig. 11-5. Pulse-height spectrum for a hypothetical 1.6 MeV (1600 keV) γ-ray emitter. Because γ-ray energy exceeds 1.022 MeV, pair-production interactions can occur in the detector. Escape peaks are due to escape of one or both annihilation photons from the detector following a pair-production interaction.

photons. If both of these photons are absorbed in the detector, the event is recorded in the photopeak. If only one is absorbed, the event is recorded in the *single escape peak*, at energy $E_\gamma - 511$ keV (Figure 11-5). If both escape, the event is recorded in the *double escape peak*, at $E_\gamma - 1022$ keV.

Scattering within or around the radiation source, or *object scatter*, changes the distribution of radiation energies striking the detector. This is especially important in counting measurements in vivo and in radionuclide imaging because substantial scattering of radiation occurs within the patient. Figure 11-6 shows spectra for ^{131}I with and without scattering material around the source. The general effect of object scatter is to add events in the lower-energy region of the spectrum. It is possible to discriminate against scattered radiation by using a pulse-height analyzer to count only events in the photopeak, as shown in Figure 11-6.

Coincidence summing can occur when a radionuclide emits two or more γ rays per nuclear disintegration. Figure 11-7 shows spectra recorded with a NaI(Tl) well counter for ^{111}In, which emits a 173 keV and

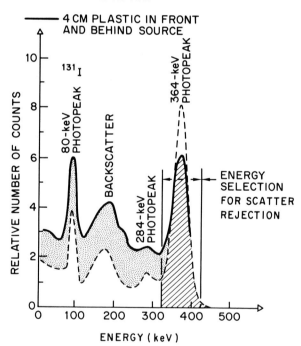

Fig. 11-6. Effect of scattering material around the source on the pulse-height spectrum for ^{131}I. Dot-shaded area, portion of spectrum due to scattered γ rays.

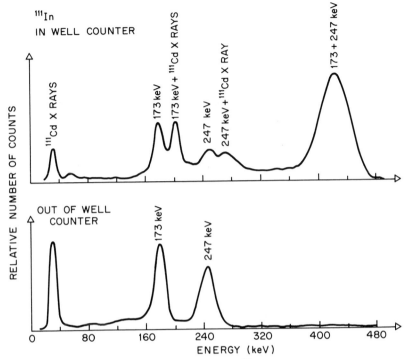

Fig. 11-7. Pulse-height spectra recorded for ^{111}In with a NaI(Tl) well counter detector. Top: Coincidence summing between the x-ray and γ-ray emissions results in additional peaks in the spectrum when the source is inside the well. Bottom: When the source is outside the well, the probability of coincidence detection decreases and the coincidence peaks disappear.

a 246 keV γ ray simultaneously. The peak at 419 keV seen when the source is inside the well counter results from simultaneous detection of these two γ rays. Summing between x rays and γ rays can also occur. With positron emitters, coincidence summing between the two 511 keV annihilation photons also may be observed. Coincidence summing is especially prominent with detector systems having a high geometric efficiency (Chapter 12, Section A.1), i.e., systems in which there is a high probability that both γ rays will be captured by the detector (e.g., well counters, Chapter 13, Section A).

3. General Effects of γ-Ray Energy

Figure 11-8 shows pulse-height spectra for a number of radionuclides emitting γ rays of different energies. The solid lines are the spectra for unscattered γ rays, and the dashed lines are the spectra for object-

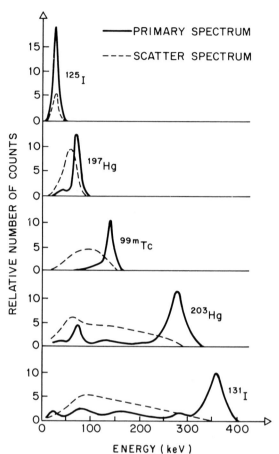

Fig. 11-8. Pulse-height spectra recorded with a NaI(Tl) detector for different γ-ray energies. Primary spectrum refers to γ rays striking the detector without scattering from objects outside the detector. Scatter spectrum refers to γ rays that have been scattered by objects outside the detector, e.g., from tissues or other materials surrounding the source distribution. [Adapted with permission from Eichling JO, Ter Pogossian MM, Rhoten ALJ: Analysis of scattered radiation encountered in lower energy diagnostic scanning, in Gottschalk A, Beck RN (eds.): Fundamentals of Scanning. Springfield, Illinois, Charles C Thomas, 1968, Fig. 19-2.]

scattered γ rays. In general, the relative number of events in the Compton versus the photopeak region becomes larger with increasing γ-ray energy because the probability of Compton versus photoelectric interactions becomes larger. Also, as γ-ray energy increases, it becomes easier to separate object scatter from the photopeak. This is because the change in γ-ray energy with Compton scattering increases with γ-ray energy (Chapter 9, Section A.2). For example, at 100 keV and at 500 keV, Compton scattering through 90° produces scattered photon energies of 84 keV and 253 keV, respectively.

4. Effects of Detector Size

The larger the detector crystal size, the more likely it is that secondary photons—i.e., Compton-scattered γ rays and annihilation photons—will be absorbed in the crystal. Thus with increasing crystal size, the number of events in the photopeak versus Compton regions increases. Figure 11-9 shows this effect on the spectrum for ^{137}Cs. For γ-ray energies greater than 1.02 MeV, the size of annihilation escape peaks also decreases with increasing crystal size.

5. Effects of Counting Rate

Distortions of the spectrum occur at high counting rates as a result of overlap of detector output pulses. Pulse pileup between two events can produce a single pulse with an amplitude equal to their sum (Chapter 5, Section B.3). Pileup between photopeak events and lower-energy events causes a general broadening of the photopeak (Figure 11-10). This is one of the causes of deadtime losses (Chapter 12, Section C). There also may be a shift of the photopeak toward lower energies because of baseline shift in the amplifier at high counting rates. Thus if a single-channel analyzer (SCA) is set up at low counting rates on the photopeak and the detector is used at very high counting rates, the photopeak can shift out of the SCA window and an incorrect reading may be recorded.

6. Energy Resolution

Sharp lines and sharp edges in the ideal spectrum (Figure 11-2B) become broadened lines and rounded edges in actual spectra (Figure 11-3). With NaI(Tl) detectors, this is caused by (1) random statistical variations in the number of scintillation light protons produced per keV of radiation energy deposited in the detector, (2) statistical variations in the number of light photons detected at the cathode of the PM tube, (3) nonuniform sensitivity to scintillation light over the area of the PM tube

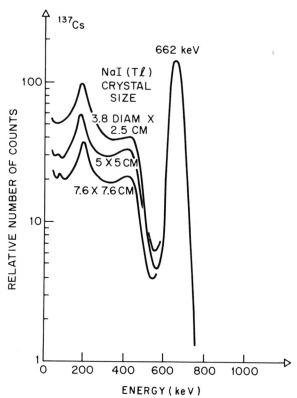

Fig. 11-9.   Effect of NaI(Tl) crystal size on the pulse-height spectrum for ^{137}Cs. The spectra have been normalized to equal photopeak heights. In practice, the photopeak height also increases somewhat with increasing detector size because of increasing detection efficiency (Chapter 12, Section A).

cathode, (4) statistical variations in the number of photoelectrons released from the photocathode, (5) statistical variations in the electron multiplication factor of the dynodes, (6) fluctuations in the high voltage applied to the PM tube, and (7) electrical noise in the PM tube.

Because of these factors, there are differences in amplitude of the signal from the detector for events in which precisely the same amount of radiation energy is deposited in the detector. With NaI(Tl) detectors, the principal source of variation is in the number of photoelectrons released from the photocathode. The average number is about three per keV of radiation energy absorbed in the NaI(Tl) crystal (Chapter 4, Section C).

Thus complete absorption of a 662 keV γ ray from ^{137}Cs results in the release of about 2000 photoelectrons from the photocathode *on the average;* however, the actual number varies from one γ ray to the next according to Poisson statistics, with a standard deviation of $\pm \sqrt{2000} \approx \pm 45$ photoelectrons, or about ± 2.3 percent (Chapter 6, Section B). Other factors mentioned above cause further variations in output pulse amplitude.

The photopeak is thus a Poisson- or Gaussian-shaped curve. The width of this curve, ΔE, measured across its points of half-maximum amplitude is the *energy resolution*. This is referred to as the full width at half maximum (FWHM). Usually the FWHM is expressed as a percentage of the photopeak energy E_γ:

$$\text{FWHM}(\%) = (\Delta E/E_\gamma) \times 100\% \qquad (11\text{-}3)$$

Figure 11-11 illustrates this computation for a ^{137}Cs spectrum.

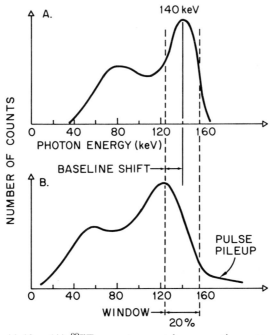

Fig. 11-10.   (A) ^{99m}Tc spectrum at low counting rate. (B) Spectral broadening and shift in apparent photopeak energy due to pulse pileup and baseline shift in the spectrometer amplifier at high counting rate.

Energy resolution becomes better [FWHM(%) becomes smaller] with increasing γ-ray energy because the number of photoelectrons released at the photocathode increases with increasing γ-ray energy, and thus the percentage statistical variation in their number decreases. Figure 11-12 shows FWHM(%) versus E_γ for a typical 5 cm × 5 cm NaI(Tl) detector.

The resolution of NaI(Tl) spectrometer systems usually is specified for the 662 keV γ rays of [137]Cs. With good quality PM tubes, energy resolution of 6.5–7 percent for ^{137}Cs is achievable. These detectors have energy resolutions of 11–13 percent for the 140 keV γ rays of [99m]Tc. With large-area crystals having multiple PM tubes (e.g., the Anger camera) the resolution for ^{99m}Tc may be 13–15 percent because of slightly different responses between PM tubes. Poor light coupling between the NaI(Tl) crystal and the PM tubes can cause a reduction in the number of photoelectrons released per keV and thus a degradation of energy resolution. This is a particular problem with multicrystal cameras (Chapter 17, Section C), which may have energy resolution values as poor as 40–50 percent for [99m]Tc. Energy resolution may be degraded by other conditions that interfere with the efficient collection of light from the crystal by the PM tube. For example, a cracked detector crystal causes internal reflections and trapping of light in the detector crystal. A sudden

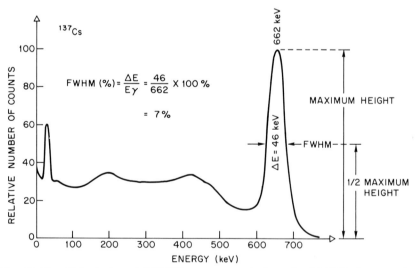

Fig. 11-11. Calculation of FWHM energy resolution of a NaI(Tl) detector for [137]Cs 662 keV γ rays.

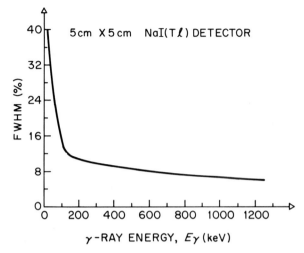

Fig. 11-12. Energy resolution [FWHM (%)] versus γ-ray energy for a 5 cm diam × 5 cm thick NaI(Tl) detector.

degradation of energy resolution and loss of output pulse amplitude are often the first symptoms of a cracked crystal. Deterioration of the optical coupling grease between the detector crystal and PM tube has similar effects.

Good energy resolution is a desirable characteristic for any spectrometer system because it permits precise identification and separation of γ rays with very similar energies, e.g., for radionuclide identification or scatter rejection. The best energy resolution is obtained with semiconductor detectors (Section C.3).

7. Energy Linearity

Energy linearity refers to the linearity of the relationship between output pulse amplitude and energy absorbed in the detector. Most NaI(Tl) systems are quite linear for energies between 0.1 and 2 MeV, and a single-source energy calibration usually is acceptable in this range; however, one can run into problems by calibrating a spectrometer with a high-energy source—e.g., ^{131}I or [137]Cs—and then attempting to use it for a much lower-energy source—e.g., [125]I (or vice versa). One or more low-energy sources should be used to calibrate a spectrometer for energies below about 100 keV.

C. SPECTROMETRY WITH OTHER DETECTORS

1. Liquid Scintillation Spectrometry

Whereas NaI(Tl) spectrometers are used in many different configurations and applications, both for in vivo and in vitro measurements, liquid scintillation (LS) spectrometers are used almost exclusively in a single configuration for in vitro sample counting (Chapter 14, Section B). Liquid scintillation detectors are used primarily for counting the low-energy β emissions from ^{3}H, ^{14}C, ^{35}S, ^{45}Ca, and ^{32}P.

Figure 11-13 shows pulse-height spectra recorded with a LS system for a γ-ray emitter, ^{137}Cs, and for a β emitter, ^{14}C. Liquid scintillators

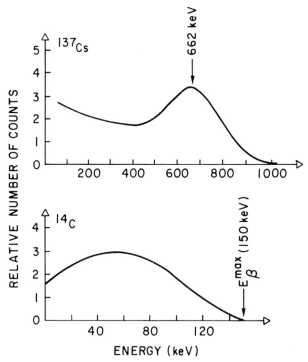

Fig. 11-13. Pulse-height spectra recorded with a liquid scintillation detector, for a γ-ray emitter, ^{137}Cs (top), and a β emitter, ^{14}C (bottom).

provide poor energy resolution for γ rays because they produce relatively few scintillation light photons per keV of energy absorbed and hence produce relatively few photoelectrons at the PM tube photocathode in comparison to NaI(Tl) (Section B.6). Another factor is the relatively poor optical coupling for transfer of light photons from the scintillator vial to the PM tubes. The spectrum for a β emitter has no sharp peak because the energy spectrum for β particles has a broad distribution from zero up to E_β^{max} for the radionuclide (compare Figure 11-13 with Figure 2-2).

2. Proportional Counter Spectrometers

Gas proportional counters (Chapter 4, Section A.3) have found limited use for spectrometry in nuclear medicine. Their energy resolution is four to ten times better than NaI(Tl), but considerably poorer than semiconductor detectors. Their major disadvantage is poor detection efficiency for γ rays (Chapter 12, Section A.2). Some applications of proportional counter spectrometry are discussed in Chapter 14, Section C.2.

3. Semiconductor Detector Spectrometers

The major advantage of semiconductor detectors (Chapter 4, Section B) is their superb energy resolution. It is typically 6–9 times better than proportional counters and 20–80 times better than NaI(Tl). Figure 11-14 shows comparative NaI(Tl) and Ge(Li) spectra for ^{99m}Tc. The superior energy resolution of Ge(Li) permits almost complete elimination of scattered radiation by pulse-height analysis and clean separation of multiple photon emissions from single or multiple sources.

The output signal from a semiconductor detector is a pulse of electrical current, the amplitude of which is proportional to the radiation energy deposited in the detector. The energy resolution of semiconductor detectors is determined by statistical variations in the number of charges in this pulse. The average number is about one charge (electron) per 3 eV of radiation energy absorbed, as compared to only three photoelectrons per keV in a NaI(Tl) detector system. The much larger number of charges produced in semiconductor detectors results in much smaller percentage statistical variations in signal amplitude and hence much better energy resolution than NaI(Tl).

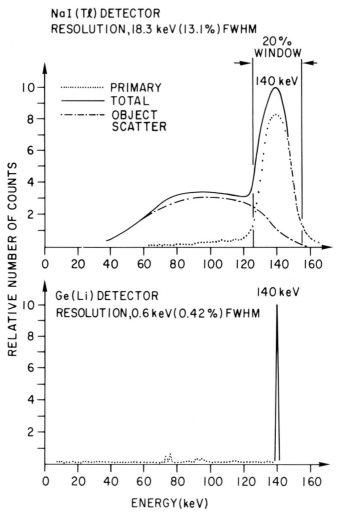

Fig. 11-14. Comparative pulse-height spectra recorded from a ^{99m}Tc source with NaI(Tl) and Ge(Li) detectors. In the NaI(Tl) spectra, primary refers to unscattered γ rays and object scatter to γ rays scattered by materials around the source. Separation of primary and object scatter spectra is much easier with the semiconductor detector.

REFERENCES

Additional discussion of NaI(Tl) pulse-height spectrometry may be found in the following:

Hine GJ: Sodium iodide scintillators, in Hine GJ (ed): *Instrumentation in Nuclear Physics in Nuclear Medicine*, vol 1. New York, Academic Press, 1967, chapter 6

Rollo FD: Detection and measurement of nuclear radiation, in Rollo FD (ed): *Nuclear Medicine Physics, Instrumentation and Agents*. St. Louis, CV Mosby Co., 1977, Chapter 5

Birks JB, *The Theory and Practice of Scintillation Counting*. New York, the MacMillan Co., 1964

Spectrometry with semiconductor detectors is discussed in:

TerPogossian MM, Phelps ME: Semiconductor detector systems. Semin Nucl Med 3:343–365, 1973

12
Problems in Radiation Detection and Measurement

Nuclear medicine studies are performed with a variety of types of radiation measurement instruments, depending on the kind of radiation source that is being measured and the type of information sought. For example, some instruments are designed for in vitro measurements, on blood samples, urine specimens, etc. Others are designed for in vivo measurements of radioactivity in patients (Chapters 13 and 14). Still others are used to obtain images of radioactive distributions in patients (Chapters 15–21).

All of these instruments have special design characteristics to optimize them for their specific tasks, as described in the chapters indicated above; however, some considerations of design characteristics and performance limitations are common to all of them. An important consideration in any radiation measurement instrument is its *detection efficiency*. Maximum detection efficiency is desirable because one thus obtains maximum information with a minimum amount of radioactivity. Also important are the instrument's *counting-rate limitations*. There are finite counting-rate limits for all counting and imaging instruments used in nuclear medicine, above which inaccurate results are obtained because of data losses and other data distortions. Nonpenetrating radiations, such as β particles, have special detection and measurement problems.

In this chapter, we discuss some of these general considerations in nuclear medicine instrumentation.

A. DETECTION EFFICIENCY

Detection efficiency refers to the efficiency with which a radiation-measuring instrument converts emissions from the radiation source into useful signals from the detector. Thus if a γ-ray emitting source of activity $A(\mu\text{Ci})$ emits η γ rays per disintegration, the emission rate ξ of that source is

$$\xi(\gamma \text{ rays/sec}) = 3.7 \times 10^4(\text{dis}/\mu\text{Ci}\cdot\text{sec}) \times A(\mu\text{Ci}) \times \eta(\gamma \text{ rays/dis}) \quad (12\text{-}1)$$

If the counting rate recorded from this source is R (counts/sec), then the detection efficiency D is for the measuring system is

$$D = R/\xi \quad (12\text{-}2)$$

or if the emission rate ξ and detection efficiency D are known, one can estimate the counting rate that will be recorded from the source from

$$R = D\xi \quad (12\text{-}3)$$

In general, it is desirable to have as large a detection efficiency as possible, so that a maximum counting rate can be obtained from a minimum amount of activity. Detection efficiency is affected by several factors, including

1. *Absorption and scatter* of radiation within the source itself, or by material between the source and the radiation detector. This is especially important for in vivo studies, in which the source activity generally is at some depth within the patient.
2. The *geometric efficiency*, or efficiency with which the detector intercepts radiation emitted from the source. This is determined mostly by detector size and distance from the source to the detector.
3. The *intrinsic efficiency* of the detector, which refers to the efficiency with which the detector absorbs incident radiation events and converts them into potentially usable detector output signals. This is primarily a function of detector thickness and composition and of the type and energy of the radiation to be detected.
4. The efficiency with which detector output signals are recorded by the counting system. This is an important factor in *energy-selective counting*, in which a pulse-height analyzer is used to select for counting only those detector output signals within a desired amplitude (energy) range.

In theory one therefore can describe detection efficiency D as a product of individual factors,

$$D = F \times g \times \varepsilon \times f \qquad (12\text{-}4)$$

where F is a factor for absorption and scattering occurring within the source or between the source and detector, g is the geometric efficiency of the detector, ε is its intrinsic efficiency, and f is the fraction of output signals from the detector that fall within the pulse-height analyzer window. Each of these factors will be considered in greater detail in this section. Most of the discussion will be related to the detection of γ rays with NaI(T1) detector systems. An additional factor with radionuclide imaging instruments is the collimator efficiency, that is, the efficiency with which the collimator transmits radiation to the detector. This is discussed in Chapter 16, Section B.

1. Geometric Efficiency

Radiation from a radioactive source is emitted *isotropically*, that is, with equal intensity in all directions. At a distance r from a point source of γ-ray emitting radioactivity, the emitted radiation passes through the surface of an imaginary sphere having a surface area $4\pi r^2$. Thus the flux I of radiation passing through the sphere per unit of surface area, in units of γ rays/sec/cm^2, is

$$I = \xi/4\pi r^2 \qquad (12\text{-}5)$$

where ξ is the emission rate of the source. As distance r increases, the flux of radiation decreases as $1/r^2$ (Figure 12-1). This behavior is known as the *inverse-square law*. It has important implications for detection efficiency and for radiation safety considerations (Chapter 23, Section C.2). The inverse-square law applies to all types of radioactive emissions.

A radiation detector of surface area a placed at a distance r from a point source of radiation and facing toward it will intercept a fraction $a/4\pi r^2$ of the emitted radiation. Thus its geometric efficiency g_p is

$$g_p = a/4\pi r^2 \qquad (12\text{-}6)$$

where the subscript p denotes a point source. Point-source geometric efficiency follows the inverse-square law.

Example 12-1.

Calculate the geometric efficiency of a $d = 7.5$ cm diameter detector at a distance of 20 cm from a point source.

Answer.

The area, *a*, of the detector is

$$a = \pi d^2/4 = \pi \, [(7.5)^2/4] \text{ cm}^2$$

Therefore from Equation 12-6

$$g_p = a/4\pi r^2$$
$$= \pi(7.5)^2/[4 \times 4\pi(20)^2]$$
$$= (7.5)^2/[16 \times (20)^2]$$
$$= 0.0088$$

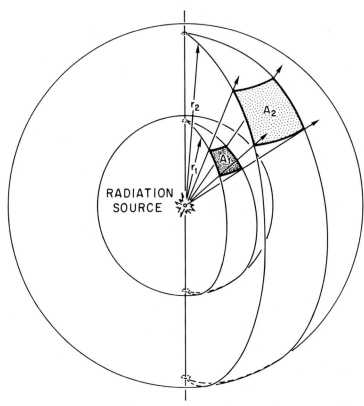

Fig. 12-1. Illustration of the inverse-square law. As the distance from the radiation source increases from r_1 to r_2, the radiations passing through A_1 are spread out over a larger area A_2. Because $A \propto r^2$, the intensity of radiation *per unit area* decreases as $1/r^2$.

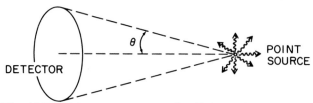

Fig. 12-2.   Point-source geometric efficiency for a circular large-area detector placed relatively close to the source depends on the angle subtended, θ (Equation 12-7).

Thus the detector described in Example 12-1 intercepts less than 1 percent of the emitted radiation and has a rather small geometric efficiency, in spite of its relatively large diameter. At 40 cm distance, the geometric efficiency is smaller by another factor of 4.

Equation 12-6 assumes that the distance from the point source to the detector is large in comparison to detector diameter. At close distances, the equation fails. For example, at $r = 0$, it predicts $g_p = \infty$. An equation that is applicable to close distances, or for circular area detectors having very large diameters, is

$$g_p = \tfrac{1}{2}(1 - \cos\theta) \tag{12-7}$$

where θ is the angle subtended between the center and edge of the detector from the source (Figure 12-2). For example, when the radiation source is in contact with the surface of the detector, $\theta = 90°$ and $g_p = \tfrac{1}{2}$ (Figure 12-3A). Geometric efficiency can be increased by making θ larger. For example, in a well counter (Chapter 13, Section A) the source is partially surrounded by the detector (Figure 12-3B) so that $\theta \approx 150°$ and $g_p \approx 0.93$. In liquid scintillation counting (Chapter 14, Section B), the

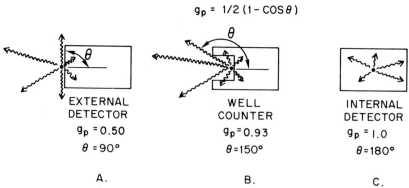

Fig. 12-3.   Examples of point-source geometric efficiencies for different source-detector geometries.

source is immersed in the detector material (scintillator fluid), so that $\theta = 180°$ and $g_p = 1$ (Figure 12-3C).

Equations 12-6 and 12-7 apply to point sources of radiation. They also can be applied to distributed sources of dimensions that are small in comparison to the source-to-detector distance; however, for larger sources (e.g., source diameter $\gtrsim 0.3r$) more complex forms, described in references 1–3, are required.

2. Intrinsic Efficiency

The fraction of radiation striking the detector that interacts with it is called the *intrinsic efficiency* ε of the detector:

$$\varepsilon = \frac{\text{No. of radiations interacting with detector}}{\text{No. of radiations striking the detector}} \quad (12\text{-}8)$$

Intrinsic efficiency ranges between 0 and 1 and depends on the type and energy of the radiation and on the attenuation coefficient and thickness of the detector. For γ-ray detectors, it is given by

$$\varepsilon = 1 - \exp[-\mu_l(E)x] \quad (12\text{-}9)$$

where $\mu_l(E)$ is the linear attenuation coefficient of the detector at the γ-ray energy of interest, E, and x is the detector thickness. In Equation 12-9 it is assumed that *any* interaction of the γ ray in the detector produces a *potentially* useful signal from the detector, although not necessarily all are recorded if energy-selective counting is used, as described in Section A.3.

Figure 9-7 shows the mass attenuation coefficient μ_m versus E for NaI(Tl). Values of μ_l for Equation 12-9 may be obtained by multiplication of μ_m by 3.67 g/cm^3, the density of NaI(Tl). Figure 12-4 shows intrinsic efficiency versus γ-ray energy for NaI(Tl) detectors of different thicknesses. For energies below about 100 keV, intrinsic efficiency is nearly unity for NaI(Tl) thicknesses greater than about 0.3 cm. For greater energies, crystal thickness effects become significant, but a 5 cm thick crystal provides $\varepsilon \approx 1$ over most of the energy range of interest in nuclear medicine.

The intrinsic efficiency of semiconductor detectors is also energy dependent. Because of its low atomic number, Si ($Z = 14$) is used primarily for low-energy γ and x rays (≤ 100 keV), whereas Ge ($Z = 32$) is preferred for higher energies. The effective atomic number of NaI(Tl) is about 49, which is greater than either Ge or Si; however, comparison to Ge is complicated by the fact that Ge has a greater density than NaI(Tl) ($\rho = 5.68$ versus 3.67 g/cm^3). The linear attenuation coefficient of NaI(Tl) is greater than that of Ge for E $\leq$ 250 keV, but at greater energies the

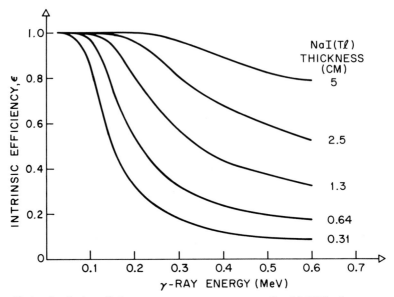

Fig. 12-4. Intrinsic efficiency versus γ-ray energy for NaI(Tl) detectors of different thicknesses.

reverse is true; however, differences in cost and available physical sizes favor NaI(Tl) over Ge or Si detectors for most applications.

Gas-filled detectors generally have reasonably good intrinsic efficiencies ($\varepsilon \approx 1$) for particle radiations (β or α) but not for γ and x rays. Linear attenuation coefficients for most gases are quite small because of their low densities (e.g., $\rho \sim 0.0013$ g/cm³ for air). In fact, most gas-filled detectors detect γ rays by the electrons they knock loose from the walls of the detector surrounding the gas volume rather than by direct interaction of γ and x rays with the gas. Intrinsic efficiencies for GM tubes, proportional counters, and ionization chambers for γ rays are typically 0.01 or less over most of the nuclear medicine energy range. Some special types of proportional counters, employing xenon gas at high pressures, achieve greater efficiencies, but they are still generally most useful for γ- and x-ray energies below about 100 keV.

3. Energy-Selective Counting

Intrinsic efficiency assumes that all γ rays that interact with the detector produce an output signal; however, not all output signals are counted if a pulse-height analyzer is used for energy-selective counting. For example, if counting is restricted to the photopeak, most of the γ rays interacting with the detector by Compton scattering are not counted.

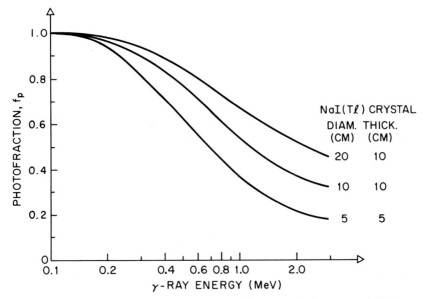

Fig. 12-5. Photofraction versus γ-ray energy for NaI(Tl) detectors of different sizes.

The fraction of detected γ rays that product output signals in the photopeak is called the *photofraction* f_p. The photofraction depends on the detector material and on the γ-ray energy, both of which affect the probability of photoelectric absorption by the detector. It depends also on crystal size (Figure 11-9) because with a larger volume detector there is a greater probability of a second interaction to absorb the scattered γ ray following a Compton scattering interaction in the detector (or of annihilation photons following pair production). Figure 12-5 shows the photofraction versus energy for NaI(Tl) detectors of different sizes.

If energy-selective counting is not used, then $f \approx 1$ is obtained. (Generally, some energy discrimination is used to reject very small amplitude noise pulses.) Full-spectrum counting provides the maximum possible counting rate and is used to advantage when a single radionuclide is counted, with little or no interference from scattered radiation. This applies, for example, to many in vitro measurements (Chapters 13 and 14).

4. Absorption and Scatter

When the radiation source is embedded at depth within an absorbing and scattering medium, (e.g., in vivo measurements) calculation of detection efficiency is complicated by corrections for absorption and scattering in the medium. Absorption generally decreases the recorded counting rate, but scattered radiation may decrease or increase the counting rate, depending on whether there is more scattering away from or toward the detector. For example, the counting rate for a source at a shallow depth in a scattering medium may be greater than for the same source in air because the added contribution from backscattering may more than compensate for a small reduction in counting rate by absorption. At greater depths absorption effects may predominate.

Calculations of absorption and scattering corrections are complicated because they depend on several factors, including the γ-ray energy, depth of the source in the absorbing and scattering medium, use of energy-selective counting, etc. Figure 12-6 shows the general effects versus γ-ray energy for a point source 7.5 cm deep in tissue-equivalent material and a NaI(Tl) counting system. The fraction of γ rays emitted from the source that reach the detector without experiencing absorption or scattering increases with γ-ray energy because absorption and scattering coefficients decrease with increasing energy. The fraction of γ rays *absorbed* in the tissue-equivalent material decreases with energy to a negligible fraction above about 100 keV.

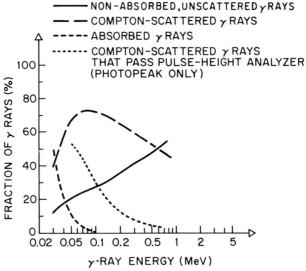

Fig. 12-6.   General effects of γ-ray energy on fraction of γ rays scattered or absorbed from a point source 7.5 cm deep in tissue and on the fraction of unscattered γ rays and scattered γ rays having sufficient energy to be recorded with a photopeak window and NaI(Tl) detector. [Reproduced with permission from: Anger HO: Radioisotope Cameras, in Instrumentation in Nuclear Medicine, Vol. 1, Hine GJ (ed.) New York, Academic Press, 1967, p. 514.]

The fraction of γ rays scattered first increases with γ-ray energy as absorption effects decrease, reaching a maximum at about 100 keV, after which it also decreases with increasing energy. If energy-selective counting is used, the fraction of Compton-scattered γ rays recorded in the photopeak decreases with increasing γ-ray energy. This reflects the increasing energy separation between scattered γ rays and the photopeak (Chapter 11, Section B.3). With semiconductor detectors (Ge or Si) this fraction is much smaller because of their ability to clearly resolve scattered γ rays from the photopeak (Figure 11-14).

5. Calibration Sources

Detection efficiencies can be determined experimentally using *calibration sources*. A calibration source is one for which the activity or emission rate is known accurately. This determination usually is made by the commercial supplier of the source. Various methods for determining absolute activity that may be applied to this determination are described in reference 4.

Detection efficiency can be determined by measuring the counting rate recorded from the calibration source and applying Equation 12-2. This method generally is satisfactory for systems in which a standard measuring configuration is used and for which the calibration source accurately simulates the shape and distribution of the sources usually measured with the system. For example, "rod standards" (Figure 12-7) are used for determining detection efficiencies of well counters for test tube samples.

Some γ-ray emitting source materials that are available as calibration standards are listed in Table 12-1. Most are quite long-lived. Detection efficiencies for short-lived radionuclides can be estimated from measurements made on a calibration standard having similar emission characteristics. For example, ^{57}Co (E_γ = 129 keV and 137 keV) is used frequently to simulate ^{99m}Tc (E_γ = 140 keV). (Cobalt-57 is sometimes called "mock ^{99m}Tc.") For most detection systems, intrinsic efficiencies at these two energies are virtually identical. Therefore the detection efficiency per emitted γ ray as calculated from Equation 12-2 would be the same for ^{99m}Tc and ^{57}Co (assuming the same energy-selective counting conditions were used, e.g., photopeak counting for both). If the detection efficiency is determined on the basis of cps/μCi, one must take into account the differing emission frequencies of the two radionuclides. Cobalt-57 emits 0.96 γ/dis, whereas ^{99m}Tc emits 0.88 γ/dis (Appendix B). Therefore the counting rate *per* μCi for ^{99m}Tc would be a factor of 0.88/0.96 = 0.92 smaller than that measured for ^{57}Co. This should be applied as a correction factor to the counting rate per μCi determined for ^{57}Co to obtain the counting rate per μCi for ^{99m}Tc.

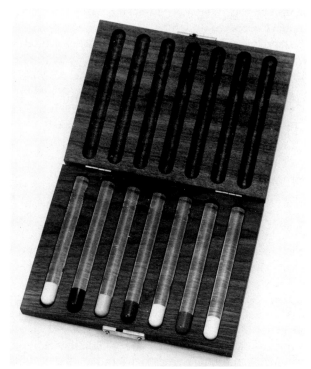

Fig. 12-7. "Rod standards" containing accurately known
quantities of different radionuclides used for determining the
detection efficiencies of well counters. The sources are
meant to simulate radioactivity in test tubes.

Calibration sources are used also in phantoms simulating the human
anatomy for estimating the detection efficiency for in vivo measurement
systems; the result is only as accurate, however, as the phantom and
source distribution are accurate for simulating human studies. For example, a 1 cm discrepancy between source depths in the phantom and in the
human subject may result in a 10–20 percent difference in counting rate
(Chapter 13, Section D).

B. PROBLEMS IN THE DETECTION AND
MEASUREMENT OF β PARTICLES

Because of their relatively short ranges in solid materials, β particles
create special detection and measurement problems. These problems are
especially severe with low-energy β-particle emitters, e.g., ^{3}H and ^{14}C.

Table 12-1
Properties of Some γ-Ray Sources Used
as Calibration Standards

Radionuclide	Half-Life	γ-Ray or X-Ray Energy (keV)†	Emission Frequency (γ rays/dis)
^{129}I	17.0×10^6 years	29.7 (K_α x ray)	0.58
		34.0 (K_β x ray)	0.13
		39.5	0.80
^{109}Cd	453 days	22.0 (K_α x ray)	0.85
		25.0 (K_β x ray)	0.16
		87.7	0.04
^{57}Co	270 days	14.4	0.10
		122.0	0.86
		136.3	0.10
^{113}Sn	115 days	24.1 (K_α x ray)	0.80
		27.5 (K_β x ray)	0.17
		391.7	0.62
^{85}Sr	65.1 days	514	0.99
^{137}Cs	30 years	32.0 (K_α x ray)	0.06
		37.0 (K_β x ray)	0.01
		661.6	0.85
^{54}Mn	312 days	834.8	1.00
^{60}Co	5.26 years	1173.2	1.00
		1332.4	1.00

† Only predominant photon emissions are listed.
Data adapted from ref. 5.

The preferred method for assay of these radionuclides is by liquid scintillation counting techniques (Chapter 4, Section C.4; Chapter 14, Section B); however, these techniques are not applicable in all situations, e.g., surveying a bench top with a survey meter to detect ^{14}C contamination (Chapter 23, Section E.1). A complete discussion of the problems arising in detection and assay of β-particle emitters is beyond the scope of this book; however, a few of the practical problems will be described briefly.

A survey meter may be used to detect surface contamination by β particle emitters provided it has an entrance window sufficiently thin to permit the β particles to enter the sensitive volume of the detector. Figure 12-8 shows relative counting rate versus entrance window thickness for two β-emitting radionuclides. Efficient detection of low-energy β emitters requires a very thin entrance window, preferably fabricated from a low-density material. A typical entrance window for a survey meter designed for ^{3}H and ^{14}C detection is 0.03 mm thick Mylar ($\sim$1.3 mg/cm^2 thick). Mica and beryllium also are used. Such thin windows are very fragile, and usually they are protected by an overlying wire screen. More energetic β particles—e.g., from ^{32}P—can be detected with much thicker and more rugged entrance windows; e.g., 0.2 mm thick aluminum ($\approx$50 mg/cm^2) provides about 50 percent detection efficiency for ^{32}P.

Geiger-Müller and proportional counters sometimes are used to assay the activities of β-emitting radionuclides in planchets or similar sample holders. Two serious problems arising in these measurements are *self-absorption* and *backscattering*, as illustrated in Figure 12-9. Self-absorption depends on the sample thickness and the β-particle energy. Figure 12-10 shows relative counting rate versus sample thickness for several β emitters. For ^{14}C and similar low-energy β emitters, self-absorption in a sample thickness of only a few mg/cm^2 is sufficient to cause a significant reduction of counting rate. (Note that for water, $\rho = 1$ g/cm^3, 1 mg/cm^2 is 0.001 cm thick.) Backscattering of β particles from the

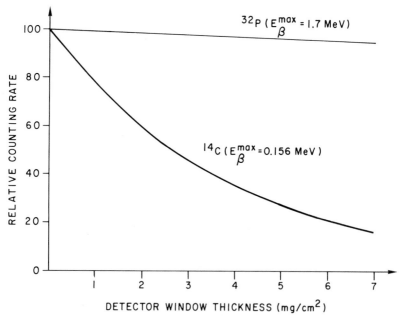

Fig. 12-8. Relative counting rate versus detector window thickness for some β-emitting radionuclides. [Adapted with permission from ref. 6: Quimby EH, Feitelberg S, Gross W: Radioactive Nuclides in Medicine and Biology. Philadelphia, Lea & Febiger, 1970, Chap 16.]

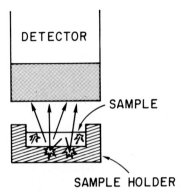

Fig. 12-9.   Self-absorption and backscattering in β-particle counting.

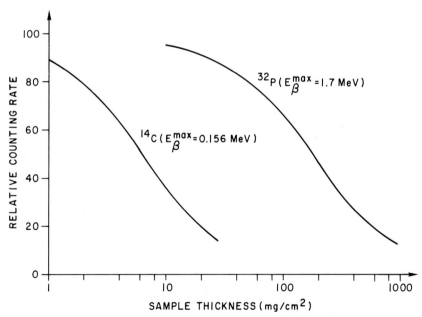

Fig. 12-10.   Effect of sample self-absorption on counting rate for some β emitters. [Adapted with permission from ref. 6: Quimby EH, Feitelberg S, Gross W: Radioactive Nuclides in Medicine and Biology. Philadelphia, Lea & Febiger, 1970, Chap 16.]

sample and sample holder tends to increase the sample counting rate and can amount to 20–30 percent of the total sample counting rate in some circumstances.

Accurate assay of β-emitting radioactive samples by external β-particle counting techniques requires very careful attention to sample preparation. If only relative counting rates are important, then it is necessary to have sample volumes and sample holders as nearly identical as possible. Other techniques for dealing with these difficult problems are discussed in reference 6.

It should also be noted that bremsstrahlung counting can be employed as an indirect method for detecting β particles using detectors that normally are sensitive only to more penetrating radiations such as x rays and γ rays, e.g., a sodium iodide well counter (Chapter 13, Section A). Bremsstrahlung counting also was employed in some early studies utilizing ^{32}P for the detection of brain tumors and still is used occasionally to map the distribution of intraperitoneal therapeutic infusions of ^{32}P-colloids administered for the control of ascites. Bremsstrahlung counting is effective only for relatively energetic β particles (e.g., ^{32}P, $E_\beta^{max} = 1.7$ MeV, but not ^{14}C, $E_\beta^{max} = 0.156$ MeV) and requires perhaps 1000 times greater activity than a γ-ray emitter because of the very low efficiency of bremsstrahlung production.

C. DEADTIME

1. Causes of Deadtime

Every radiation counting system exhibits a characteristic *deadtime* or *pulse resolving time* τ that is related to the time required to process individual detected events. The pulses produced by a radiation detector have a finite time duration (Table 5-1), so that if a second pulse occurs before the first has disappeared, the two pulses will overlap to form a single distorted pulse. With GM detectors, the overlap may occur in the detector itself, so that the second pulse does not produce a detectable output signal and is lost. With energy-sensitive detectors (scintillation, semiconductor, proportional counter), the overlap usually occurs in the pulse amplifier, causing baseline shift and pulse pileup (Chapter 5, Section B.3). Shifted or overlapped pulse amplitudes may fall outside the selected analyzer window, again resulting in a loss of valid events. Such losses are called *deadtime losses*. The shorter the deadtime, the smaller the deadtime losses. The deadtime for a GM tube is typically 50–200 μsec. Sodium iodide and semiconductor detector systems typically have deadtimes in the range 0.5–5 μsec. Gas proportional counters and liquid scintillation systems have deadtimes of 0.1–1 μsec.

Deadtime losses also occur in pulse-height analyzers, scalers, computer interfaces, and other components which process pulse signals. Generally scalers and single-channel analyzers have deadtimes of much less than 1 μsec, whereas multichannel analyzer and computer interface deadtimes are on the order of 10 μsec. Usually the deadtime is given for the counting system as whole; however, if one of the components has a deadtime that is long in comparison to the other components, then system deadtime is determined by that component.

2. Mathematical Models

Counting systems usually are classified as being of the paralyzable or nonparalyzable type. A *nonparalyzable system* is one for which, if an event occurs during the deadtime τ of a preceding event, then the second event is simply ignored, with no effect on subsequently occurring events (Figure 12-11). Scalers, pulse-height analyzers, and computer interfaces frequently behave as nonparalyzable systems. A *paralyzable system* is one for which each event introduces a deadtime τ whether or not that event actually was counted. Thus an event occurring during the deadtime of a preceding event would not be counted but still would introduce its own deadtime during which subsequent events could not be recorded. A paralyzable system may be thought of as one with an "extendable" deadtime. Most radiation detectors behave as paralyzable systems.

Because of deadtime losses, the *observed* counting rate R_o (cps) is less than the *true* counting rate R_t (cps), where the latter is the counting rate that would be recorded if $τ = 0$. The relationship between R_o, R_t, and τ depends on the type of deadtime. For nonparalyzable systems,

$$R_o = R_t/(1 + R_t τ) \qquad (12\text{-}10)$$

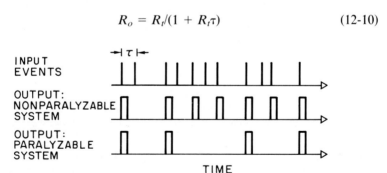

Fig. 12-11. Difference in output signals between nonparalyzable and paralyzable systems, both with deadtime τ. With a nonparalyzable system events are lost if they occur within a time τ of a preceding *recorded* event, whereas with a paralyzable system events are lost if they occur within a time τ of *any* preceding event, whether or not that event has been recorded.

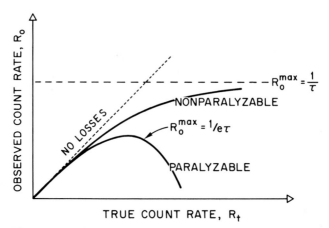

Fig. 12-12. Observed (R_o) versus true (R_t) counting rate
curves for paralyzable and nonparalyzable systems having
the same deadtime τ.

$$R_t = R_o/(1 - R_o\tau) \tag{12-11}$$

where τ is given in seconds. If the system has a paralyzable deadtime,
then

$$R_o = R_t e^{-R_t\tau} \tag{12-12}$$

There is no analytic equation for R_t as a function of R_o in the paralyzable
case.

Figure 12-12 shows R_o versus R_t for the two types of systems. The
nonparalyzable system increases asymptotically toward a maximum
value

$$R_o^{max} = 1/\tau \tag{12-13}$$

At very high true counting rates, greater than one count per deadtime
interval, the system simply records one event per deadtime interval,
ignoring all the others that occur during the deadtime interval between
counted events.

For a paralyzable system, the observed counting rate rises to a
maximum value given by

$$R_o^{max} = 1/e\tau \tag{12-14}$$

where e (= 2.718 . . .) is the base of natural logarithms. Then the
observed counting rate actually *decreases* with a further increase in true

counting rate. This is because additional events serve only to extend the already long deadtime intervals without contributing to additional events in the observed counting rate. At very high true counting rates, the observed counting rate actually approaches zero. This is called *counter paralysis*.

Deadtime losses are given by the difference between observed and true counting rates, $R_t - R_o$, and *percentage losses* are given by

$$\text{percentage losses} = [(R_t - R_o)/R_t] \times 100\% \qquad (12\text{-}15)$$

When the product $R_t\tau$ is "small" (≤ 0.1), the percentage losses are "small" (i.e., ≤ 10 percent), and they can be described by the same equation for both paralyzable and nonparalyzable systems:

$$\text{percentage losses} \approx (R_t\tau) \times 100\% \qquad (12\text{-}16)$$

Example 12-2.

Calculate the percentage losses for a counting system having a deadtime of 10 μsec at true counting rates of 10,000 and 100,000 cps.

Answer.

At 10,000 cps, $R_t\tau = 10^4$ cps $\times 10^{-5}$ sec $= 0.1$. Because the losses are "small," Equation 12-16 can be used:

$$\text{Percentage losses} \approx (0.1) \times 100\%$$

$$\approx 10\%$$

The observed counting rate would therefore be approximately 9000 cps; i.e., 10 percent less than the true counting rate of 10,000 cps. At 100,000 cps, $R_t\tau = 10^5$ cps $\times 10^{-5}$ sec $= 1.0$; thus the losses are not small. For a nonparalyzable system, the observed counting rate would be (Equation 12-10)

$$R_o = 100,000/(1 + 1.0) \text{ cps}$$

$$= 50,000 \text{ cps}$$

i.e., the losses would be 50 percent. For a paralyzable system (Equation 12-12)

$$R_o = 10^5 e^{-1.0} \text{ cps}$$

$$= 100,000 \times 0.368 \text{ cps}$$

$$= 36,800 \text{ cps}$$

The losses are therefore 100,000 − 36,800 cps = 63,200 cps, or 63.2 percent (of 100,000 cps).

Example 12-2 illustrates that for a given deadtime and true counting rate, the deadtime losses for a paralyzable system are greater than those of a nonparalyzable system. This is shown also by Figure 12-12.

3. Window Fraction Effects

It should be noted that with NaI(Tl) and other detectors used for energy-selective counting, any detected event can cause pileup with any other event in the pulse-height spectrum. Thus if a pulse-height analyzer is used, the number of events lost depends on the *total-spectrum counting rate*, not just on the counting rate within the selected analyzer window. With such systems, the apparent deadtime may appear to change with pulse-height analyzer window setting. For example, if a certain fraction of detected events are lost with a given window setting, the same *fraction* will be lost when the analyzer window is narrowed, making it appear that the deadtime *per event in the analyzer window* is longer when the narrower window is used. An approximate equation for apparent deadtime is[7]

$$\tau_a = \tau/w_f \qquad (12\text{-}17)$$

where τ is the actual deadtime per detected event and w_f is the *window fraction*, i.e., the fraction of detected events occurring within the selected analyzer window. For example, if a NaI(Tl) detector system has a deadtime of 1 μsec (amplifier pulse duration) but a narrow window is used so that only 25 percent of detected events are within the window (w_f), the apparent deadtime will be 1/0.25 = 4 μsec. Window fractions also change with the amount of scattered radiation recorded by the detector because this also changes the energy spectrum of events recorded by the detector. In general, increased amounts of scattered radiation decrease the window fraction recorded with a photopeak window (see Figure 11-6). The window fraction effect must be considered in specifying and comparing deadtime values for systems using pulse-height analysis for energy-selective counting.

4. Deadtime Correction Methods

Measurements made on systems with a standardized measuring configuration, with little or no variation in window fraction from one measurement to the next, can be corrected for deadtime losses using the mathematical models described in Section C.2. Some in vitro counting

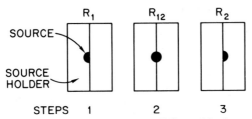

STEPS   1   2   3

Fig. 12-13.   Illustration of the steps followed in determining deadtime by the two-source method.

systems are in this category. Given an observed counting rate R_o and a deadtime τ, the true counting rate can be determined from Equation 12-11 if the system is nonparalyzable or by graphical or approximation methods (Equation 12-12, Figure 12-12) if it is paralyzable.

Deadtime τ can be determined using the *two-source method*. Two radioactive sources of similar activities, for which the deadtime losses are expected to be 10–20 percent, are needed (Figure 12-13). The counting rate for source 1 is determined, R_1 (cps). Without disturbing the position of source 1 (so as not to change the detection efficiency for source 1), source 2 is placed in position for counting and the counting rate for the two sources together is determined, R_{12} (cps). Then source 1 is removed (again, without disturbing source 2), and the counting rate for source 2 alone is determined, R_2 (cps). If the system is nonparalyzable, the deadtime τ_n in seconds is given by

$$\tau_n \approx (R_1 + R_2 - R_{12})/(R_{12}^2 - R_1^2 - R_2^2) \qquad (12\text{-}18)$$

If the system is paralyzable, then

$$\tau_p \approx [2R_{12}/(R_1 + R_2)^2]\ \mathrm{ln}[(R_1 + R_2)/R_{12}] \qquad (12\text{-}19)$$

If a short-lived radionuclide is used, decay corrections can be avoided by making the three measurements R_1, R_{12}, and R_2, separated by equal time intervals.†

Which of Equations 12-18 or 12-19 is to be used must be determined from additional measurements. For example, a graph of observed counting rate versus activity might be constructed to determine which of the two curves in Figure 12-12 describes the system.

For measurements in which the window fraction is variable (e.g.,

---

† Some texts recommend also that a background measurement be made; however, background counting rates generally are negligibly small in comparison to the counting rates used in these tests.

most in vivo measurements), the equations given in Section C.2 can be used only if the window fraction is known. Another approach is to use a fixed-rate pulser connected to the preamplifier of the radiation detector. The pulser injects pulses of fixed amplitude (usually larger than the photopeak pulses of interest) into the circuitry, and the counting rate for these events is monitored using a separate single-channel analyzer window (Figure 12-14). The fractional loss of pulser events is equal to the fractional loss of radiation events because both are subject to the same loss mechanisms. The observed counting rate R_o from the γ-ray source is corrected by the ratio of true to observed pulser counting rates, P_t/P_o, to obtain the true γ-ray counting rate,

$$R_t = R_o (P_t/P_o) \qquad (12\text{-}20)$$

Deadtime losses also affect counting statistics. For example, the standard deviation in observed counts, N_o, is not given by $\sqrt{N_o}$ if there are substantial deadtime losses. Detailed discussions of counting statistics with deadtime losses are given in references 8–10.

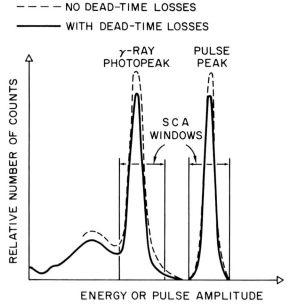

Fig. 12-14. Principles of deadtime correction using the fixed-rate pulser method. The fractional loss of events in the pulse peak (from the fixed-rate pulser) is assumed to equal the fractional losses of radiation events in the γ-ray photopeak window.

D. QUALITY ASSURANCE FOR RADIATION MEASUREMENT SYSTEMS

Radiation measurement systems are subject to various types of malfunctions that can lead to sudden or gradual changes in their performance characteristics. For example, electronic components and detectors can fail or experience a progressive deterioration of function, leading to changes in detection efficiency, increased background, etc.

To ensure consistently accurate results, *quality assurance* procedures should be employed on a regular basis for all radiation measurement systems. These would include (1) daily (or as often as the system is used) measurement of the system's response to a standard radiation source (e.g., a calibration "rod standard" for a well counter or a "check source" for a survey meter), (2) daily measurement of background levels, and (3) for systems with pulse-height analysis capabilities a periodic (e.g., monthly) measurement of system energy resolution. Additional tests may be devised to evaluate other important characteristics on specific measuring systems. The results should be recorded in a log book for analysis when problems are suspected. In some cases, it is helpful to plot the results on graph paper (e.g., counting rate for a standard source or for background), with tolerance limits (e.g., plus-minus two standard deviations, ± 2 SD) to detect subtle, progressive changes in performance.

Quality assurance procedures also are used for imaging systems as described in Chapter 18, Section E.

REFERENCES

1. Jaffey AH: Solid angle subtended by a circular aperture at point and spread sources: Formulas and some tables. Rev Sci Instrum 25(4):349–354, 1954
2. Maskitt AVH, Macklin RL, Schmitt HW: Tables of solid angles and activations. I. Solid angle subtended by a circular disc. II. Solid angle subtended by a cylinder. III. Activation of a cylinder by a point source. Oak Ridge, Tenn., Oak Ridge National Laboratory, U.S.A.E.C., ORNL-2170, Physics, 1956
3. Steyn JJ, Nargolivall SS: Detectors, in Kriegers J (ed): Instrumentation in Applied Nuclear Chemistry. New York, Plenum Press, 1973, pp 98–101
4. Orvis AL: Assay of radiopharmaceuticals, in Hine GJ, Sorenson JA (eds): Instrumentation in Nuclear Medicine (vol. 2). New York, Academic Press, 1974, Chap 13
5. Lederer CM, Hollander JM, Perlman I: Table of Isotopes. New York, John Wiley and Sons, 1967, pp. 562–563.
6. Quimby EH, Feitelberg S, Gross W: Radioactive Nuclides in Medicine and Biology. Philadelphia, Lea & Febiger, 1970, Chap 16

7. Wicks R, Blau M: The effects of window fraction on the deadtime of Anger cameras. J Nucl Med 18:732–735, 1977
8. Evans RD: The Atomic Nucleus. New York, McGraw-Hill, 1955, pp 785–793
9. Budinger TF: Quantitative nuclear medicine imaging: Application of computers to the gamma camera and whole body scanner, in Lawrence JH (ed): Recent Advances in Nuclear Medicine (vol 4). New York, Grune & Stratton, 1974, pp 41–129
10. Heiss WD, Prosenz P, Roszucky A: Technical considerations in the use of a gamma camera 1600-channel analyzer system for the measurement of regional cerebral blood flow. J. Nucl Med 13:534–543, 1972

13
Counting Systems—Part I

Radiation counting systems are used for a variety of purposes in nuclear medicine. *In vitro* (from Latin, meaning "in glass") *counting systems* are employed to measure radioactivity in tissue, blood, and urine samples, for radioimmunoassay and competitive protein binding assay of drugs, hormones, and other biologically active compounds, and for radionuclide identification, quality control, and radioactivity assays in radiopharmacy and radiochemistry. In vitro counting systems range from relatively simple, manually operated, single-sample, single-detector instruments to automated systems capable of processing 100–200 samples in a batch with computer processing of the resulting data.

In vivo (from Latin, meaning "in the living subject") *counting systems* are employed for measuring radioactivity in human subjects or experimentally in animals. Different in vivo systems are designed for measuring localized concentrations in single organs (e.g., thyroid, kidney) and for measurements of whole-body content of radioactivity.

Most nuclear medicine counting systems are comprised of the basic components shown in Figure 5-1: a detector and HV supply, preamplifier, amplifier, one or more single-channel analyzers or a multichannel analyzer ("data analysis"), and a scaler-timer, ratemeter, or other data readout device. Some of the more sophisticated systems may employ a computer or microprocessor capability for data analysis and readout.

At present, the most efficient and economical detector for counting γ-ray emissions† is NaI(Tl). The characteristics of various NaI(Tl)

---

† In this chapter the term γ-ray emission will also be meant to include other forms of electromagnetic radiation, e.g., x rays, bremsstrahlung, and annihilation radiation.

counting systems will be discussed in this chapter. A discussion of counting systems employing other types of detectors for γ-ray counting and for particle (β, α, etc.) counting is presented in Chapter 14.

A. NaI(Tl) WELL COUNTER

1. Detector Characteristics

The detector for a NaI(Tl) well counter is a single crystal of NaI(Tl) with a hole in one end of the crystal for the insertion of the sample (Figure 13-1A). Dimensions of the most commonly used well detectors are given in Table 13-1. The 4.5 cm diam × 5 cm long crystal with 1.6 cm diam × 3.8 cm deep well, the *standard well counter* detector, is the most frequently used in nuclear medicine. It is designed for counting of samples in standard-sized test tubes. Very large well counter detectors, up to 13 cm diam × 25 cm length, have been employed for counting very small quantities of high-energy γ-ray emitters (e.g., ^{40}K and ^{137}Cs). Most well counter systems employ 5 cm or greater thickness of lead around the detector, to reduce background counting levels (Figure 13-1B).

Light transfer between the NaI(Tl) crystal and the PM tube is less than optimal with well-type detectors because of reflecting and scattering

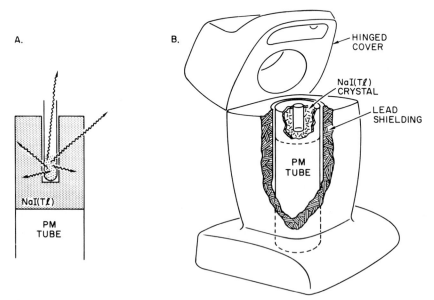

Fig. 13-1. (A) Cross-sectional view of a well counter detector containing a radioactive sample. (B) Well counter detector and shielding.

Table 13-1
Dimensions of Typical NaI(Tl) Well Counter Detectors

Crystal Dimensions (cm)		Well Dimensions (cm)	
Diameter	Length	Diameter	Depth
4.5†	5.0†	1.6†	3.8†
5.0	5.0	1.6	3.8
7.5	7.5	1.7	5.2
10.0	10.0	3.8	7.0
12.7	12.7	3.8	7.0

† "Standard" well counter detector.

of light by the well surface inside the detector crystal. Energy resolution is therefore poorer (10–15 percent FWHM for ^{137}Cs) than obtained with optimized NaI(Tl) detector designs (6.5–7 percent FWHM, Chapter 11, Section B.6).

2. Detection Efficiency

The detection efficiency D (Chapter 12, Section A) of the NaI(Tl) well counter for most γ-ray emitters is quite high, primarily because of their near 100 percent *geometric efficiency g*. The combination of high detection efficiency and low background counting levels makes the well counter very suitable for counting samples containing very small quantities (nCi–μCi) of γ-ray emitting activity. The geometric efficiency for small (≤ 1 ml) samples in the standard well counter is about 95 percent (Figure 12-3).

The *intrinsic efficiency* ε (Equation 12-8) of well-counter detectors depends on the γ-ray energy and on the thickness of NaI(Tl) surrounding the sample; however, the calculation of intrinsic efficiency is complicated because different thicknesses of detector are traversed by γ rays at different angles around the source. Calculated intrinsic efficiencies (i.e., all pulses counted) versus γ-ray energy for 1 ml sample volumes and for different NaI(Tl) well counter detectors are shown in Figure 13-2. Intrinsic efficiency is close to 100 percent for 1.3–4.5 cm wall thickness and $E_\gamma \leq 150$ keV, but at 500 keV the intrinsic efficiencies range from 39 to 82 percent.

Intrinsic efficiency can be used to calculate the counting rate per μCi for a radionuclide if all pulses from the detector are counted; however, if only photopeak events are recorded, then the *photofraction f_p* must also be considered (Chapter 12, Section A.3). The photofraction decreases

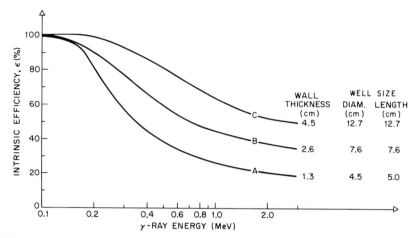

Fig. 13-2.   Intrinsic efficiency (γ-ray absorption efficiency, Equation 12-8) versus γ-ray energy for different NaI(Tl) well counter detectors.

with increasing γ-ray energy and increases with increasing well detector size (Figure 13-3). At 100 keV, $f_p \approx 100$ percent for all detector sizes. At 500 keV, f_p ranges from 48 to 83 percent from the smallest to the largest common detector sizes (Table 13-1).

The *intrinsic photopeak efficiency* ε_p is the product of the intrinsic efficiency and photofraction:

$$\varepsilon_p = \varepsilon f_p \tag{13-2}$$

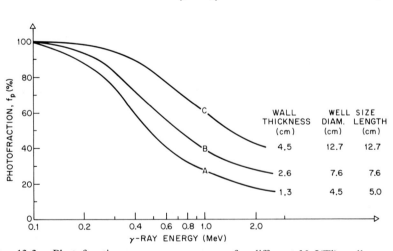

Fig. 13-3.   Photofraction versus γ-ray energy for different NaI(Tl) well counter detectors.

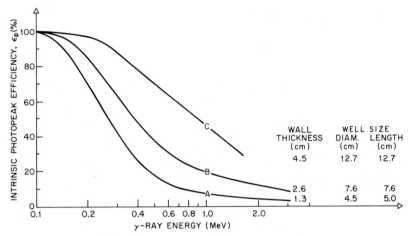

Fig. 13-4. Intrinsic photopeak efficiency versus γ-ray energy for different NaI(Tl) well counter detectors.

This may be used to estimate photopeak counting rates. Figure 13-4 shows ε_p versus γ-ray energy.

Table 13-2 lists some detection efficiencies, expressed as cpm/μCi, for full-spectrum counting of different radionuclides in the standard well counter. These values apply to 1 ml samples in standard-size test tubes.

3. Sample Volume Effects

The fraction of γ rays escaping through the hole at the end of the well depends on the position of the source in the well. The fraction is only about 5 percent near the bottom of the well but increases to 50 percent near the top and is even larger for sources outside the well (Figure 12-3). Thus the geometric efficiency of a well counter depends on sample positioning. If a small volume of radioactive solution of *constant activity* in a test tube is diluted progressively by adding water to it, the counting rate recorded from the sample in a standard well detector progressively decreases, even though total activity in the sample remains constant (Figure 13-5A). In essence, the geometric efficiency for the sample decreases as portions of the activity are displaced to the top of the well.

If the volume of a sample is increased by adding radioactive solution at a *constant* concentration, the counting rate first increases linearly with sample volume (or activity) but the proportionality is lost as the volume approaches and then exceeds the top of the well. Eventually there is very little change with increasing sample volume although the total activity is increasing (Figure 13-5B). For example, an increase of sample volume in

Table 13-2

Counting Efficiency for 1 ml Samples in a
Standard Sodium Iodide Well Counter
(Assuming All Pulses Counted)

Radioisotope	γ-Ray Energies (MeV) (Percent per Disintegration)	Counting Efficiency per Disintegration (%)	Counts per Minute per Microcurie
^{51}Cr	0.320 (8%)	4.3	95,500
^{60}Co	1.17 (100%), 1.33 (100%)	43	955,000
^{198}Au	0.411 (96.1%), 0.68 (1.1%), 1.09 (0.26%)	43.5	965.000
^{199}Au	0.051 (0.3%), 0.158 (41%), 0.209 (9%)	46	1,020,000
^{131}I	0.08 (2%), 0.28 (5%), 0.36 (80%), 0.64 (9%), 0.72 (3%)	48.3	1,070,000
^{59}Fe	0.19 (2.8%), 1.10 (57%), 1.29 (43%)	27.3	606,000
^{203}He	0.073 (17%), 0.279 (83%)	67	1,490,000
^{42}K	1.53 (18%)	4.0	89,000
^{22}Na	0.511 (200%), 1.28 (100%)	81	1,800,000
^{24}Na	1.37 (100%), 2.75 (100%)	38	844,000

Adapted with permission from ref. 1.

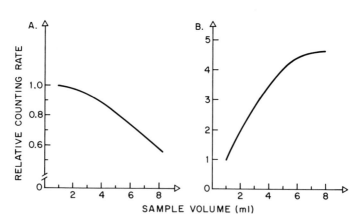

Fig. 13-5. (A) Change in counting rate in a standard NaI(Tl) well counter for a
sample of constant *activity* but diluted to increasing sample volume in a test tube.
(B) Change in counting rate with volume for constant *concentration*.

266

a standard-size test tube from 7 to 8 ml, a 14 percent increase in volume, increases the counting rate by only about 1 percent.

Thus sample volume has significant effects on counting rate with well counters. Sample volumes should be the same when comparing two samples. One technique that is used when adequate sample volumes are available is to fill the test tubes to capacity because with full test tubes small differences in total volume have only minor effects on counting rate (Figure 13-5B); however, this requires that identical test tubes be used for all samples, so that the volume of activity inside the well itself does not differ between samples.

Absorption of γ rays within the sample volume or by the walls of the test tube is not a major factor except when low-energy sources, such as ^{125}I (27–35 keV) are counted. Identical test tubes and carefully prepared samples of equal volume should be used when comparing samples of these radionuclides.

4. Assay of Absolute Activity

A standard NaI(Tl) well counter can be used for assay of absolute activity (μCi or μCi/ml) in samples of unknown activity using the calibration data given in Table 13-2. Alternatively, one can compare the counting rate of the unknown sample to that of a calibration source (Chapter 12, Section A.5). "Mock" sources containing long-lived radionuclides are used to simulate short-lived radionuclides—e.g., a mixture of ^{133}Ba (356 and 384 keV γ rays) and ^{137}Cs (662 keV γ rays) for "mock ^{131}I." Frequently, such standards are calibrated in terms of "equivalent activity" of the radionuclide they are meant to simulate. Thus if the activity of a "mock ^{131}I" standard is given as "A (μCi) of ^{131}I," then the activity of a sample of ^{131}I of unknown activity X would be obtained from

$$X(\mu\text{Ci}) = A(\mu\text{Ci}) \times [R(^{131}\text{I})/R(\text{mock }^{131}\text{I})] \qquad (13\text{-}2)$$

where $R(^{131}I)$ and $R(\text{mock }^{131}I)$ are the counting rates recorded in the well counter for the sample and the calibration standard, respectively.

Another commonly used mock standard is ^{57}Co (129 and 137 keV) for ^{99m}Tc (140 keV). If the ^{57}Co is calibrated in "equivalent μCi of ^{99m}Tc," then Equation 13-2 can be used for ^{99m}Tc calibrations also. If it is calibrated in μCi of ^{57}Co, however, one must correct for the differing emission frequencies between ^{57}Co and ^{99m}Tc (0.96 γ rays/dis versus 0.88 γ rays/dis, respectively). The activity X of a sample of ^{99m}Tc of unknown activity would then be given by

$$X(\mu\text{Ci}) = A(\mu\text{Ci}) \times [R(^{99m}\text{Tc})/R(^{57}\text{Co})] \times (0.96/0.88) \qquad (13\text{-}3)$$

where A is the calibrated activity of the ^{57}Co standard and $R(^{99m}$Tc) and $R(^{57}$Co) are the counting rates recorded from the ^{99m}Tc sample and the ^{57}Co standard, respectively.

5. Shielding and Background

It is desirable to keep counting rates from background radiation as low as possible with the well counter in order to minimize statistical uncertainties in counting measurements (Chapter 6, Section D.4). Sources of background include cosmic rays, natural radioactivity in the detector (e.g., ^{40}K) and surrounding shielding materials (e.g., radionuclides of Rn, Th, and U in lead), and other radiation sources in the room. Additional sources of background in a hospital environment are radiation therapy units, which, even though located some distance from the counter, can produce significant and variable sources of background. External sources of background radiation are minimized by surrounding the detector with lead (Figure 13-1B). The thickness of the lead is typically 2.5–7.5 cm; however, even with lead shielding it is still advisable to keep the counting area as free as possible of unnecessary radioactive samples.

In well counters with automatic multiple-sample changers it is important to determine if high-activity samples are producing significant backgrounds for low activity samples in the same counting rack. In many nuclear medicine procedures background counting rates are measured between samples, but if the background counting rate becomes large (e.g., from a radioactive spill or contamination of the detector) it can produce significant statistical errors even when properly subtracted from the sample counting rate.

6. Energy Calibration

For routine operation and calibration, it is desirable to adjust the amplification factor of the pulse amplifier system so the SCA dial settings can be read directly in keV. For example, the gain could be adjusted so that the ten-turn 1000-division dials commonly used on SCAs could be read as 1 keV per division (1 MeV full scale). A simple method to obtain this calibration is to insert a standard source, such as ^{137}Cs, in the well counter. The lower-level setting of the SCA is then set to 642 divisions and the window width to 40 divisions. [If the SCA has an upper-level discriminator (ULD) instead of a window adjustment, the ULD should be set at 682 keV.] The center of this setting at 662 divisions corresponds to the energy of the ^{137}Cs γ ray in keV. By adjusting the high voltage or amplifier settings until a maximum counting rate is observed, one will

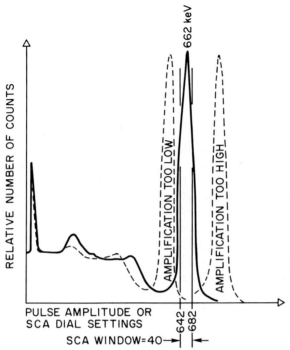

Fig. 13-6. Calibration of a pulse-height analyzer using ^{137}Cs. Amplifier gain is adjusted until a maximum counting rate is observed with the window setting from 642 to 682.

calibrate the dial readings in keV (1 keV per division), since the 662 keV γ ray will be centered at 662 divisions (Figure 13-6). This calibration procedure can be used also for in vivo detection systems.

The dials of the SCA can now be set to the γ ray energy of interest. For example, to count the 364 keV photopeak of ^{131}I, the lower level dial and window can be set to 324 and 80 divisions, respectively, corresponding to an energy window of 324–404 keV (~20 percent window centered on the photopeak). This calibration might not be accurate for energies below about 100 keV because of the nonlinear energy response of NaI(Tl) detectors. For example, if ^{125}I is to be counted the ^{137}Cs calibration should be used only as a rough approximation. The calibration procedure should be repeated using an actual ^{125}I or mock ^{125}I (^{129}I) source for accurate results.

Many commercial systems have pushbutton selection of the SCA window settings for different radionuclides. In these systems compensation has been made by the manufacturer for the nonlinear energy response of the NaI(Tl) detector; however, because of possible drifts in the electronics with time these settings should be checked periodically. Usually this is done by counting a long-lived standard source, such as ^{137}Cs, on a daily basis as a quality assurance check. If the counting rate varies for the standard source, the SCA calibration (or some other factor affecting detection efficiency) has changed.

7. Multiple Radionuclide Source Counting

When multiple radionuclides are counted simultaneously (e.g., from tracer studies with double labels) there is "crosstalk" interference because of overlap of the γ-ray spectra of the two sources, as shown in Figure 13-7 for ^{99m}Tc and [51]Cr. If SCA windows are positioned on the [99m]Tc (window 1) and [51]Cr (window 2) photopeaks, a correction for the interference can be applied as follows: A sample containing only ^{51}Cr is counted and the ratio R_{12} of counts in window 1 to counts in window 2 is determined. Similarly, a sample containing only ^{99m}Tc is counted and the ratio R_{21} of counts in window 2 to counts in window 1 is determined. Suppose then that a mixed sample containing unknown proportions of ^{99m}Tc and ^{51}Cr is counted, and that N_1 counts are recorded in the [99m]Tc

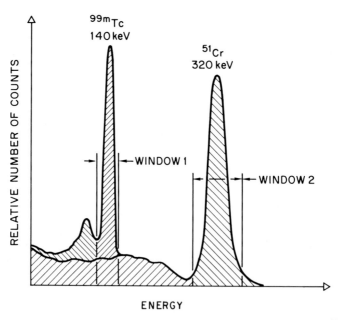

Fig. 13-7. Window settings used for simultaneous measurement of ^{99m}Tc and ^{51}Cr in a sample. Crosstalk from ^{51}Cr into the ^{99m}Tc window must be corrected for, using methods described in the text.

window (window 1) and that N_2 counts are recorded in the ^{51}Cr window 1 (window 2). Suppose further that room and instrument background counts are negligible or have been subtracted from N_1 and N_2. Then the number of counts from ^{99m}Tc in window 1 can be calculated from

$$N(^{99m}Tc) = (N_1 - R_{12}N_2)/(1 - R_{12}R_{21}) \qquad (13\text{-}4)$$

and the number of counts from ^{51}Cr in window 2 from

$$N(^{51}Cr) = (N_2 - R_{21}N_1)/(1 - R_{12}R_{21}) \qquad (13\text{-}5)$$

Equations 13-4 and 13-5 permit calculation of the number of counts that would be recorded in the photopeak window for each radionuclide in the absence of crosstalk interference from the other radionuclide. The equations can be used for other combinations of radionuclides and window settings with appropriate changes in symbols. For greatest accuracy, the ratios R_{12} and R_{21} should be determined to a high degree of statistical accuracy (e.g., ±1 percent) so that they do not add significantly to the uncertainties in the calculated results. The technique is most accurate when crosstalk is small, i.e., R_{12} and/or $R_{21} \ll 1$. Generally, the technique is *not* reliable for in vivo measurements because of varying amounts of crosstalk due to Compton scattering within body tissue.

Example 13-1.
    A mixed sample containing ^{99m}Tc and ^{51}Cr provides 18000 counts in the ^{99m}Tc window and 8000 counts in the ^{51}Cr window. A sample containing ^{51}Cr alone gives 25000 counts in the ^{51}Cr window and 15000 crosstalk counts in the ^{99m}Tc window whereas a sample containing ^{99m}Tc alone gives 20000 counts in the ^{99m}Tc window and 1000 crosstalk counts in the ^{51}Cr window. What are the counts due to each radionuclide in their respective photopeak windows? Assume that background counts are negligible.
Answer.
    The crosstalk interference factors are, for ^{51}Cr crosstalk in the ^{99m}Tc window

$$R_{12} = 15000/25000 = 0.6$$

and for ^{99m}Tc crosstalk in the ^{51}C window

$$R_{21} = 1000/20000 = 0.05$$

Therefore, the counts in the ^{99m}Tc window from ^{99m}Tc are (Equation 13-4)

$$N_1(^{99m}Tc) = (18000 - 0.6 \times 8000)/(1 - 0.6 \times 0.05)$$

$$= 13200/0.97$$

$$\approx 13608 \text{ counts}$$

and the counts in the ^{51}Cr window from ^{51}Cr are (Equation 13-5)

$$N_2(^{51}Cr) = (8000 - 0.05 \times 18000)/(1 - 0.6 \times 0.05)$$

$$= 7100/0.97$$

$$\approx 7320 \text{ counts}$$

---

8. Deadtime

Because NaI(Tl) well counters have such high detection efficiency, only small amounts of activity can be counted (typically fractions of a μCi). If higher levels of activity are employed, serious deadtime problems can be encountered (Chapter 12, Section C). For example, if the deadtime for the system is 4 μsec and 1 μCi of activity emitting one γ ray per disintegration is counted with 100 percent detection efficiency, then the true counting rate is 37,000 cps; however, the recorded counting rate would be about 32,000 cps because of 15 percent deadtime losses (Equation 12-12).

9. Automatic Multiple-Sample Systems

Samples with high counting rates require short counting times and provide good statistical accuracy with little interference from normal background radiation. If only a few samples must be counted, they can be counted quickly and conveniently using manual techniques; however, with long counting times and/or large numbers of samples, the counting procedures become time-consuming and cumbersome. Systems with automatic sample changers have been developed to alleviate this problem (Figure 13-8). Typically, these systems can accommodate 100 or more samples.

Systems with automatic sample changers not only save time but also allow samples to be counted repeatedly to detect variations caused by malfunction of the detector or electronic equipment or changes in background counting rates. Background counting rates can be recorded automatically by alternating sample and blank counting vials. In these systems, counting vials loaded into a tray or carriage are selected automatically and placed sequentially in the NaI(Tl) well counter. Mea-

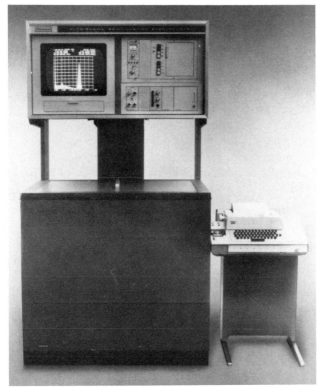

Fig. 13-8. A modern NaI(Tl) well counter with automatic
sample-changing capabilities. This system also incorporates
a multi-channel analyzer for spectral analysis. [Courtesy,
Packard Instrument Company, Inc.]

surements are taken for a preset time or a preset number of counts
selected by the user. The well counter is shielded usually with 5–7.5 cm
of lead, with a small hole in the lead shielding over the detector for
insertion of the sample. One disadvantage of automatic systems is that
there is no lead shielding directly over the top of the sample being
counted. Therefore the system is not as well shielded as a manual well
counter (Figure 13-1B), which can cause an increase in background
counting rates, particularly from the other samples in the carriage. This
can be a problem when low-activity samples are counted with high-
activity samples in the carriage.

Commercial systems usually have one to three SCAs, although some
systems incorporate MCAs to allow the selection of many different
counting windows. The MCA also can be used to display the entire
spectrum recorded by the NaI(Tl) detector on a CRT display scope. The

displayed spectrum allows the user to inspect visually and select the positions of the single-channel windows for counting and to examine crosstalk interference when multiple radionuclides are counted simultaneously. It is also very useful for quickly and reliably checking to see if there are any significant photopeaks in the spectrum from background sources, which could indicate a radioactive spill or contamination, or for checking the general condition of the NaI(Tl) detector.

Many modern well counter systems are interfaced to minicomputers or have electronic circuits that can perform programmed operations of background subtraction, radioactive decay corrections, a variety of arithmetic operations, statistical analysis, calculation of parameters for radioimmunoassay, etc. Data from these systems are displayed with printers, scalers, and other visual display devices.

10. Applications

NaI(Tl) well counters are used almost exclusively to count x- or γ-ray emitting radionuclides. Radionuclides with β emissions can be counted by detecting bremsstrahlung radiation, but the counting rate per μCi is small because efficiency of bremsstrahlung production is very small. Well counters are used primarily for radioimmunoassays (e.g., T_3 and T_4 tests), assay of radioactivity in blood and urine samples, radiochemical assays, and radiopharmaceutical quality control. Systems with multiple SCAs or MCAs allow multiple radionuclide sources to be counted simultaneously. These capabilities combined with automatic sampling changing and automatic data processing make the NaI(Tl) well counter a major tool for nuclear medicine in vitro assays.

B. COUNTING WITH CONVENTIONAL NaI(Tl) DETECTORS

The principle restriction on the use of most NaI(Tl) well counters is that they are useful only for small sample volumes (a few ml, typically) and small amounts of activity (≤ 1 μCi). For activities greater than about 1 μCi of most radionuclides the counting rate becomes so high that deadtime losses may become excessive. Large sample volumes and larger amounts of activity can be counted using a conventional NaI(Tl) detector with the sample at some distance from the detector. Placing the sample at a distance from the detector decreases the geometric efficiency (see Example 12-1) and allows higher levels of activity to be counted than with the well detector. The sample-to-detector distance can be adjusted to accommodate the level of activity to be measured. Typically, shielding from background sources with these arrangements is not as good as with the well counter because the front of the detector is exposed; however, owing to the high-counting-rate applications of these systems, background counting rates usually are not significant unless there are other high-activity samples in the immediate vicinity.

The detection efficiency of a conventional detector depends upon a number of factors, such as detector-to-sample distance, detector diameter, and sample size (Chapter 12, Section A). If the sample-to-detector distance is large compared to the sample diameter, then usually the counting efficiency is relatively constant as the sample size is increased; however, this can not always be assumed to be true and sample size effects should be evaluated experimentally for specific counting conditions to be employed.

C. LIQUID AND GAS-FLOW COUNTING

NaI(Tl) detectors are used frequently as γ-ray monitors in conjunction with gas or liquid chromatographs. Chromatographs are used to separate and identify different chemical compounds by selective retention or movement of chemical species in certain media. By comparing the flow of radioactivity with the flow of chemical species, one can determine the radiochemical identity of different radioactive species (Figure 13-9). The SCA typically is used to count only the photopeak to reduce background due to scattered radiation from activity in the flow line outside the

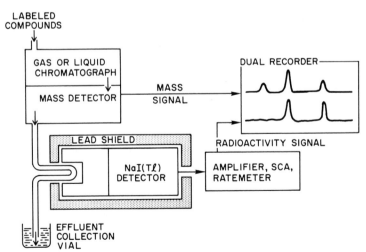

Fig. 13-9. NaI(Tl) detector system used in conjunction with a gas or liquid chromatograph. The "mass detector" is used to detect chemical species and the radiation detector the radioactivity associated with these species for radiochemical identification.

detector and in the chromatograph. MCAs or multiple SCAs also can be employed to detect multiple radionuclides simultaneously.

With simple systems the data output from the SCA is recorded with a ratemeter (digital or analog) and plotted on a strip-chart recorder. With more sophisticated systems the data are collected with small computers that have extended capability for data analysis.

D. IN VIVO COUNTING SYSTEMS

In vivo counting systems are used to measure radioactive concentrations in patients and, occasionally, in experimental animals. Systems designed to monitor radioactivity in single organs or in localized parts of the body are called *probe systems*. For example, *single-probe* systems, employing only one detector, are used for measuring thyroidal uptake of radioactive iodine and for obtaining cardiac output curves. *Multiprobe* systems are used for renal function studies, for lung clearance studies, for obtaining washout curves from the brain, etc. In general, probe systems provide some degree of measurement localization but without the detail of imaging techniques (Chapters 15–21).

The simplest probe system consists of a collimated NaI(Tl) detector mounted on a stationary or mobile stand that can be oriented and positioned over an area of interest on the patient (Figure 13-10). The detector is connected to the usual NaI(Tl) electronics, including a SCA for energy selection and a scaler-timer and/or ratemeter-chart recorder for data readout. A typical probe system employs a 5 cm diam × 5 cm thick NaI(Tl) crystal, with a cylindrical or conically shaped collimator, 15–25 cm long, in front of the detector. More complex systems may employ more detectors, possibly arranged in banks, with more complex data processing and readout devices (e.g., computers).

When calibrating a probe system for in vivo measurements, it is important to remember the effects of attenuation and scatter on the recorded counting rate (Chapter 12, Section A.4). Usually, the depth of the source distribution within the patient is not known accurately. Since the linear attenuation coefficient for soft tissue is in the range $\mu_l = 0.1$–0.2 cm^{-1} for most γ-ray energies in nuclear medicine, a 1–2 cm difference in source depth can result in a 10–40 percent difference in recorded counting rate. The intensity of scattered radiation is another important variable. For example, a source lying outside the direct field of view of the collimator can contribute to the recorded counting rate by Compton scattering in the tissues surrounding the source distribution. To minimize the contribution from scattered radiation, measurements usually are made with the SCA window set on the photopeak of the γ-ray emission to be

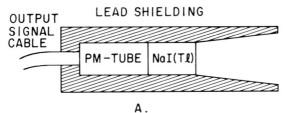

Fig. 13-10. (A) Schematic representation of a NaI(Tl) probe system with collimator.

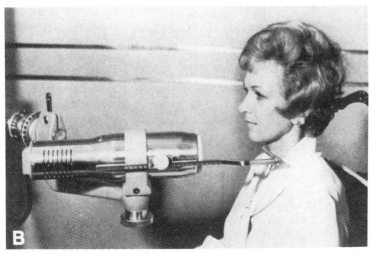

Fig. 13-10. (B) Typical probe system for measuring thyroid uptake. [From ref. 2: Hine GJ, Williams JB: Thyroid radioiodine uptake measurements, in Hine GJ (ed): Instrumentation in Nuclear Medicine (vol 1). New York, Academic Press, 1967, p. 345. With permission.]

counted. Even this is not completely effective for eliminating all of the variable effects of scattered radiation on the measurement, however, especially when low-energy γ rays are counted (see Figures 11-6 and 11-8).

Another class of in vivo measurement systems are *whole-body counters*, which are designed to measure the total amount of radioactivity in the body, with no attempt at localization of the activity distribution. Many (but not all) of these systems employ NaI(Tl) detectors. They are used for studying retention, turnover, and clearance rates with such nuclides as ^{60}Co and ^{57}Co (labeled vitamin B$_{12}$), ^{24}Na, ^{42}K, ^{47}Ca, and ^{59}Fe. Most of these radionuclides emit high-energy γ rays, and several have quite long half-lives. Thus it is important that a whole-body counter have

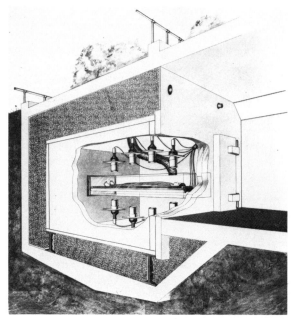

Fig. 13-11. Cross-section through Oak Ridge whole-body counter. From the outside in, shielding consists of earth, concrete, dunite (a natural rock), steel, and lead. [From ref. 3: Sorenson JA: Quantitative measurement of radioactivity in vivo by whole-body counting, in Hine GJ, Sorenson JA (eds): Instrumentation in Nuclear Medicine (vol 2). New York, Academic Press, 1974, p. 338. With permission.]

good detection efficiency, so that very small amounts of activity ($\leqslant 1$ μCi) can be detected and measured accurately. Another application for whole-body counting is the measurement of naturally occurring ^{40}K, which can be used to estimate total body potassium content. This is another high-energy γ emitter present in very small quantities, requiring good detection efficiency for accurate measurement.

Most whole-body counters employ relatively large NaI(Tl) detectors, 15–30 cm diam × 5–10 cm thick to obtain good geometric efficiency as well as good intrinsic efficiency for high-energy γ rays. Several such detectors may be employed. Also the "counting chamber" is well-shielded with lead, concrete, steel, and other materials to obtain minimal background levels, thus ensuring minimum statistical error due to background counting rates (Chapter 6, Section D.4). Shielding materials are selected carefully for minimum contamination with background radioactivity.

Figure 13-11 shows a cutaway view of the Oak Ridge whole-body counter. This system uses multiple detectors positioned above and below the patient support table. Other arrangements of detectors above and below the patient also have been used for whole-body counting. The Anger camera with pinhole collimator (Chapter 15) has been employed as a whole-body counter for monitoring therapeutic levels of ^{131}I.

REFERENCES

1. Hine GJ: γ-Ray sample counting, in Hine GJ (ed): Instrumentation in Nuclear Medicine (vol 1). New York, Academic Press, 1967, Chap 12 (gives a detailed discussion of NaI(Tl) well counters)
2. Hine GJ, Williams JB: Thyroid radioiodine uptake measurements, in Hine GJ (ed): Instrumentation in Nuclear Medicine (vol 1). New York, Academic Press, 1967, chap 14 (discusses systems for thyroid uptake measurements)
3. Sorenson JA: Quantitative measurement of radioactivity in vivo by whole-body counting, in Hine GJ, Sorenson JA (eds): Instrumentation in Nuclear Medicine (vol 2). New York, Academic Press, 1974, Chap 9 (discusses whole-body counters)

14

Counting Systems—Part II

Although NaI(Tl) systems are suitable for many applications in nuclear medicine, there are some applications that require other detector systems. For example, studies requiring especially good energy resolution may be performed using semiconductor detectors. Liquid scintillation counters are used for counting β emitters, such as ^{3}H and ^{14}C, and emitters of low-energy x and γ rays, which cannot be detected efficiently with NaI(Tl) or semiconductor detectors because of the thickness of canning material required around the detector. Gas-filled detectors also are used for particle detection and for applications not requiring the relatively high intrinsic detection efficiency or energy discrimination capabilities of NaI(Tl) or other more sophisticated detector systems, e.g., for dose calibrators.

Some characteristics of these systems will be described in this chapter. Survey meters, another instrument category employing gas-filled detectors, are discussed in Chapter 23, Section E.1.

A. SEMICONDUCTOR DETECTOR SYSTEMS

1. System Components

Semiconductor detectors (Ge and Si; Chapter 4, Section B) created revolutionary advances in nuclear physics, nuclear chemistry, radiation chemistry, nondestructive materials analysis (e.g., x-ray fluorescence and neutron activation), and other fields. To date, however, they have not had a major impact on nuclear medicine. Their disadvantages of small size and high cost outweigh their advantage of superior energy resolution in comparison to other detection systems—e.g., NaI(Tl)—for general-purpose applications; however, the energy resolution of semiconductor detectors allows the separation of γ rays differing in energy by only a few keV as opposed to 20–80 keV with NaI(Tl) (Figure 14-1; see also Figure 11-14). Therefore in applications where energy resolution is the critical factor and the relatively small size of the semiconductor detector is not completely restrictive, Ge or Si detectors are the system of choice.

Semiconductor detectors are used extensively as charged particle and γ-ray spectrometers in physics. Fluorescence scanning (Chapter 17, Section D) and radionuclide purity evaluation are their principle applications in nuclear medicine. Silicon has a lower atomic number and density than Ge and therefore a lower intrinsic detection efficiency for γ rays with energies ≥ 40 keV (Chapter 12, Section A.2). Thus Si detectors are used primarily for detection of low-energy x rays and Ge for γ rays.

The basic configuration of a semiconductor system for in vitro analysis is shown in Figure 4-13. Except for a special low-noise high-voltage supply, preamplifier, and amplifier, the system components are the same as those of NaI(Tl) counting systems. Usually a multichannel analyzer (MCA) is employed rather than a SCA with semiconductor detectors because often the detectors are used to resolve complex spectra of multiple emissions and multiple radionuclides (Figure 14-1).

The superior energy resolution of semiconductor detectors may result in a significant advantage in sensitivity (i.e., minimum detectable activity, MDA; Chapter 6, Sections D.4 and D.5) in comparison to NaI(Tl) detectors for some applications. Minimum detectable activity depends on the ratio $S/\sqrt{B}$, where S is the net sample counting rate and B is the background counting rate. Because the energy resolution of a semiconductor detector is 20–80 times better than NaI(Tl), a photopeak window 20–80 times narrower can be used, resulting in typically 20–80 times smaller background counting rate. Considering background alone, then, the MDA for a semiconductor detector could be a factor $\sqrt{20}$ to $\sqrt{80}$ smaller than a NaI(Tl) detector of comparable size. This advantage is partially offset by the larger available detector sizes with NaI(Tl), and, above about 200 keV, by the greater intrinsic photopeak efficiency of NaI(Tl) for comparable detector thicknesses (Chapter 12, Section A.2); however, for lower-energy γ rays, measured in a configuration having a high geometric efficiency (e.g., sample placed directly against the detector), there is usually an advantage in MDA favoring the semiconductor detector.

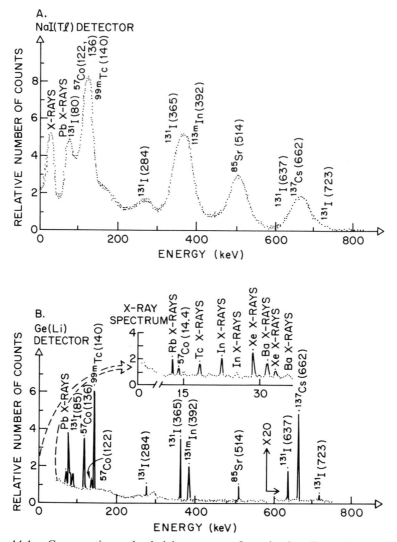

Fig. 14-1. Comparative pulse-height spectra of a mixed radionuclide sample recorded with (A) NaI(Tl) and (B) Ge(Li) detectors. Because of its superior energy resolution, the Ge(Li) detector clearly resolved multiple γ rays of similar energies that appear as single peaks with NaI(Tl).

2. Applications

The major in vitro applications of semiconductor detectors in nuclear medicine have been for tracer studies employing many radionuclides simultaneously, and for the assay of radionuclidic purity of radiopharmaceuticals. In both of these applications the superior energy resolution of semiconductor detectors, illustrated by Figure 14-1, offers a distinct advantage. The energy resolution of the Ge detector allows unequivocal identification of radionuclides, whereas the NaI(Tl) spectrum is ambiguous. Other applications of semiconductor detectors are for analysis of samples in neutron activation analysis (Chapter 7, Section A.2) and fluorescence excitation scanning (Chapter 17, Section D). Reference 1 contains an extensive description of semiconductor detectors and their application in nuclear medicine.

B. LIQUID SCINTILLATION COUNTERS

1. General Characteristics

With *liquid scintillation counters* (LSC) the radioactive sample is dissolved in a scintillator solution contained in a counting vial, which is then placed between two PM tubes in a darkened counting chamber (Figure 14-2).

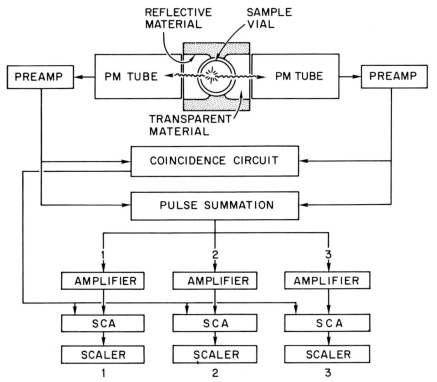

Fig. 14-2.   Basic components of a liquid scintillation counter.

Table 14-1
Radionuclides Commonly Counted With Liquid
Scintillation Detectors

Radionuclide	Half-Life	Maximum β Energy (MeV)
^{3}H	12.3 Years	0.018
^{14}C	5730 years	0.156
^{35}S	87.0 days	0.167
^{45}Ca	163 days	0.257
^{65}Zn	243 days	0.325
^{59}Fe	45 days	0.467
^{22}Na	2.6 years	0.546
^{131}I	8.06 days	0.606
^{36}Cl	3×10^5 years	0.714
^{40}K	1.3×10^9 years	1.300
^{24}Na	15.0 hours	1.392
^{32}P	14.3 days	1.710

The LS solution has a low atomic number ($Z\sim6$–8) and density ($\rho \sim 1$) in comparison to other scintillators, e.g., NaI(Tl). Therefore it has relatively poor efficiency for detecting x- or γ-rays of energies $\gtrsim 40$ keV. Thus it is used primarily for the detection of low-energy x and γ rays and β particles. Because the radioactivity is in direct contact with the scintillator, LS counting is the preferred method for the detection of low-energy β-emitting radionuclides, such as ^{3}H and ^{14}C. Numerous other β-emitting radionuclides including some (β,γ) emitters, also are counted with LSC (Table 14-1).

Since LSC systems are used primarily to count very low-energy particles, the system must have a very low electronic noise levels. For example, with ^{3}H, the energy range of the β particle is 0–18 keV. Under optimal conditions, β particles from ^{3}H decay produce only 0–25 photoelectrons at the PM tube photocathode, with an average of only about 8 ($\overline{E}_\beta \approx \frac{1}{3}E_\beta^{max}$). Background electronic noise is due mainly to *spontaneous thermal emission* of electrons from the photocathode of the PM tube. Background noise also is present from exposure to light of the scintillator solution during sample preparation. This exposure can produce light emission (phosphorescence), which persists for long periods of time (i.e., hours).

Several methods are employed in LS detectors to reduce this noise or background count rate. Thermal emission is reduced by *refrigeration* of the counting chamber to maintain the PM tubes at a constant low temperature (typically about $-10°C$). Constant PM tube temperature is important because the photocathode efficiency and electronic gain of the PM tube are temperature dependent and variations in temperature produce variation in the amplitude of the output signal.

Pulse-height analysis may also be used to discriminate against noise because true radiation events usually produce larger signals than thermal emission noise; however, thermal emission noise is still superimposed on the radiation signals, which can cause deterioration of the energy resolution and linearity of the system.

The most effective reduction of noise is achieved by *coincidence detection* techniques (Figure 14-2). When a scintillation event occurs in the scintillator, light is emitted in all directions. Optical reflectors placed around the counting vial reflect the light into two opposing PM tubes to maximize light collection efficiency. Pulses from each of the PM tubes are routed to separate preamplifiers and a *coincidence circuit*. The coincidence circuit rejects any pulse that does not arrive simultaneously (i.e., within about 0.3 μsec) with a pulse from the other PM tube. Noise pulses are distributed randomly in time; therefore the probability of two noise pulses occurring simultaneously in the two PM tubes is very small. Random coincidence rates R_r (cps) can be determined from

$$R_r = (2\tau)R_n^2 \tag{14-1}$$

where 2τ is the resolving time of the coincidence circuit and R_n is the noise pulse rate for each PM tube (assumed to be equal) due to PM tube noise and phosphorescence in the sample. For $2\tau = 0.03$ μsec and $R_n = 1000$ cps, one obtains $R_r = 3 \times 10^{-8} \times (10^3)^2 = 0.03$ cps. Thus most of the noise pulses are rejected by the coincidence circuit.

The output signals from the two PM tubes and preamplifiers are fed into the coincidence circuit as described above and also into a summation circuit, which adds the two signals together to produce an output signal proportional to the total energy of the detected event (Figure 14-2). The output signals from the summing circuit are sent to three separate amplifiers. The amplified signals are routed to separate SCAs for energy analysis. The output from the coincidence circuit is fed to each of the SCAs to enable their output only when both PM tubes have registered a pulse and thus to reject noise. Output signals from the SCAs are recorded with scalers and can be printed out or processed by automated data processing systems or by a computer.

Multiple SCAs allow the user to perform simultaneous counting of two or more radionuclides in the scintillator solution or to perform quench corrections, as discussed in Section B.5.

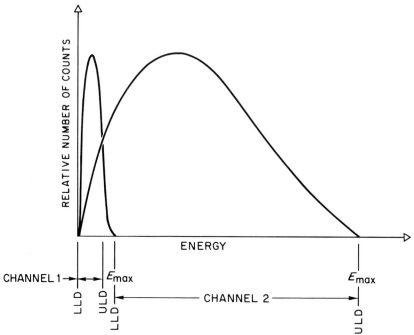

Fig. 14-3.   Example of pulse-height spectra obtained from ^{3}H and ^{14}C by liquid scintillation counting.

2. Pulse-Height Spectrometry

Pulse-height analysis is used with LS counting to reduce the background counting rate by selecting only the energy region corresponding to the radiation of interest or to select different energy regions when simultaneous sources are being counted. An example of two-channel analysis for a source containing ^{3}H and ^{14}C is shown in Figure 14-3. Because of the continuous energy distribution in β decay pulse-height analysis cannot separate completely the two spectra, and there is cross-talk interference. Methods to correct for this are discussed in Section B.4.

3. Counting Vials

Counting vials containing the radioactivity and the liquid scintillator solution usually are made of polyethylene or low-potassium-content glass. The low-potassium-content glass is used to avoid the natural background of ^{40}K. When standard laboratory glass vials (lime glass) are used, the background for ^{3}H and ^{14}C is increased by 30–40 cpm due to ^{40}K in the glass. Polyethylene vials frequently are used to avoid this problem and also to increase light transmission from the liquid scintillator to the PM tubes. Polyethylene vials are excellent for dioxane solvents but should not be used with toluene as the scintillator solvent because toluene will cause the vials to distort and swell, which may jam the sample changer. Materials such as quartz, vicor, and others also are used for counting vials.

Exposure of the vial and liquid scintillator solution to strong sunlight will produce a background of phosphorescence that may take hours to decay; therefore samples frequently are stored temporarily in a darkened container before counting. This is referred to as "dark adaption" of samples.

4. Energy and Efficiency Calibration

Beta emission results in a continuous spectrum of β-particle energies from zero to a maximum β-particle energy E_β^{max} that is characteristic of the nuclide, with a mean value at about $\frac{1}{3}E_\beta^{max}$. Usually, the SCA window is set to include most of the spectrum, resulting in detection efficiencies of 80 percent or better for most β-emitting radionuclides. An exception is ^3H. The low-energy β emission of ^3H ($E_\beta^{max} = 18$ keV) reduces the counting efficiency to about 40–60 percent because some of the events produce pulses below typical noise pulse amplitudes that must be rejected by pulse-height analysis (Section B.1).

Most LS counters have three SCA channels (Figure 14-2). The following procedure can be used to set up the system for optimal counting: First, the amplifier gains for all three channels are adjusted to have the same gain factor. On the first SCA (channel 1) the lower-level discriminator (LLD) is set to the lowest value that eliminates electronic noise. Electronic noise is detected at LLD values for which high counting rates are obtained with no sample in the counter. The upper-level discriminator (ULD) is set to its highest value, i.e., widest possible window setting. The LLD on the second SCA (channel 2) is set to the same value as the first SCA, while the ULD is set at one-third of the maximum setting. The LLD on the third SCA (channel 3) is set to one-third of the maximum setting and the ULD is set to the maximum value. The vial of scintillation solution containing a β-emitting radionuclide is then placed in the LS counter and the amplifier gains are adjusted until the counting rate in channel 2 is approximately equal to the counting rate in channel 3. Then $\frac{1}{3}E_\beta^{max}$ is approximately at the dividing line between channels 2 and 3 (Figure 14-4). Channel 1 is then used to determine total counting rate, and channels 2 and 3 are used for quench corrections (Section B.5).

Frequently, samples containing a mixture of two radionuclides (e.g.,

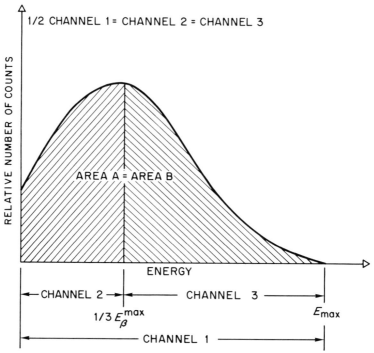

Fig. 14-4. Pulse-height spectrometer settings frequently used for mixed sample counting and quench corrections.

³H and ¹⁴C) are counted. By placing separate SCA windows on each of the β spectra (Figure 14-3), the activities of each of the radionuclides can be determined. The optimal window for each radionuclide is determined individually by using separate ³H and ¹⁴C sources. If possible the SCAs should be adjusted so that counts from the lower-energy emitter are not included in the channel used for the higher-energy emitter. The method and equations used to correct for crosstalk interference—described in Chapter 13, Section A.7 for well counter applications—can be used on the LS counter.

5. Quench Corrections

Quenching refers to any process that reduces the amount of scintil-lation light produced by the sample or detected by the PM tubes. The causes of quenching in LS counting were described in Chapter 4, Section C.4. The principle effect of quenching is to cause an apparent shift of the energy spectrum to lower energies (Figure 14-5). This results in a loss of

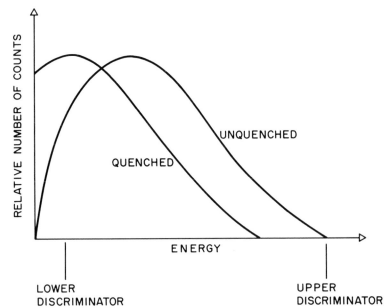

Fig. 14-5.   Effect of quenching on a liquid scintillation counter pulse-height
spectrum.

counts because some events are shifted below the LLD limit set to reject
noise. Thus inaccurate counting rates are recorded. The error depends on
the amount of quenching, which may vary from one sample to the next.

To obtain accurate results, it is necessary to correct the observed
counting rate for quench-caused spectral shifts. Several methods have
been developed.

With the *internal standardization method,* the sample counting rate is
determined; then a known quantity of the radionuclide of interest (from a
calibrated standard solution) is added to the sample and it is recounted.
The counting efficiency is calculated by

$$\text{eff} = \frac{\text{cpm (STD + sample)} - \text{cpm (sample)}}{\mu\text{Ci standard}} \qquad (14\text{-}2)$$

From the efficiency, the activity of the sample is obtained from

$$\mu\text{Ci sample} = \frac{\text{cpm sample}}{\text{eff}} \qquad (14\text{-}3)$$

With the internal standardization, the sample must be counted twice and the added activity of the standard must be distributed in the scintillator solution in the same manner as the sample. The method is not accurate if the sample and standard are not dissolved in the same way in the scintillator. Also, self-absorption of the emitted β particle by the labeled molecule might not be accounted for unless the standard is also in the form of the labeled molecule.

A second approach is called the *channel ratio method*. One channel is set to count an unquenched sample as efficiently as possible (i.e., channel 1 in Figure 14-4), and a second channel is set to accumulate counts in the lower-energy region of the spectrum (channel 2 in Figure 14-4). When the spectrum shifts to the left due to quenching the lower channel gains counts while the upper channel loses counts, and the ratio of counts in the two channels changes. A series of standards of known activity are counted, each quenched deliberately a little more than the preceding one by adding a quenching agent, to obtain a *quench curve* relating counting efficiency (cpm/μCi) to the channel ratio. Then for subsequently measured samples, the channel ratio is used to determine the quench-corrected counting efficiency.

Once the correction curve has been obtained, only one (dual channel) counting measurement per sample is required to determine counting efficiency. All causes of quenching are corrected by the channel ratio method. A disadvantage of the method is that at very low counting rates statistical errors in the value determined for the channel ratio may be large, which may result in significant errors in the estimated quench correction factor. Longer counting times may be employed to minimize this source of error.

A third approach is called the *automatic external standardization (AES) method*. This method incorporates features of both internal standardization and channel ratio. The sample is first counted, and then recounted (usually for 1 min or less) with an external standard γ-ray source (usually ^{137}Cs) placed close to the sample (some counters count the sample plus standard first). Positioning of the standard is automatic. Compton recoil electrons produced by interactions of the γ rays with the scintillator solution are counted in two channels and a channel ratio determined, or

$$\text{AES (ratio)} = \frac{\text{cpm (sample + STD)} - \text{cpm sample channel 2}}{\text{cpm (sample + STD)} - \text{cpm sample channel 1}} \qquad (14\text{-}4)$$

where STD refers to the standard γ-ray source and channels 1 and 2 are as indicated in Figure 14-4.

A series of quenched standards containing known amounts of the radionuclide of interest is prepared, and counting efficiency is related to the AES ratio. The AES ratio is then used to correct for quenching on subsequently measured samples.

The external standard method generally provides a high counting rate and thus small statistical errors in the determination of the quench correction factor while maintaining the sensitivity of the channel ratio method for detecting quenching effects. The disadvantage of the AES method is that only chemical and color quenching are corrected; beta-particle self-absorption effects or losses due to sample distribution effects are not. For example, the AES method might not be accurate with multiphase solutions in which the sample is not soluble in the counting solution.

AES quench curves and crosstalk correction factors are shown in Figure 14-6 for ^{14}C and ^{3}H for double-label studies, i.e., both radionuclides counted simultaneously. It is apparent from Figure 14-6 that as quenching increases (AES ratio decreases) the efficiency for counting both ^{14}C and ^{3}H decreases. Thus even though the true efficiency may be determined accurately from the quench correction curve, counting efficiency deteriorates with increased quenching, resulting in increased statistical errors.

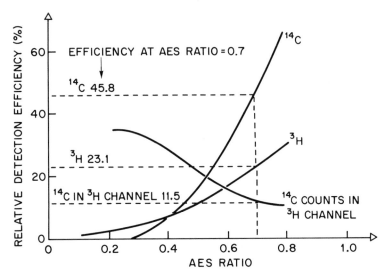

Fig. 14-6. Quench correction curves based on the automatic external standardization method for counting mixed ^{14}C–^{3}H samples. For example, with an AES ratio of 0.7 (dashed line) counts in the ^{3}H channel must first be corrected for ^{14}C crosstalk by 11.5 percent of the counts in the ^{14}C channel. The counting efficiency for the corrected ^{3}H counts is 23.1 percent and for the ^{14}C counts is 45.8 percent relative to an unquenched sample. Note that the AES ratio *decreases* with increasing quenching.

6. Sample Preparation Techniques

Samples can be combined with scintillator solution in several different ways. Nonpolar compounds (i.e., lipids), steroids, many hydrocarbons, and other organic compounds can be dissolved directly in the scintillator solution, which is also a nonpolar solution. Polar compounds (i.e., H_2O-soluble compounds) frequently can be dissolved by adding small amounts of ethanol, anisole, cellosolves, 1,4-dioxane, and certain other liquids that act as a common solvent for both the nonpolar scintillator solutions and polar compounds. Polar compounds also can be used by forming insoluble suspensions. For example, $^{14}CO_2$ can be precipitated as barium carbonate and then suspended in the scintillator solution with the addition of thixatropic jelling agents. Silica gels from thin-layer chromatography also can be counted in this manner. Water-soluble compounds also can be added to scintillator solutions with the addition of a small amount of detergent. This results in the formation of a suspension of small water droplets (containing the labeled compound) throughout the solution. Samples deposited on filter paper such as from paper chromatography frequently are counted by placing the paper strip in the liquid scintillator. The scintillator solution also can be dissolved or suspended in the sample itself.

Another straightforward approach to counting complicated organic compounds such as proteins or sections of acrylamide gel columns with high efficiency is to combust the sample. The $^{14}CO_2$ and ^3H_2O released may be collected, dissolved in scintillator solution, and then counted.

Numerous other techniques have been developed for LS sample preparation. A detailed discussion of these techniques is presented in references 2 and 3. Careful sample preparation is critical for accurate application of the LS technique.

7. Liquid and Gas Flow Counting

In addition to counting individual samples, LS systems also are used for continuous monitoring of gas streams or flowing liquids. In these systems the vial of liquid scintillation solution is replaced with a cell filled with finely dispersed solid scintillator crystals through which the radioactively labeled gas or liquid is allowed to flow. The most common scintillator material for this purpose is the organic scintillator anthracene. This technique is used primarily for β-emitting radionuclides, typically ^{14}C and ^3H. The β particles interact with the anthracene crystals, and the resulting scintillation is detected in the same manner as from the liquid scintillation vial.

These systems have been used for monitoring the effluent from amino acid analyzers, liquid chromatographs, and gas chromatographs. In order to monitor the effluent from gas chromatographs, the compounds usually are passed through a gas combustion furnace to convert them into $^{14}CO_2$ or ^3H_3O (vapor). Carrier gas from the gas chromatograph (i.e., He) is used to sweep the $^{14}CO_2$ or ^3H_2O through the counting cell.

Counting rates in these systems depend upon the activity concentration and the flow rate. If fast flow rates and low-activity concentrations are required, the result may be data of poor statistical quality.

Data from flow counting represent the time course of some process and usually are displayed as time histogram curves using ratemeters and strip-chart recorders or computer displays. A computer may also be used for curve analysis, background subtraction, peak ratios, efficiency corrections, etc.

8. Automatic Multiple-Sample LS Counters

Liquid scintillation counting may be used for counting large numbers of samples or for counting low-level samples for long counting times. To expedite this and to remove the tedious job of manually counting multiple samples, automatic multiple-sample LSC systems have been developed. These systems have automatic sample changers that frequently can handle 100 or more counting vials (Figure 14-7). A number of different sample-changing mechanisms have been developed, but the most common ones employ either trays or an endless belt for transport of the

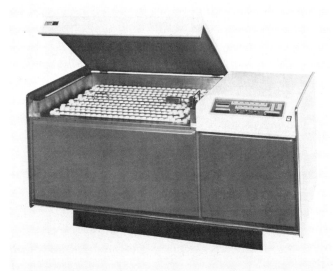

Fig. 14-7. A multi-sample changer liquid scintillation counter. Samples are transported to the counting chamber by an endless loop conveyor belt. [Courtesy of Tracor Analytic, Elk Grove, Ill.].

samples. Sample vials are selected automatically and loaded into the light-tight LS counting chamber. The samples are counted sequentially in serial fashion. Empty positions in the sample changer can be bypassed, and samples below a selectable low-level counting rate may be rejected automatically to avoid long counting times on samples that contain an insignificant amount of activity when preset counts are selected. Most LS counter systems are provided with three SCAs for multiple radionuclide counting and for applying quenching corrections. Scalers and timers also are provided for visual inspection of the counting rate in each channel.

Modern automatic multiple-sample LSC systems are provided with many different ways of handling and presenting the recorded data. The recorded counting rate can be printed out serially with sample number, time, counting time, and number of recorded counts for each or all SCA channels. Computer-based systems allow automatic implementation of quench corrections, efficiency corrections, background subtraction, statistical analysis, and calculations of parameters for radioimmunoassay or other assay analysis.

9. Applications

The use of LSC systems in nuclear medicine has increased significantly in recent years because of their usefulness for radioimmunoassays and protein-binding assays of drugs, hormones, and other biologically active compounds. Liquid scintillation counter systems also are commonly used in studies of metabolic or physiologic processes with ^{3}H- or ^{14}C-labeled metabolic substrates or other physiologically important molecules.

C. GAS-FILLED DETECTORS

1. Dose Calibrators

Although they are inefficient detectors for most γ-ray energies encountered in nuclear medicine, gas-filled detectors still find some specialized applications. A *dose calibrator* is essentially a well-type ionization chamber that is used for assaying relatively large quantities (i.e., mCi range) of γ-ray-emitting radioactivity (Figure 14-8). Dose calibrators are used for measuring or verifying the activity of generator eluates, patient preparations, shipments of radioactivity received from suppliers, and similar quantities of activity too large for assay with NaI(Tl) detector systems.

The detector element for a dose calibrator is an air-filled ionization

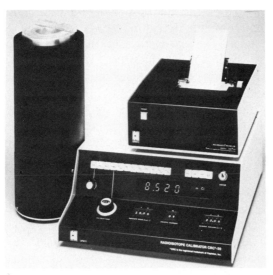

Fig. 14-8. An ionization chamber dose calibrator. Samples are inserted into the well in the sealed ionization chamber (left). Activity is displayed and printed out on the electrometer readout (right). Readout is in mCi of sample activity for specific radionuclides selected by pushbutton control. [Courtesy Capintec, Inc., Montvali, N.J.]

chamber, sealed to avoid variations in response with ambient temperature and atmospheric pressure changes. Ionization chamber dose calibrators assay the total amount of activity present by measuring the total amount of ionization produced by the sample. Plug-in resistor modules, pushbuttons, or other selector mechanisms are used to adjust the elec-trometer readout to display the activity of the selected radionuclide directly in mCi or μCi units. Because ionization chambers have no inherent ability for energy discrimination, they cannot be used to select electronically different γ-ray energies for measurement, as is possible with detectors having pulse-height analysis capabilities. One approach that is used to distinguish low-energy versus high-energy activity (e.g., ^{99m}Tc versus ^{99}Mo) is to measure the sample with and without a few millimeters of lead shielding around the source. Effectively, only the activity of the high-energy emitter is recorded with the shielding in place, whereas the total activity of both emitters is recorded with the shielding absent. This technique can be used to detect μCi quantities of ^{99}Mo in the presence of tens or even hundreds of millicuries of ^{99m}Tc.

As with the NaI(Tl) well counter (Chapter 13, Section A.3), dose calibrators are subject to sample volume effects. These effects should be investigated experimentally when a new dose calibrator is acquired, so that correction factors can be applied in its use, if necessary. For example, a quantity of activity can be measured in a very small volume (e.g., 0.1 ml in a 1 ml syringe), and that activity can be diluted progressively to larger volumes in larger syringes and then in beakers, etc. to determine the amount by which the instrument reading changes with sample volume.

Another parameter worth evaluating is linearity of response versus sample activity. This may be determined conveniently by recording the reading for a ^{99m}Tc source of moderately high activity (e.g. 100 mCi, or whatever the approximate maximum amount of activity the dose calibrator will be used to assay), then recording the readings over a 24–48 hour period (4–8 half-lives) to determine whether or not they follow the expected decay curve for ^{99m}Tc. Deviations from the expected decay curve may indicate instrument electronic nonlinearities requiring attention from the serviceman or correction of readings. In applying this technique it is necessary to correct for ^{99}Mo contamination using the

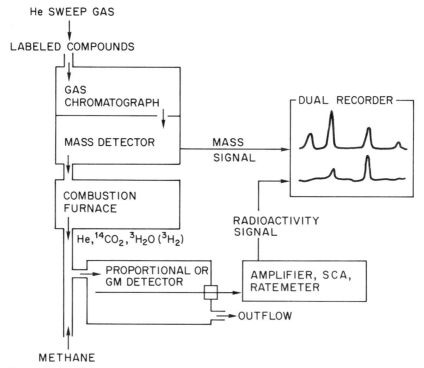

Fig. 14-9. Schematic representation of a gas flow counter used in conjunction with a mass spectrometer for radiochemical analysis.

shielding technique described above, especially after several ^{99m}Tc half-lives have elapsed.

2. Gas Flow Counters

Gas-filled detectors also are used in gas flow counters, primarily for measurement of β-emitting activity. The detector in these systems usually can be operated in either proportional counter or GM mode. The most frequent application for these systems in nuclear medicine is for monitoring the effluent from gas chromatographs (Figure 14-9). Gases labeled with ^{3}H or ^{14}C in helium carrier gas from the chromatograph are passed through a combustion furnace to convert them to ^{3}H$_2$O or ^{14}CO$_2$, which then is allowed to flow through the counter gas volume itself with the counting gas (usually 90 percent He plus 10 percent methane). This permits a time-course analysis of the outflow from the chromatograph. These systems have good geometric and intrinsic detection efficiencies for low-energy β emitters, such as ^{3}H and ^{14}C; however, their intrinsic efficiency for γ-ray detection is only about 1 percent.

REFERENCES

1. TerPogossian MM, Phelps ME: Semiconductor detector systems. Semin Nucl Med 3:343–365, 1975.

    Additional discussion of liquid scintillation counting systems may be found in the following:

2. Rapkin E: Preparation of samples for liquid scintillation counting, in Hine GF (ed): Instrumentation in Nuclear Medicine. New York, Academic Press, 1967, pp 181–220
3. Bransome ED Jr: The Current Status of Liquid Scintillation Counting. New York, Grune & Stratton, 1970, chaps 16–27

15

The Anger Camera: Basic Principles

Radionuclide imaging is one of the most important applications of radioactivity in medicine. Radionuclide imaging laboratories are found in almost every hospital, performing hundreds and even thousands of imaging procedures per month in larger institutions.

In this chapter, we will discuss briefly some general aspects of radionuclide imaging and its historical development, and we will describe the basic principles of the most widely used imaging device, the Anger camera. The performance characteristics of this instrument are discussed in Chapter 16. Other imaging devices are described in Chapters 17 and 20 and general problems in radionuclide imaging in Chapter 18.

A. GENERAL CONCEPTS OF RADIONUCLIDE IMAGING AND HISTORICAL DEVELOPMENT

The purpose of radionuclide imaging is to obtain a picture of the distribution of a radioactively labeled substance within the body after it has been administered (e.g., by intravenous injection) to a patient. This is accomplished by recording the emissions from the radioactivity, with external radiation detectors placed at different locations outside the patient. The preferred emissions for this application are γ rays in the approximate energy range 80–500 keV (or annihilation photons, 511 keV). Gamma rays of these energies are sufficiently penetrating in body tissues to be detected from deep-lying organs but are shielded adequately with reasonable thicknesses of lead. Alpha particles and electrons (β particles,

Auger and conversion electrons) are of little use because they cannot penetrate more than a few millimeters of tissue and therefore cannot get outside the body to the radiation detector, except from very superficial tissues. Bremsstrahlung generated by electron emissions is more penetrating, but the intensity of this radiation generally is very weak.

Imaging system detectors must therefore have good detection efficiency for γ rays. It is also desirable that they have energy discrimination capability, so that γ rays that have lost energy by Compton scattering within the body can be rejected. Sodium iodide provides both of these features at a reasonable cost; for this reason it is currently the detector material of choice for imaging systems.

The first attempts at radionuclide "imaging" occurred in the late 1940s. An array of radiation detectors was positioned on a matrix of measuring points around the head. Alternatively, a single detector was positioned manually for separate measurements at each point in the matrix. These devices were tedious to use and provided only very crude mappings of the distribution of radioactivity in the head, e.g., left-side versus right-side asymmetries.

A significant advance occurred in the early 1950s with the introduction of the rectilinear scanner by Ben Cassen. With this instrument, the detector was scanned mechanically in a rasterlike pattern over the area of interest. The image was a pattern of dots imprinted on a sheet of paper by a mechanical printer that followed the scanning motion of the detector, printing the dots as the γ rays were detected. The design of this instrument was subsequently improved, and rectilinear scanners still find some use today, as described in Chapter 17, Section A.

The principal disadvantage of the rectilinear scanner is its long imaging time (typically many minutes) because the image is formed by sequential measurements at many individual points within the imaged area. The first γ-ray "camera" capable of recording at all points in the image at one time was described by Hal Anger in 1953. He used a pinhole aperture in a sheet of lead to project a γ-ray image of the radioactive distribution onto a radiation detector comprised of a NaI(Tl) screen and a sheet of x-ray film. The film was exposed by the scintillation light flashes generated by the γ rays in the NaI(Tl) screen. Unfortunately, this detection system (especially the film component) was so inefficient that hour-long exposures and therapeutic levels of administered radioactivity were needed to obtain satisfactory images.

In the late 1950s, Anger replaced the film-screen combination with a single, large-area, NaI(Tl) crystal and a photomultiplier tube assembly to greatly increase the detection efficiency of his "camera" concept. This instrument, the *Anger scintillation camera*, has been substantially refined and improved since that time. Although many other ideas for imaging instruments have come along since then, (see Chapter 17), none has matched the Anger camera for a balance of image quality, detection efficiency, and ease of use in a hospital environment. The Anger camera has thus become the standard nuclear imaging instrument for clinical applications and seems likely to remain so for the foreseeable future.

B. BASIC PRINCIPLES OF THE ANGER CAMERA

1. System Components

Figure 15-1 illustrates the basic principles of image formation with the Anger camera. A γ-ray image is projected by the *collimator* onto the NaI(Tl) *detector crystal*, creating a pattern of scintillations in the crystal that outlines the distribution of radioactivity in front of the collimator. A *photomultiplier (PM) tube array* viewing the back surface of the crystal, and electronic *position logic circuits*, determine the location of each scintillation event as it occurs in the crystal. Individual events also are analyzed for energy by *pulse-height analyzer* circuits. When an event falls within the selected energy window, the electron beam in a *cathode ray tube (CRT) display* is deflected by X- and Y-position signals to a location on the CRT face corresponding to the location at which the scintillation event occurred in the crystal, and the beam is turned on momentarily, causing a flash of light to appear at that point on the display. Thus the CRT display shows a pattern of light flashes corresponding to the pattern of scintillation events occurring in the detector crystal. The CRT display flashes are much brighter, however, and can be recorded photographically. Time exposures lasting from fractions of a second to several minutes are recorded, typically on Polaroid or transparency film.

The Anger camera can be used for *static* imaging studies, in which an image of an unchanging radionuclide distribution can be recorded over an extended imaging time, e.g., minutes. It can also be used for *dynamic* imaging studies, in which changes in the radionuclide distribution can be observed, as rapidly as several images per second. Dynamic imaging generally requires the availability of an automatic film advancing mechanism (Section B.4) or a digital image storage system (Chapter 21).

Stationary cameras are designed to be used at a fixed location (Figure 15-2). The detector crystal, photomultiplier tubes, collimator, and a portion of the electronics are housed in a *detector stand*, with operating controls, a CRT display, and photographic camera for recording images from the CRT housed in a separate *control console*. Additional image recording devices that are capable of providing better quality images than are provided by the CRT system in the control console are available for some systems.

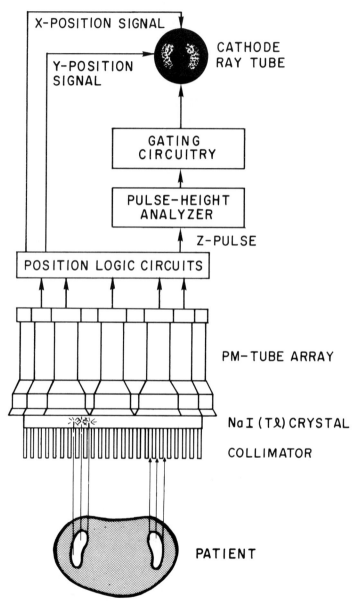

Fig. 15-1. Basic principles and components of the Anger camera.

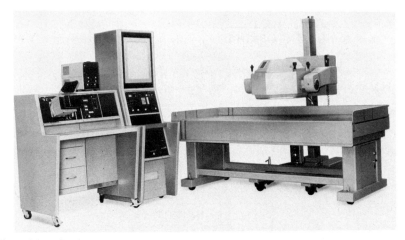

Fig. 15-2.   Stationary Anger camera system, designed for use at a fixed location. Operating controls and electronics are housed in a control console (left). Also on the control console is a CRT with Polaroid camera for image recording. Adjacent to the control console is a multiformat imaging device (Section B.5). At right is the detector stand and patient support table. The table in this example is of the type used in the "scanning camera" (Section B.5). [Courtesy Searle Radiographics.]

Mobile cameras have all of the above components mounted on a motor-driven stand that can be moved from one room to the next or to the patient's bedside for studies. Some mobile cameras, such as the example shown in Figure 15-3, are designed specifically for cardiac applications. They have relatively small detector heads and include dedicated computer hardware built into the mobile console for this application (Chapter 21, Section A).

2. Detector System and Electronics

The Anger camera employs a single, large-area, NaI(Tl) dectector crystal, usually 1.25 cm thick × 30–50 cm in diameter. Generally, larger-diameter crystals are used on stationary cameras and those with smaller diameters on mobile units. Some cameras, designed specifically for use with low-energy radionuclides, such as ^{99m}Tc, have crystal thicknesses of only 6–8 mm. As discussed in Chapter 16, Section A.4, relatively thin detector crystals are preferred for the Anger camera, even at the expense of somewhat less efficient radiation detection, because of their ability to provide better intrinsic resolution and some improvement in image detail. For lower-energy γ emitters, such as ^{99m}Tc and ^{201}Tl, however, detection efficiency is adequate even with 6 mm thick detector crystals.

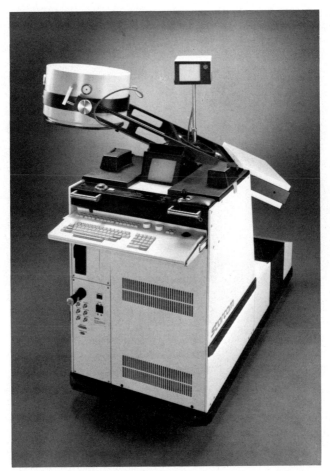

Fig. 15-3. Mobile camera has all components mounted on a moveable motor-driven stand. (Courtesy GE Medical Systems).

An array of photomultiplier tubes is coupled optically to the back face of the crystal with a silicone fluid or grease. Some manufacturers employ lucite light pipes between the detector crystal and PM tubes, whereas others couple directly to the crystal. Most modern cameras employ 37, 61, 75, or 91 tubes, arranged in a hexagonal pattern. Figure 15-4 shows a 37-tube model. Some cameras have round PM tubes, whereas in others, they are square or hexagonal for better packing. Older models with nineteen 7.5 cm diameter PM tubes may also still be found in use. The detector crystal and PM tube array are enclosed in a light-tight, lead-lined protective housing. In most modern cameras, part of the signal

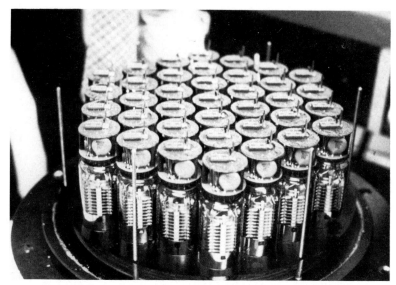

Fig. 15-4. Thirty-seven PM tubes mounted in a hexagonal array on the back of an Anger camera detector crystal. [Courtesy Richard Van Tuinen.]

processing circuitry (preamplifiers, pulse-height analyzers, automatic gain control, pulse pileup rejection circuits, etc.) are mounted directly on the individual PM tube bases in the detector housing to minimize signal distortions that can occur in long cable runs between the detector head and control console.

Figure 15-5 is a schematic drawing for a seven PM tube version of the Anger camera and will be used to illustrate the principles of scintillation event localization. Note that the outputs of tubes numbered 1, 3, 4, 5, and 6 are combined in a *summing matrix circuit* (SMC) to form a composite signal X^+, and tubes 1, 2, 3, 6, and 7 are combined to form a signal X^-. Similarly, the PM tube array is divided into vertical halves to obtain signals Y^+ and Y^-. In separate circuitry, the outputs of all seven PM tubes are combined to form a Z signal. The Z signal is proportional in amplitude to the total amount of light produced by a scintillation event in the crystal and is used for pulse-height analysis.

Suppose that a scintillation event occurs at point A in the crystal. The PM tubes closest to the event will receive the greatest amount of light and thus will provide output signals of the greatest amplitude. Therefore in the example shown in Figure 15-5, the X^+ signal will be larger than the X^- signal because the event occurred in the right-hand half of the crystal, and the Y^- signal will be larger than the Y^+ signal because the event occurred in the lower half. The summing matrix circuits combine the signals from

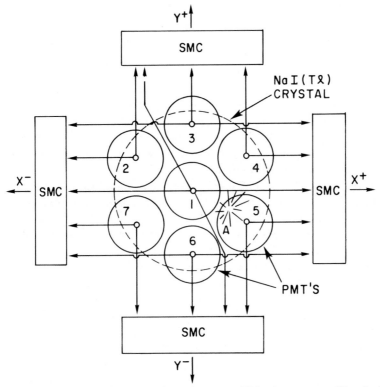

Fig. 15-5. Schematic representation of a seven PM tube camera. Signals from individual PM tubes are combined in summing matrix circuits (SMC) to obtain X^+, X^-, Y^+, and Y^- signals, which in turn are used to generate X- and Y-position signals.

the individual PM tubes in such a way that the relative amplitudes of the X^+ and X^- signals, and of the Y^+ and Y^- signals, are proportional to the distance of the scintillation event from the center line of the crystal. These four signals, therefore, can be used to determine the location at which the scintillation event occurred, and the Z signal can be used to determine its energy.

The X^+, X^-, Y^+, and Y^- signals are then combined to obtain *X-position* and *Y-position* signals, which are used to position the electron beam on the CRT display. The X-position signal is the difference between the X^+ and X^- signals divided by the total light signal (Z signal),

$$X = k(X^+ - X^-)/Z \qquad (15\text{-}1)$$

and similarly for the Y-position signal,

$$Y = k(Y^+ - Y^-)/Z \qquad (15\text{-}2)$$

In Equations 15-1 and 15-2, k is a scale factor adjusted for the deflection voltage requirements of the CRT. The X and Y signals are stretched to a length of 2–4 μsec to hold the beam momentarily in position on the CRT display. If the Z signal is accepted within the selected energy window of the pulse-height analyzer, the beam is turned on for 1–3 μsec to create a light flash at the appropriate location on the CRT display. The connection of X and Y signals to the CRT deflection plates can be interchanged using *orientation controls* on the console to provide rotation or reversal ("mirror image") of the image on the CRT.

Equations 15-1 and 15-2 do not give a true mapping of source position because the PM tubes are not "point" detectors. This gives rise to a "pincushion" artifact, which is discussed in Chapter 16, Section A.1.

The X- and Y-position signals must be normalized to the total light signal Z as described in Equations 15-1 and 15-2. Otherwise, low-energy γ-ray-emitting radionuclides, such as ^{133}Xe(81 keV) or ^{201}Tl(70–80 keV), which generate smaller amounts of light per scintillation event, would produce smaller position signals (X^+, X^-, Y^+, Y^-)—and thus smaller images on the CRT display—than a high-energy radionuclide, e.g., ^{131}I(364 keV). Normalization for energy also permits the use of dual- or even triple-window pulse-height analyzers for imaging multiple-energy γ-ray emitters, e.g., ^{67}Ga.

Energy selection (pulse-height analyzer window) is accomplished using a *range selector* or *isotope selector* on the control console. Some instruments have push buttons to select automatically the appropriate energy window for different radionuclides. A visual display of the selected energy window may be provided in one (or both) of two formats. In *Z-pulse display*, multiple Z pulses are displayed simultaneously on a CRT (Figure 15-6). The vertical axis is pulse amplitude and the horizontal axis is time. A photopeak in the spectrum is a bright band in the display, representing a "cluster" of pulses of nearly identical amplitude, with pulses above or below this band representing events of higher or lower energy, respectively. To indicate the location of the pulse-height analyzer window in the spectrum, pulses accepted within the window are "blanked" momentarily, creating a blank "box" on the display. The operator adjusts controls on the control console (usually connected to the amplifier gain adjustments) until the blank box appears to be centered in the brightened band, indicating proper centering of the analyzer window on the photopeak.

More exact adjustment is possible with a *multichannel analyzer display* (Figure 15-6). The spectrum is obtained with multichannel ana-

Tc-99m PULSE HEIGHT SPECTRA

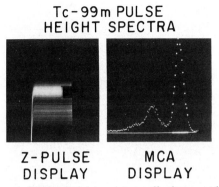

Z-PULSE DISPLAY   MCA DISPLAY

Fig. 15-6.   Two types of pulse-height spectrum displays used on Anger cameras.

lyzer circuitry (Chapter 5, Section C.4) and displayed in the conventional counts versus pulse-amplitude format. The position of the analyzer window is indicated by intensified dots on or below the display. For most studies, a 20 percent window, centered on the photopeak, is used.

Image exposure time is selected by scaler and timer controls on the console. Generally, both *preset count* and *preset time* options are available. Both the elapsed time and total counts accumulated in the image are shown on a digital display. Some cameras are provided with a ratemeter to show counting rate within the analyzer window. Another option sometimes provided is *divided crystal* counting rate, which permits separate counting of events on the right-hand ($X^+ > X^-$ signal) and left-hand ($X^- > X^+$ signal) sides of the detector crystal.

3. Collimators

To obtain an image with an Anger camera, it is necessary to project γ rays from the source distribution onto the camera detector. Gamma rays cannot be focused; thus a "lens" principle similar to that used in photography cannot be applied. Therefore, most practical γ-ray imaging systems employ the principle of *absorptive collimation* for image formation.† An absorptive collimator projects an image of the source distribution onto the detector by allowing only those γ rays traveling along certain directions to reach the detector. Gamma rays not traveling in the proper direction are absorbed by the collimator before they reach the detector. This "projection by absorption" technique is an inherently inefficient method for utilizing radiation because most of the potentially

---

† Annihilation coincidence detection (ACD) systems, discussed in Chapter 20, Section D, are an exception.

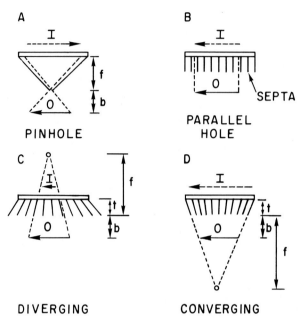

Fig. 15-7. Four types of collimators used to project "γ-ray images" onto the detector of an Anger camera. *O*, radioactive object; *I*, its projected image.

useful radiation traveling toward the detector actually is stopped by the collimator. This is one of the underlying reasons for the relatively poor quality of radionuclide images (e.g., as compared to radiographic images), as discussed in Chapter 18.

Four basic collimator types are used with the Anger camera and similar camera-type imaging devices: pinhole, parallel-hole, diverging, and converging.

A *pinhole* collimator (Figure 15-7A) consists of a small pinhole aperture in a lead, tungsten, platinum, or other heavy-metal absorber. The pinhole is located at the end of a lead cone, typically 20–25 cm from the detector. The size of the pinhole can be chosen by using removable inserts and is typically a few millimeters in diameter.

The imaging principle of a pinhole collimator is the same as that employed with inexpensive "box cameras." Gamma rays passing through the pinhole project an inverted image of the source distribution onto the detector crystal. The image is magnified when the distance *b* from the source to the pinhole is smaller than the collimator cone length *f*; it is minified when the source distribution is farther away. The image size *I* and object (source) size *O* are related according to

$$I/O = f/b \qquad (15\text{-}3)$$

The size of the imaged area also changes with distance from the pinhole collimator. If the detector diameter is D and the magnification (or minification) factor is I/O (Equation 15-3), the diameter of the image area projected onto the detector D', is

$$D' = \frac{D}{(I/O)} \qquad (15\text{-}4)$$

Thus a large magnification factor, obtained at close source-to-collimator distances, results in a small imaged area.

Image size changes with distance b. Therefore the pinhole collimator provides a somewhat distorted image of three-dimensional objects because source planes at different distances from the collimator are magnified by different amounts. Pinhole collimators are used primarily for magnification imaging of small organs (e.g., thyroid and heart).

Another type of pinhole collimator, the *multi-pinhole collimator*, has an array of multiple pinholes, typically seven, arranged in a hexagonal pattern. This collimator has been employed for tomographic imaging; however, this type of tomography is now seldom used (Chapter 20, Section A).

The *parallel-hole collimator* (Figure 15-7B) is the "workhorse" collimator in most imaging laboratories. Parallel holes are drilled or cast in lead or are shaped from lead foils. The lead walls between the holes are called collimator *septa*. Septal thickness is chosen to prevent γ rays from crossing from one hole to the next (Chapter 16, Section B.2). The parallel-hole collimator projects a γ-ray image of the same size as the source distribution onto the detector. A variation of the parallel-hole collimator is the *slant-hole collimator*, in which all of the holes are parallel to each other but angled, typically by about 25°, from the perpendicular direction. This type of collimator has characteristics that are similar to those of the parallel-hole type. Because it views the source distribution from an angle rather than directly on, it can be positioned closer to the patient for better image detail in some imaging studies, e.g., LAO cardiac views.

A *diverging collimator* (Figure 15-7C) has holes that diverge from the detector face. The holes diverge from a point typically 40–50 cm behind the collimator. This projects a *minified* image of the source distribution onto the detector. The degree of minification depends on the distance f from the front of the collimator to the convergence point, the distance b from the front of the collimator to the object (source), and the collimator thickness t:

$$I/O = (f - t)/(f + b) \qquad (15\text{-}5)$$

where I and O are image and object size, respectively. The useful image area becomes larger as the image becomes more minified (Equation 15-4).

Example 15-1.

What is the minification factor for a diverging collimator 5 cm thick, with $f = 45$ cm, and a source distribution 15 cm from the collimator? If the detector diameter is 30 cm, what is the imaged area at this distance?

Answer.

From Equation 15-5,

$$I/O \text{ (minification factor)} = (45 - 5)/(45 + 15) = 0.67$$

From Equation 15-4,

$$\text{Diameter of imaged area} = 30 \text{ cm}/0.67 = 40 \text{ cm}$$

As shown by Example 15-1, a typical diverging collimator decreases the size of the image on the detector, and increases the diameter of the imaged area, by about one-third as compared to a parallel-hole collimator. As with the pinhole collimator, image size changes with distance; thus there is a certain amount of image distortion. Diverging collimators are used primarily on cameras with smaller detectors to permit imaging of large organs such as the liver or lungs on a single view.

A *converging collimator* (Figure 15-7D) has holes that converge to a point 40–50 cm in front of the collimator. For objects between the collimator face and the convergence point, the converging collimator projects a *magnified*, noninverted image of the source distribution. Image size I and object size O are related according to

$$I/O = (f + t)/(f + t - b) \tag{15-6}$$

where f is the distance from the collimator face to the convergence point, b is the distance from the collimator face to the object, and t is collimator thickness.

Some manufacturers provide a single, invertible collimator insert that can be used in either converging or diverging mode.

Example 15-2.

Suppose the collimator described in Example 15-1 is inverted and used as a converging collimator to image a source distribtion 15 cm in front of the collimator, also with a 30 cm diameter detector.

What are the image magnification factor and the size of the imaged area?

Answer.

When the collimator is inverted, the back face becomes the front face, and the convergence distance f becomes $(45 - 5\ \mathrm{cm}) = 40\ \mathrm{cm}$. Thus from Equation 15-6

$$\text{I/O (magnification factor)} = (40 + 5)/(40 + 5 - 15) = 1.5$$

and from Equation 15-4

$$\text{Diameter of imaged area} = 30\ \mathrm{cm}/1.5 = 20\ \mathrm{cm}$$

Again, because magnification depends on distance, there is some image distortion with the converging collimator (Figure 15-8). Converging collimators are used primarily with cameras having large-area detectors to permit full utilization of the available detector area for imaging of small organs.

Converging collimators project an inverted, magnified image when the object is located between the convergence point and twice the convergence length of the collimator, and an inverted minified image beyond that distance; however, they are used rarely at distances beyond the convergence point.

4. Image Display and Recording Systems

Anger camera images generally are recorded on Polaroid or transparency film from a cathode ray tube (CRT) display (Chapter 5, Section G). Two basic types of CRTs are used. A *persistence* CRT displays light

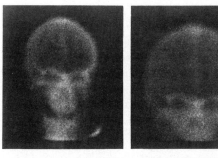

PARALLEL HOLE   CONVERGING
COLLIMATOR   COLLIMATOR

Fig. 15-8.   Example of geometric image distortions created by the converging collimator.

spots that do not fade immediately. The fading time of the spots can be adjusted from fractions of a second to several minutes using a *duration* control, and the brightness of the individual spots is adjusted using an *intensity* control. Thus the image on a persistence display is "built up" over an adjustable period of time. This is especially helpful to the camera operator during patient setup procedures; however, the image provided is of relatively poor quality (poor contrast and detail) and generally is not suitable for diagnostic interpretation.

More satisfactory images are obtained by photographic recording from a conventional, nonpersistence CRT. A specially designed photographic camera attaches directly to the CRT housing (Figure 15-2). To record an image, the camera shutter is opened, and the display is activated for a timed exposure lasting from fractions of a second to many minutes. Exposure time is determined on the basis of "preset time" or "preset count" settings on the control console. *Focus, astigmatism*, and *intensity* controls on the CRT are used to obtain sharply defined, round light spots of the proper brightness for photographic recording. Images may be recorded on transparency roll film (usually 35 mm or 70 mm sizes) or on Polaroid film. Roll-film cameras with automatic film-advancing mechanisms are available, permitting images to be obtained in rapid sequences (up to two or three frames per second).

Polaroid film is convenient to use because it requires no special processing facilities. The final image is available within 15–20 sec, so that the need for repeat images or additional images can be determined immediately. Polaroid film, however, is much more expensive than transparency roll film, and it is less suitable for rapid sequence imaging. It also has inferior photographic characteristics in comparison to transparency film. Figure 15-9 shows characteristic curves (optical density versus log exposure†) for Polaroid and transparency films that are commonly used in nuclear medicine.

Note that the Polaroid film is a *positive* film type, i.e., greater intensity of exposure results in a brighter (lower optical density) image, whereas the transparency film is a *negative* film type, for which greater exposure results in a darker (higher optical density) image. Polaroid film

---

† *Optical density* D refers to the fraction of incident light reflected (Polaroid film) or transmitted (transparency film), expressed on a logarithmic scale: $D = \log_{10}(I_0/I)$, where I_0 and I are incident and reflected or transmitted light intensities. Thus a film that reflects (or transmits) 10 percent of incident light has an optical density $D = \log_{10} 1.0/0.1 = \log_{10} 10 = 1.0$. *Exposure* in Figure 15-9 refers to the intensity of light to which the film is exposed. With normal lighting and viewing conditions, an optical density of 0 is perceived as clear or "bright", a density of 1 as "medium grey", and a density of 2 as "dark". Densities greater than about 2.5 are perceived as black or opaque, and usually require bright backlighting for visibility of details on transparency films.

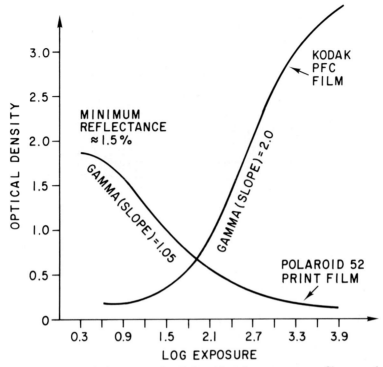

Fig. 15-9. Characteristic curves for Polaroid and transparency films used for Anger camera imaging. The limited optical density range of Polaroid film limits both its contrast (gamma, or slope of curve) and latitude (range of useful exposure values). [Courtesy Brent S. Baxter.]

is capable of displaying only a limited range of optical densities because Polaroid paper reflects at most 100 percent, and at least 1–2 percent, of incident light, giving it a useful range of only 1.7–2 optical density units. Transparency film, on the other hand, transmits from virtually 100 percent down to less than 0.1 percent of incident light, giving it a much wider density range (>3 optical density units). Most transparency films used for recording nuclear medicine images are *single-emulsion* types, i.e., coated with emulsion only on one side of the film base, to preserve image detail.

Because of its limited density range, Polaroid film has a quite limited *latitude* (range of exposures providing optical densities within the useful density range of the film). As a result, exposure time and CRT intensity adjustments generally are quite critical with Polaroid film. For this reason, Polaroid cameras used with Anger camera CRT displays often have three separate lenses, each with a different lens aperture opening, to

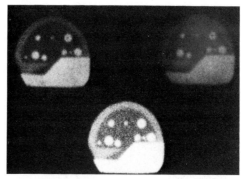

Fig. 15-10.   Example of images recorded with a triple-lens camera. Images of three different densities are obtained simultaneously through three different lens apertures.

provide simultaneously images of three different densities on a single film. Images are reduced in size as a result (Figure 15-10), but generally at least one of the three images is of satisfactory density.

Polaroid images also have less *contrast* than transparency film images, as can be seen from the relative slopes of the characteristic curves shown in Figure 15-9. (A steeper curve provides greater image contrast.) This statement may be somewhat surprising because, visually, Polaroid images have a very "contrasty" appearance; however, this is only another result of the limited dynamic range of Polaroid film. There is not much difference in reflected light between areas on a Polaroid image that look "completely black" versus "completely white," and this is what gives them a "contrasty" appearance.

Another class of image recording devices are the *multiformat* imaging systems. These devices record multiple images, also from a CRT display, on a single sheet of x-ray film, typically of 8 × 10 or 11 × 14 inch size. Usually, they stand separate from the camera control console (Figure 15-2).

Recently, multiformat cameras that use scanning laser beams to print the images under microprocessor control onto transparency film have become available. These cameras provide very high quality images, because of the capability for very precise control of the intensity and size of the laser beam; however, they are considerably more expensive than CRT-based cameras. They also require special red-sensitive film types to match the output spectrum of most lasers. These film types cannot be handled under the usual red or yellow darkroom safe-lights.

Multiformat systems can be programmed to record from one "full-size" image up to as many as 64 images of reduced size (in an 8 × 8 array)

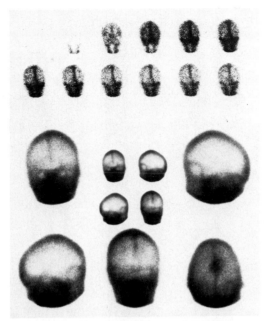

Fig. 15-11. Example of a series of brain images recorded on a single sheet of transparency film using a multiformat image recording device.

on a single sheet of film. A complete study, consisting, for example, of a rapid sequence series and several static images, may be recorded on one sheet of film (Figure 15-11). The photographic characteristics of x-ray film are similar to those of transparency roll film (Figure 15-9). Some users prefer to use single-emulsion film types rather than ordinary x-ray film, which has emulsion coated on both side of the film base, because the single-emulsion types provide clearer, sharper images. X-ray film and Polaroid film are comparable in cost; however, the ability to record many images on a single sheet gives the multiformat systems a cost advantage over Polaroid systems.

5. The Scanning Camera

A modification of the Anger camera, called the *scanning camera*, is used to obtain whole-body images on a single sheet of film. On a scanning camera, the detector passes linearly, head-to-foot, above (or below) the patient's body, recording and displaying a conventional Anger camera image on a CRT display. Alternatively, the patient support table may pass linearly in front of the camera detector (Figure 15-2). The image moves

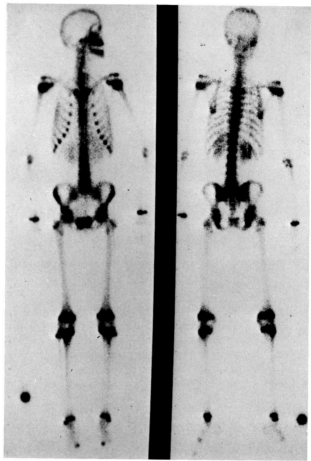

Fig. 15-12. Whole-body bone scan images obtained with a scanning Anger camera. Left: Anterior view. Right: Posterior view. Note "strip" artefact between adjacent scan passes. [Courtesy Paul E. Christian.]

from top-to-bottom of the CRT in synchrony with the motion of the detector head. Thus, a whole-body image can be recorded on a single film (Figure 15-12).

Some systems employ a parallel-hole collimator, which does not have quite a wide enough field-of-view to cover the entire width of the body. These systems generally use two or three adjacent scan passes to cover the required width. As illustrated by Figure 15-12, a "strip" artefact is sometimes seen on these images between the adjacent scan passes. Other systems employ a diverging collimator, which covers the entire width of the patient in a single scan but with some loss of resolution and collimator efficiency in comparison to the parallel-hole types (Chapter 16, Section C).

REFERENCES

The principles of the Anger camera are discussed in greater detail in the following:

Anger RT: The Anger scintillation camera-A review, in Rao DV, Chandra R, Graham MC (eds): Physics of Nuclear Medicine, Recent Advances, New York, American Institute of Physics, 1984, pp. 32–58

Rao DV, Chandra R, Graham MC (eds): Physics of Nuclear Medicine, Recent Advances, New York, American Institute of Physics, 1984, pp. 209–331

Richardson RL: Anger scintillation camera, in Rollo FD (ed): Nuclear Medicine Physics, Instrumentation, and Agents, St. Louis, C.V. Mosby Co., 1977, chap 6

Zimmerman RE: Recent developments in Anger cameras, in Rao DV, Chandra R, Graham MC (eds): Physics of Nuclear Medicine, Recent Advances, New York, American Institute of Physics, 1984, pp. 59–67

16
The Anger Camera: Performance Characteristics

The Anger camera is not capable of producing "perfect" images of a radionuclide distribution. There are certain inherent imperfections that arise from the performance characteristics of the detector and its associated electronic circuitry and of the collimator. Image artefacts also can be caused by malfunctions of various camera components. In this chapter, we describe the causes of these imperfections and their effects on Anger camera images.

A. LIMITATIONS OF THE DETECTOR SYSTEM AND ELECTRONICS

1. Image Nonlinearity

A basic problem arising in the detector and electronics is image *nonlinearity*. Straight-line objects appear as curved line images. An inward "bowing" of line images is called *pincushion distortion*; an outward bowing is called *barrel distortion* (Figure 16-1). Nonlinearities result when the X- and Y-position signals do not change linearly with displacement distance of a radiation source across the face of the detector. For example, when a source is moved from the edge of one of the PM tubes toward its center, the light collection efficiency of that PM tube increases more rapidly than the distance the source is moved. This causes the image of a line source crossing in front of a PM tube to be

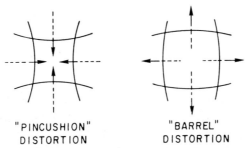

"PINCUSHION"   "BARREL"
DISTORTION   DISTORTION

Fig. 16-1. Appearance of straight-line objects with "pincushion" and "barrel" distortions.

bowed toward its center. The result is a characteristic pincushion distortion in areas of an Anger camera image lying directly in front of the PM tubes and barrel distortion between them. Differences in sensitivity among the PM tubes, nonuniformities in optical light guides, as well as PM-tube or electronic malfunctions, also can cause nonlinearities.

Figure 16-2 shows images of straight-line "test patterns" recorded on two different cameras to demonstrate the general appearance of Anger camera nonlinearities. On properly functioning cameras, the nonlinearities themselves (including the pincushion distortions in front of PM tubes) are barely perceptible and rarely interfere directly with image interpretation; however, they can have significant effects on image nonuniformities, as discussed below.

2. Image Nonuniformity

A more noticeable problem is image *nonuniformity*. Exposing the detector crystal to a uniform flux of radiation produces an image with small but noticeable nonuniformities in intensity, even with a properly

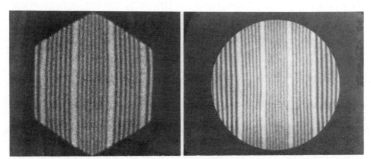

Fig. 16-2. Illustration of nonlinearities in images of straight-line test patterns obtained with an Anger camera. Image at left demonstrates barrel distortion; image at right demonstrates "wavy" line distortion.

FLOOD-FIELD IMAGES

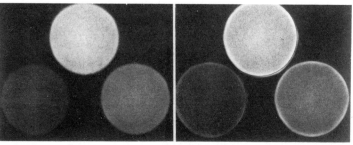

With Collimator attached   Without Collimator

Fig. 16-3. Flood-field images obtained by exposing the camera to a uniform radiation field. Image at left, with collimator attached, demonstrates a large-area "hot spot" near its center. Image at right, with collimator removed, demonstrates in addition the edge-packing artefact.

functioning camera (Figure 16-3). These variations may be equivalent to counting rate variations of ±10 percent or more.

There are two primary causes of Anger camera nonuniformities. The first is *nonuniform detection efficiency* arising mainly from small differences in the pulse-height spectrum for different PM tubes. It is virtually impossible to select and tune all of the PM tubes of an Anger camera to have exactly the same output response. If a fixed pulse-height window is used for all output pulses, this results in an apparent difference in detection efficiency due to differences in the "window fraction" for different areas of the crystal (Figure 16-4).

The second and more severe cause of nonuniformities are image *nonlinearities* described above. In areas of pincushion distortion events are crowded toward the center of the distortion, causing an apparent "hot spot," whereas in areas of barrel distortion events are pushed outward from the center, causing an apparent "cold spot" (Figure 16-1). Because of the characteristic pincushion distortions occurring in front of PM tubes, it is common to see a pattern of hot spots at the locations of the PM tubes on an otherwise uniform Anger camera image. Other causes of nonlinearities—e.g., instrument malfunctions—also can result in nonuniformities, as can nonuniform CRT display brightness, fingerprints on the CRT face, etc. Another characteristic nonuniformity is a bright ring around the edge of the image (Figure 16-3). The artefact, called *edge packing*, results from a somewhat greater light collection efficiency for events near the edge versus central regions of the detector crystal, as a result of internal reflections of scintillation light from the sides of the

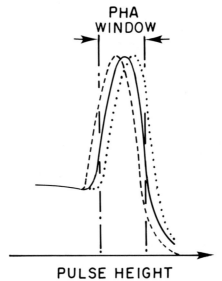

PULSE HEIGHT

Fig. 16-4. Pulse-height spectra for different PM tubes in Anger camera. If a fixed pulse-height window is used, different spectra can cause apparent differences in sensitivity in different parts of the detector, leading to image nonuniformities.

detector crystal back into the PM tubes near the edge. Also, for events occurring toward the center of the crystal, there are always PM tubes on either side of the event location, whereas at the edges of the crystal there are PM tubes only to one side. Thus events at the very edges are not distributed uniformly but are ''pulled'' toward the center, compounding the edge-packing artefact.

The part of the image demonstrating this artefact usually is masked on the CRT display and therefore is not a part of the useful imaging area. Typically, 5 cm or more of the detector diameter is eliminated by the mask. When specifying Anger camera detector diameter, it is important to distinguish between the physical diameter of the crystal and the diameter of the useful imaging area.

3. Nonuniformity Correction Techniques

Several techniques have been developed to correct or compensate for image nonuniformities. One approach that is used in some camera ''tuning'' procedures to partially correct for image nonuniformities is to adjust individual PM tube gains so that greater or lesser portions of the photopeak are included within the selected pulse-height analyzer window over different areas of the detector crystal. In effect, this adjusts detection efficiency to compensate for nonuniformities; however, if the camera is used with an energy window other than the one at which the PM tube gain adjustments were made, the portions of the photopeak that are included in different areas of the detector are changed, and striking nonuniformities may appear (Figure 16-5). Because of this, it is advisable to check for image nonuniformities before employing ''offset'' or other nonstandard energy window settings on an Anger camera.

Some cameras incorporate microprocessor-based computer circuitry to correct for image nonuniformities. With these cameras, a test image of a uniform radiation field, obtained prior to patient studies, is divided into a matrix of small, square elements (e.g. 64 × 64 elements) and stored in digital format (counts/area) in the microprocessor device. The test image is used to generate a matrix of ''correction factors'', similar to the approach employed with Anger camera computer systems (Chapter 21), except that the microprocessor performs the corrections in ''real time'' as the image data are collected, rather than by post-processing of the image.

In one scheme, the test image is first normalized relative to the image matrix element having the smallest number of counts, i.e., the ''coldest'' matrix element in the image. This element is assigned to a relative intensity of 100. Other elements are assigned greater values, depending on their relative intensities in the uniform field image. In subsequent patient

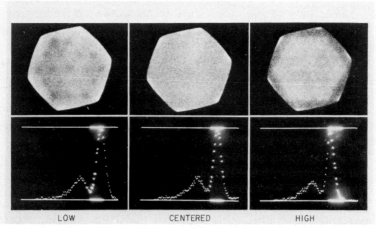

Fig. 16-5. Image nonuniformities introduced on some Anger cameras by the use of offset windows.

imaging procedures, a certain fraction of the counts recorded in each element are thrown out, depending on the relative intensity of that area in the test image. For example, if an element has relative intensity 110, 10 of every 100 counts recorded in that element in patient imaging procedures are not displayed. This is refered to as "count skimming". A variation of this technique is to "add" counts in "cold" areas, by double exposing dots on the display for a certain fraction of the counts recorded. Yet another approach to compensate for nonuniformities is to adjust the duration of the unblanking pulse and hence of the brightness of the light flashes for individual events on the CRT display.

Each of the above methods is essentially a cosmetic approach to correcting Anger camera nonuniformities. They do nothing to correct the principal underlying cause, i.e., camera nonlinearities. Recently, with the development of economical microprocessor circuits, it has become practical to attack the nonlinearity problem as well. In the most advanced technique, the camera is provided with a set of microprocessors that are used to store correction matrices for regional differences in pulse-height spectra and for position distortions. The correction matrices are programmed into the microprocessor using calibration measurements performed at the factory before installation of the camera. The calibrations involve precise measurements using line sources of pulse-height spectra for individual PM tubes and of position distortions over the entire area of the detector crystal. In subsequent imaging procedures the correction matrices are used on an event-by-event basis to compensate for regional differences in sensitivity by adjusting either the system gain or the pulse-height window, and to compensate for nonlinearities by accurately repositioning each event.

In comparison to count skimming/adding and other cosmetic corrections the pulse-height and position correction methods described above have two important advantages. First, they provide a quantitatively correct image, in which the number of events recorded per unit area is represented accurately over the entire image. By comparison, count skimming/adding results in an inaccurate image because events are superficially added or subtracted from different areas of the image. Count skimming/adding can transform a camera with 2–3% sensitivity variations into one with 8–9% variations in order to achieve the appearance of "uniformity"; thus, the "corrected" image may be inaccurate for quantitative studies.

The second advantage of using the pulse-height/position and correction method is that, once obtained, the correction matrices are relatively stable with time and applicable for all radionuclides and imaging conditions, whereas the count skimming/adding techniques require different correction matrices for different radionuclides, different energy windows, different scattering conditions, etc.

Improved techniques for nonlinearity and nonuniformity corrections provide not only more uniform and more accurate images, but also permit greater design flexibility for the camera detector. This has contributed directly to improved intrinsic resolution, as discussed in the next section.

4. Intrinsic Spatial Resolution Limits

Another limitation of the Anger camera is the detail or *spatial resolution* of the images that it produces. Sharp edges or small, point objects produce blurred rather than sharply defined images. Part of the blurring arises from collimator characteristics, discussed in Section B, and part arises in the detector and positioning electronics. The limit of spatial resolution achievable by the detector and the electronics is called the *intrinsic resolution* of the camera.

Intrinsic resolution is limited primarily by two factors. The first is *multiple scattering* of photons within the detector. If a photon undergoes Compton scattering within the detector crystal and the residual scattered photon also is detected but at some distance away, the two events are recorded as a single event at a location somewhere between them. This is not a serious cause of degraded resolution at photon energies used in nuclear medicine. Anger has calculated that less than 10% of photons are misplaced by more than 2.5 mm due to multiple scattering events at 662 keV (1). For ^{99m}Tc (140 keV), the photofraction is even larger and the effect is negligibly small.

The primary cause of limited intrinsic resolution is *statistical fluctuation in the distribution of light photons* between PM tubes from one scintillation event to the next. The problem is exactly analogous to the statistical fluctuations observed in radioactive decay, discussed in Chapter 6. If a certain PM tube records, on the average, N light photons from scintillation events occurring at a certain location in the detector crystal, the actual number recorded from one event to the next varies with a standard deviation given by $\sqrt{N}$. Thus if a very fine beam of γ rays is directed at the detector, the light flashes appearing on the CRT screen are not all placed at precisely the same location but are distributed over a certain area, the size of that area depending on the magnitude of these statistical fluctuations.

Methods for measuring and characterizing spatial resolution are discussed in Chapter 18. One method is to obtain images of "bar patterns," which consist of strips of lead separated from each other by spaces equal to the widths of the strips. Images are obtained by exposing the detector crystal through the bar pattern with a uniform radiation field,

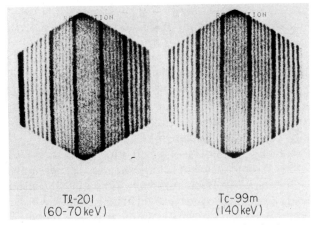

Fig. 16-6. Demonstration of Anger camera intrinsic resolution limits using a bar pattern and ^{201}Tl and ^{99m}Tc radiation sources.

e.g., a sheet source of radioactivity or a point source at a distance. The intrinsic resolution limits of modern Anger cameras permit them to resolve 3–5 mm bar patterns—i.e., lead strips 3–5 mm wide, separated from each other by 3–5 mm intervals—for ^{99m}Tc (140 keV) radiation (Figure 16-6).

Intrinsic resolution also depends on detector crystal thickness, because with thicker detectors there is greater spreading of scintillation light before it reaches the PM tubes. This is the primary reason why Anger cameras use relatively thin detectors in comparison to many other NaI(Tl) systems.

Intrinsic resolution becomes worse with decreasing γ-ray energy because lower-energy γ rays produce fewer light photons per scintillation event, and smaller numbers of light photons result in larger relative statistical fluctuations in their distribution (Chapter 6, Section B.1). As a rule of thumb, intrinsic resolution is proportional to $1/\sqrt{E}$, where E is the γ-ray energy, because the number of scintillation light photons produced, N, is proportional to E and the relative statistical fluctuations in their distribution are proportional to $1/\sqrt{N}$. This causes noticeably greater blurring at lower γ-ray energies (Figure 16-6).

Intrinsic resolution improves with increased light collection and detection efficiency of scintillation light. Modern cameras are substantially improved over earlier versions in this regard because of the use of more efficient PM tubes and of better techniques for optical coupling between the detector crystal and the PM tubes. The use of greater numbers of smaller PM tubes (e.g., 37 tubes of 2 inch diameter versus 19 tubes of 3 inch diameter), and improved electronics also have contributed to this improvement.

Improvements in camera uniformity described in Section A.3 above have contributed directly to improvements in intrinsic resolution. Earlier camera designs used relatively thick light pipes and large-diameter PM tubes to achieve satisfactory uniformity at the expense of degraded intrinsic resolution. This limitation has been overcome with effective nonuniformity correction techniques. Camera designs now use thinner light pipes and large numbers of small PM tubes that provide more accurate determination of event locations and, hence, better intrinsic resolution. The same developments have permitted the use of thinner detector crystals, which also have provided improved intrinsic resolution. Further improvements in intrinsic resolution may be possible, particularly by increasing light collection efficiency and PM-tube sensitivity. Another potential future development is the "all-digital" camera, in which the location of each event will be determined by digitizing and analyzing the individual signals from each PM tube. By carefully mapping the response of the camera and using microprocessor-based electronics, it should be possible to determine the location of each event to an accuracy limited only by the statistics of the light photons collected. However, significant improvements beyond about 2mm FWHM for ^{99m}Tc will be difficult to achieve, due to the ultimate limitation of the light photon yield of NaI(Tl).

5. Detection Efficiency

The Anger camera employs a sodium iodide crystal that is relatively thin in comparison to most other sodium iodide systems used in nuclear medicine, 6–12 mm versus 2–5 cm for probe counting systems, scanners, etc. As a result, the *detection efficiency* of the Anger camera detector is somewhat less than would be desirable at higher γ-ray energies. Figure 16-7 shows photopeak counting efficiency versus γ-ray energy for the Anger camera detector and for thicker NaI(Tl) crystals. The Anger camera is nearly 100 percent efficient for energies up to about 100 keV, but then shows a rather marked decrease in efficiency with increasing energy. At about 500 keV, the Anger camera is only 10–20 percent efficient at converting incident γ rays into photopeak pulses.

Decreasing detection efficiency (as well as increasing collimator septal penetration; Section B.2) is a limiting factor on Anger camera performance at higher γ-ray energies. Deteriorating intrinsic resolution is a limiting factor at lower energies. Because of these factors, the optimal γ-ray energy range is ~100–200 keV for the Anger camera.

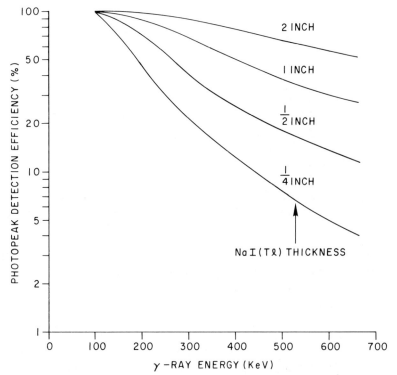

Fig. 16-7. Photopeak detection efficiency versus γ-ray energy for NaI(Tl) detectors of different thicknesses. [Adapted from ref. 1: Anger HO: Radioisotope cameras, in Hine GJ (ed): Instrumentation in Nuclear Medicine (vol 1). New York, Academic Press, p. 506 1967.

6. Problems at High Counting Rates

The Anger camera, like any other sodium iodide counting system, experiences counting losses at high counting rates. The principle cause of counting losses is *pulse pileup* (Figure 5-6)—that is, two γ-ray events are detected so close together in time that they are perceived by the electronic circuitry to be a single event. If one (or both) of the events was originally a valid photopeak event, the combined apparent energy of the two events may exceed the acceptable limit of the selected energy window, and thus both events are rejected.

Pulse pileup can occur between any two events in the pulse-height spectrum. Thus system counting losses are determined by total-spectrum counting rates. Most Anger cameras behave as paralyzable systems (Chapter 12, Section C). The apparent deadtime for a selected energy window depends on the *window fraction*, that is, the fraction of the total

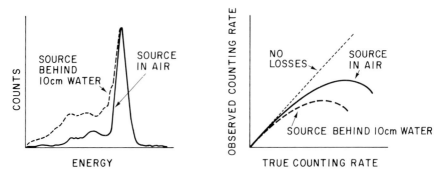

Fig. 16-8.   Effect of scattered radiation on counting losses. Scattered radiation decreases the window fraction recorded with a photopeak window (left), thus causing an apparent increase in deadtime counting losses (right).

spectrum counting rate occurring within that window. The smaller the window fraction, the larger the apparent deadtime. Thus the deadtime is longer when a photopeak window is used than when a "full spectrum" window is used. The deadtime is longer when scattering material is present around the radiation source than when no scattering material is present because scattered radiation decreases the window fraction (Figure 16-8). When specifying Anger camera deadtime it is important to note the conditions of measurement. Deadtime values as small as 1–2 μsec may be obtained in the absence of scattering material with a full-spectrum window; however, under clinically realistic conditions (^{99m}Tc source in scattering material, 20 percent photopeak window) deadtimes of 5–10 μsec are more typical. For a deadtime of 10 μsec, counting losses are about 10 percent for a counting rate of 10^4 cps. Deadtime losses are not serious in most static imaging studies, but they may be important in certain high-counting-rate dynamic studies, e.g., first-pass cardiac flow studies with counting rates up to 5×10^4 cps.

Pulse pileup also causes image distortions at high counting rates. Two separate events occurring simultaneously in the Compton portion of the spectrum, which individually would occur below the energy window and be rejected, may be added to form a single photopeak event by the camera electronics. This produces a single event on the image display at a location somewhere between the locations of the two individual events. Figure 16-9 shows images of two point sources obtained at high counting rates, demonstrating pulse pileup events. The general effect of the pulse pileup artefact is to cause a loss of image contrast and detail, as illustrated by Figure 16-10. Image distortions as well as counting-rate losses should be considered when evaluating the performance characteristics of an Anger camera at high counting rates. The images in Figure 16-10 also

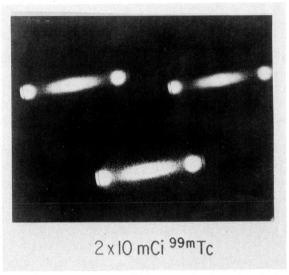

$$2 \times 10 \text{ mCi } ^{99m}\text{Tc}$$

Fig. 16-9. Images of two ^{99m}Tc point sources of relatively high activities. Events appearing in the band between the two point sources are mispositioned pileup events.

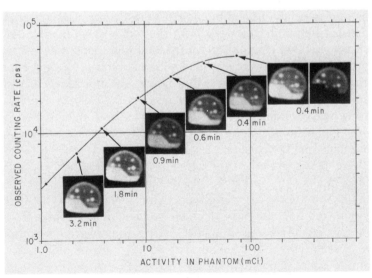

Fig. 16-10. Demonstration of pileup effects on image quality. At very high counting rates there is a loss of image contrast, which can be restored by shielding useless high-activity areas from the detector (top righthand image). Times required to record 1.2×10^6 counts are indicated.

demonstrate the improvement in image quality that can be obtained when high-activity areas outside the imaging area of interest are shielded from the detector (e.g., with a thin sheet of lead).

Recent design improvements have improved the performance characteristics of the Anger camera at high counting rates. Pileup rejection circuits (Chapter 5, Section B.3) are used to minimize pileup artefacts. It should be noted that whereas this improves image quality, it also provides an apparently *longer* deadtime and *smaller* maximum achievable counting rate. This is because a camera without pileup rejection circuits will record and display *mispositioned pileup events* that in fact should *not* be recorded (2). Comparisons of deadtime values between different cameras should be made with this consideration in mind.

Camera deadtime can be shortened by the use of *analog buffers*, or *derandomizers*. These are electronic circuits that "hold" a voltage level or pulse from one circuit component, e.g., an amplifier, until the next circuit in the pulse-processing sequence, e.g., the pulse-height analyzer, is ready to receive it. It also is possible to shorten the apparent deadtime of the camera by shortening the effective charge integration time for the output signals from the PM tubes. This can be accomplished by differentiating the output voltage pulses from the PM tubes (see Figures 5-3 and 5-4); however, this also has the effect of decreasing the amount of signal available for determining event location. This is equivalent to decreasing the amount of light collected by the PM tubes, and causes a degradation of intrinsic resolution. Other means for shortening deadtime are to bypass the pileup rejection circuits and the nonuniformity and other correction circuits. Some cameras are provided with an optional "high count rate" mode of operation in which these techniques are activated by a switch on the control panel. This mode is intended specifically for applications requiring high counting rates, e.g., first-pass cardiac studies. For routine imaging applications, "normal mode" operation is used to obtain the desired high-quality images.

Table 16-1 summarizes the performance characteristics at different counting rates of one commercially manufactured Anger camera. They represent state-of-the-art performance for mid 1980s. The observed maximum counting rate, as well as the incident counting rate producing 20% losses, usually are used to characterize counting rate performance. Values given for flood-field uniformity refer to "integral" uniformity, i.e., magnitude of local nonuniformities relative to average counts/area for entire detector. CFOV refers to central portion of detector crystal. UFOV refers to entire useful detector area, excluding edge-packing areas. The data are for a 75–PM tube camera, with 6 mm thick crystal, and 38.7 cm UFOV.

Table 16-1
Representative Performance Characteristics Relating to
Counting Rate for an Anger Camera*

Parameter	Worst-Case Value		Comments
Incident count rate producing 20% loss	140 Kcps		"High count rate" switch on, 20% analyzer window
Observed maximum counting rate	200 Kcps		
	CFOV	**UFOV**	
Intrinsic spatial resolution (FWHM)	<3.6 mm	<3.7 mm <3.9 mm	At low count rate At 75 Kcps
Intrinsic flood-field uniformity	±4.0%	±5.0%	

*See text for definitions of terms.
Adapted with permission from The Orbital Gamma Camera Systems Data, Siemens, Inc.

B. DESIGN AND PERFORMANCE CHARACTERISTICS OF PARALLEL-HOLE COLLIMATORS

1. Basic Limitations in Collimator Performance

The collimator is a "weak link" for the performance of an Anger camera system, as indeed it is in any nuclear medicine imaging system employing the principles of *absorptive collimation. Collimator efficiency*, defined as the fraction of γ rays striking the collimator that actually pass through it to project the γ-ray image onto the detector, is typically only a few percent or less. *Collimator resolution*, which refers to the sharpness or detail of the γ-ray image projected onto the detector, also is rather poor, generally worse than the intrinsic resolution of the camera detector and electronics.

Because it is a limiting factor in camera system performance, it is important that the collimator be designed carefully. Poor design can result only in poorer overall performance. Design considerations for parallel-hole collimators will be discussed in this section. Design characteristics for converging and diverging collimators are similar to those of the parallel-hole type. Design characteristics of pinhole collimators will not be discussed in detail here but are described in references listed at the end of the chapter. The analysis to be presented for parallel-hole collimators is similar to that presented by Anger in reference 1, which may be consulted for a more detailed discussion.

2. Septal Thickness

A primary consideration in collimator design is to ensure that *septal penetration* by γ rays crossing from one collimator hole into another is negligibly small. This is essential if an accurate γ-ray image is to be projected by the collimator onto the camera detector. No thickness of septal material is sufficient to stop *all* γ rays, so the usual criteria is to accept some reasonably small level of septal penetration, e.g., ~5 percent.

The required septal thickness may be determined by analysis of Figure 16-11. The shortest path length for γ rays to travel from one hole to the next is w. Septal thickness t is related to w, and to the length l and diameter d of the collimator holes, by[1]

$$t = 2dw/(l - w) \qquad (16\text{-}1)$$

If septal penetration is to be less than 5 percent, the transmission factor for the thickness w must be

$$e^{-\mu w} \lesssim 0.05 \qquad (16\text{-}2)$$

where μ is the linear attenuation coefficient of the septal material. Since $e^{-3} \sim 0.05$, this implies

$$\mu w \gtrsim 3 \qquad (16\text{-}3)$$
$$w > 3/\mu \qquad (16\text{-}4)$$

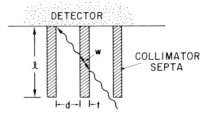

Fig. 16-11.   Minimum path length w for a γ ray passing through the collimator septa from one hole to the next depends on length l and diameter d of the collimator holes and on septal thicknesses t.

and thus

$$t \gtrsim \frac{6d/\mu}{1 - (3/\mu)} \qquad (16\text{-}5)$$

It is desirable that septal thickness t be as small as possible so that the collimator septa obstruct the smallest possible area of detector surface and collimator efficiency is maximized. This objective is realized by using a material with a large value of μ for the collimator septa. Materials of high atomic number Z and high density ρ are preferred. Lead ($Z = 82$, $\rho = 11.34$ g/cm^3) is the material of choice for reasons of cost and availability; however, other materials, including tantalum ($Z = 73$, $\rho = 16.6$ g/cm^3), tungsten ($Z = 74$, $\rho = 19.4$ g/cm^3), and even gold ($Z = 79$, $\rho = 19.3$ g/cm^3) have been employed in experimental applications.

Attenuation coefficients of heavy elements depend strongly on γ-ray energy in the nuclear medicine energy range (Chapter 9, Section B.1). Thus the required septal thickness also depends strongly on the γ-ray energy for which the collimator is designed to be used. Commercially available collimators are categorized according to the maximum γ-ray energy for which their septal thickness is considered to be adequate. *Low-energy collimators* generally have an upper limit of about 150 keV and *medium-energy collimators* about 400 keV. High-energy collimators (e.g., 1 MeV) are not available commercially except by special order.

Example 16-1.
Calculate the septal thickness required for low-energy (150 keV) and medium-energy (400 keV) lead collimators having hole diameters 0.25 cm and lengths 2.5 cm.

Answer.
The linear attenuation coefficient of lead at 150 keV is $\mu_l = 1.89$ cm^2/g $\times$ 11.34 g/cm^3 = 21.43 cm^{-1} and at 400 keV is $\mu_l = 0.22$ cm^2/g $\times$ 11.34 g/cm^3 = 2.49 cm^{-1} (Appendix D). Therefore from Equation 16-5 for the low-energy collimator

$$t \gtrsim \frac{6 \times 0.25/21.43}{2.5 - \dfrac{3}{21.43}}$$

$$\gtrsim 0.030 \text{ cm}$$

and for the medium-energy collimator

$$t \gtrsim \frac{6 \times 0.25/2.49}{2.5 - \dfrac{3}{2.49}}$$

$$\gtrsim 0.465 \text{ cm}$$

Thickness needed for low-energy collimators are only a few tenths of a millimeter, which is in the range of lead "foil" thicknesses and approaches the limits of lead thicknesses that can be used without loss of necessary mechanical strength. Indeed, low-energy collimators generally are quite fragile, and their septa can be damaged easily by mechanical abuse (dropping, stacking on sharp objects, etc.). Medium-energy collimators require substantially greater thicknesses, typically a few millimeters of lead.

Low-energy γ-ray emitters (e.g., ^{99m}Tc, 140 keV) can be imaged using medium-energy collimators. This is done, however, with an unnecessary sacrifice of collimator efficiency because the collimator septa are unnecessarily thick. (See Table 16-2 for comparative efficiencies of low- and medium-energy collimators.) Low-energy collimators are used whenever possible to obtain maximum collimator efficiency. When choosing a collimator, however, one must consider not only the energy of the γ rays to be imaged but also the energies of any other γ rays emitted by the radionuclide of interest or by other radionuclides that may be present as well, e.g., residual activity from another study or radionuclide impurities. Higher-energy γ rays may be recorded by Compton downscatter into a lower-energy analyzer window. If the collimator septa are too thin, the collimator may be virtually transparent to higher-energy γ rays, causing a relatively intense "foggy" background image to be superimposed on the desired image, with a resulting loss of image contrast. Whether or not a low-energy collimator can be used when higher-energy γ rays are present depends on the energy and intensity of those emissions and requires experimental evaluation in specific cases.

3. Geometry of Collimator Holes

Collimator performance also is affected by the geometry of the collimator holes, specifically, their *shape, length*, and *diameter*.

The preferred hole shape, to maximize the exposed area of detector surface for a given septal thickness, is round or hexagonal, with the holes arranged in a close-packed hexagonal array. Square and triangular holes also have been used.

Collimator hole length and diameter affect strongly both collimator resolution and collimator efficiency. Collimator resolution R_c is defined as the full width at half-maximum (FWHM) of the radiation profile from a point or line source of radiation projected by the collimator onto the detector (Figure 16-12). This profile is also called the *point* or *line spread function* (PSF or LSF). Collimator resolution R_c is given by†

$$R_c \approx d(l_e + b)/l_e \qquad (16\text{-}6)$$

where b is the distance from the radiation source to the collimator, and d is the diameter and $l_e = l - 2\mu^{-1}$ the "effective length" of the collimator holes (Figure 16-12). Here μ is the linear attenuation coefficient of the collimator material. The effective length of the collimator holes is somewhat less than their actual length due to septal penetration. From Example 16-1 it can be seen that for low-energy collimators (150 keV), the difference between effective and actual length is about 0.1 cm whereas for medium-energy collimators it is about 0.8 cm.

---

† It should be noted that some versions of Equation 16-6 include additional correction terms involving the thickness of the detector crystal, reflecting the fact that the image actually is formed at some depth within the detector crystal. Because photons of different energies penetrate to different average depths within the crystal, the correction actually is photon-energy dependent, a point not noted by most authors. The correction is small and for simplicity is omitted from Equation 16-6, as well as from Equations 16-10 and 16-13 for the converging and diverging collimators presented later in this chapter.

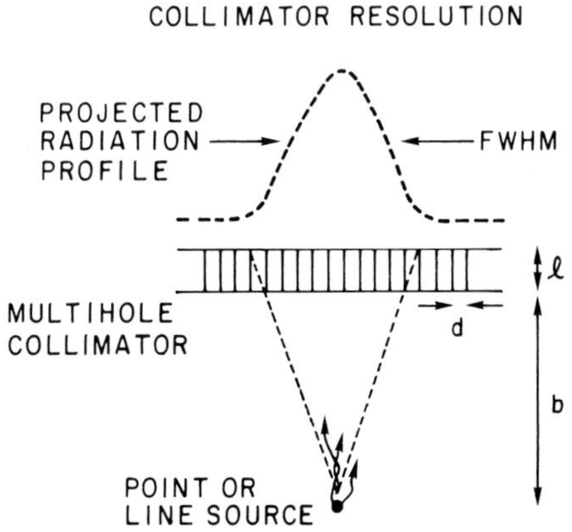

COLLIMATOR RESOLUTION

Fig. 16-12. Radiation profile (point or line spread function, PSF or LSF) for a parallel-hole collimator. The FWHM (full width at half-maximum) of the profile is used to characterize collimator resolution.

Example 16-2.
Calculate the resolution (FWHM) of the low-energy collimator described in Example 16-1, at source depths $b = 0$ and $b = 10$ cm, assuming it has a septal thickness of 0.03 cm.

Answer.
The effective length of the collimator is

$$l_e = 2.5 \text{ cm} - (2/21.43) \text{ cm}$$

$$\approx 2.4 \text{ cm}$$

Thus, for $b = 0$

$$R_c \approx 0.25(2.4 + 0)/2.4 \text{ cm}$$

$$\approx 0.25 \text{ cm}$$

and at $b = 10$ cm

$$R_c \approx 0.25(2.4 + 10)/2.4 \text{ cm}$$

$$\approx 1.3 \text{ cm}$$

This example illustrates the strong dependence of collimator resolution on source distance from the collimator.

Collimator efficiency g, defined as the fraction of γ rays passing through the collimator per γ ray emitted by the source, is given by

$$g \approx K^2(d/l_e)^2[d^2/(d + t)^2] \qquad (16\text{-}7)$$

where t is septal thickness and K is a constant that depends on hole shape ($\sim$0.24 for round holes in a hexagonal array, $\sim$0.26 for hexagonal holes in a hexagonal array, $\sim$0.28 for square holes in a square array)[1]

Equation 16-7 applies to a source *in air* and assumes no attenuation of radiation by intervening body tissues.

Several aspects of Equations 16-6 and 16-7 should be noted. First, resolution improves as the ratio of hole diameter to effective length (d/l_e') is made smaller. Long, narrow holes provide image with the best resolution; however, collimator efficiency decreases approximately as the *square* of the ratio of hole diameter to length, $(d/l_e')^2$. Thus an approximate relationship between collimator resolution R_c and efficiency g is

$$g \propto R_c^2 \qquad (16\text{-}8)$$

Example 16-3.
Calculate the efficiency g of the collimator described in Examples 16-1 and 16-2, assuming it has hexagonal holes in an hexagonal array.

Answer.
For hexagonal holes in a hexagonal array, $K = 0.26$

$$g \approx (0.26)^2 \ (0.25/2.4)^2 \ [(0.25)^2 \ / \ (0.25 + 0.03)^2]$$

$$\approx (0.0676) \times (0.0109) \times (0.797)$$

$$\approx 5.85 \times 10^{-4} \ \text{(photons transmitted/photons emitted)}$$

This example illustrates the relatively small fraction of emitted γ rays that are transmitted by a typical Anger camera collimator.

Therefore, for a given septal thickness, collimator resolution is improved only at the expense of decreased collimator efficiency, and vice versa. The implications of this important tradeoff in collimator design are discussed further in Chapter 18, Section C.2.

Equation 16-7 also demonstrates the effect of septal thickness on efficiency. As noted in Section B.1, medium-energy collimators have lower efficiencies than low-energy collimators because of their greater septal thicknesses.

In addition to providing low- and medium-energy collimators, manufacturers of Anger camera systems also provide a selection of collimators with different combinations of resolution and efficiency. Those with good resolution but poor efficiency generally are described as "high resolution" collimators, whereas those with the opposite characteristics are described as "high sensitivity" collimators. Those with characteristics intermediate to the extremes are referred to as "general purpose," "all purpose," or by other similar names.

Equation 16-6 indicates that collimator resolution becomes poorer as source-to-collimator distance b increases. Thus structures closest to the collimator are imaged with sharpest detail. Figure 16-13 shows graphically the relationship between collimator resolution and source-to-collimator distance for three different collimators provided by one commercial manufacturer. Typically, collimator resolution deteriorates by a factor of 2 at a distance of 4–5 cm from the collimator.

On the other hand, according to Equation 16-7, collimator efficiency for a source in air is independent of source-to-collimator distance b. This rather surprising result is obtained provided the counting rate for the entire detector area is measured. The reason for this is illustrated by Figure 16-14. As the source is moved farther away from the collimator, the efficiency with which radiation is transmitted through any one collimator hole decreases in proportion to $1/b^2$ (inverse-square law), but the number of holes through which radiation can pass to reach the detector increases in proportion to b^2. The two effects cancel each other, with the result that total counting rate—and thus collimator efficiency—does not change with source-to-collimator distance. Another illustration of this effect is shown in Figure 16-15. As source-to-collimator distance increases, the maximum height of the PSF or LSF decreases, but the width increases (and resolution becomes poorer), so that the total area under the curve (total detector counting rate) does not change.

Invariance of collimator efficiency with source-to-collimator distance applies to point sources, line sources, and uniform sheet sources in air with parallel-hole collimators; however, it applies only to uniform sheet sources with converging, diverging, or pinhole collimators (Section C). When the source is embedded at different depths in the patient, attenuation effects also must be considered. Septal penetration and scatter of photons from the walls of the collimator holes also are not considered in the above analysis.

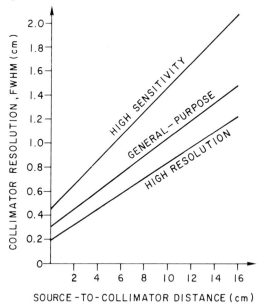

Fig. 16-13. Collimator resolution versus source-to-collimator distance for three different collimators. [Adapted from ref. 4: Hine GJ, Paras D, Warr CP: Recent advances in gamma-camera imaging. Proc SPIE 152:123, 1978, permission of the author and SPIE.]

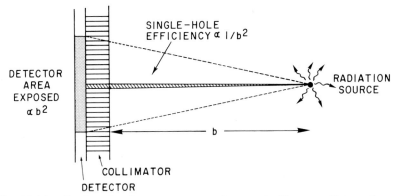

Fig. 16-14. Explanation for constant counting rate (collimator efficiency) versus source-to-collimator distance for a point source in air and a parallel-hole collimator. Efficiency for a single hole decreases as $1/b^2$, but number of holes passing radiation (area of detector exposed) increases as b^2.

Table 16-2 summarizes the performance characteristics of a number of collimators provided by one commercial manufacturer. Collimator resolution is the FWHM for a source at 10 cm from the face of the collimator. Collimator efficiency g refers to the relative number of γ rays transmitted by the collimator per γ ray emitted by the source. Note that the approximate relationship between collimator efficiency and resolution

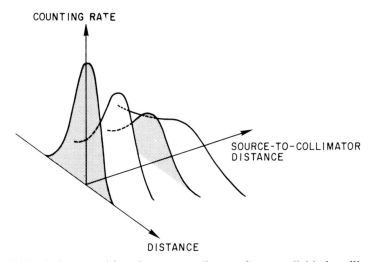

Fig. 16-15. Point spread functions versus distance for a parallel-hole collimator. Area under curve is proportional to collimator efficiency and does not change with distance.

given by Equation 16-8 is verified by these data. Note also the relatively small values of collimator efficiency.

4. System Resolution

The sharpness of images recorded with an Anger camera is limited by several factors, including intrinsic resolution, collimator resolution, scattered radiation, and septal penetration. In terms of the FWHM of a point or line spread function, the most important factors are the intrinsic resolution R_i of the detector and electronics and the collimator resolution R_c. The combined effect of these two factors is to produce a *system resolution* R_s that is somewhat worse than either one alone. System resolution R_s (FWHM) is given by

$$R_s = \sqrt{R_i^2 + R_c^2} \tag{16-9}$$

Because collimator resolution depends on source-to-collimator distance, system resolution also depends on this parameter. Figure 16-16 shows system resolution versus source-to-collimator distance for a typical parallel-hole collimator and different values of intrinsic resolution. At a distance of 5–10 cm (typical depth of organs inside the body), *system resolution* is much poorer than intrinsic resolution and is determined primarily by *collimator resolution*. There are significant differences between system resolutions for cameras having substantially different intrinsic resolutions (e.g., 4 mm versus 8 mm), but the difference in system resolutions for cameras having small differences in intrinsic resolutions (e.g., 4 mm versus 5 mm) is minor and not clinically

Table 16-2
Performance Characteristics of Some Typical
Commercially Manufactured Parallel-Hole Collimators

Collimator Type	Suggested Maximum Energy (keV)	Efficiency g	Resolution R (FWHM at 10 cm)
Low energy, high resolution	150	1.84×10^{-4}	7.4 mm
Low energy, general purpose	150	2.68×10^{-4}	9.1 mm
Low energy, high sensitivity	150	5.74×10^{-4}	13.2 mm
Medium energy, high sensitivity	400	1.72×10^{-4}	13.4 mm

Adapted from ref. 3: Hine GJ, Erickson JJ: Advances in scintigraphic instruments, in Hine GJ, Sorenson JA (eds): Instrumentation in Nuclear Medicine (vol 2). New York, Academic Press, 1974. With permission.

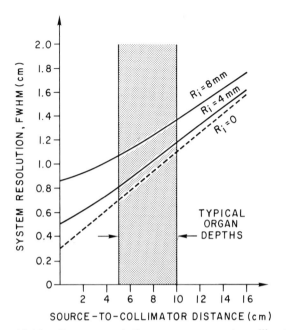

Fig. 16-16. System resolution versus source-to-collimator distance for a typical parallel-hole collimator and for different values of intrinsic resolution. At most typical organ depths, system resolution is determined primarily by collimator resolution.

significant. Small differences in intrinsic resolution may be apparent on bar pattern images or on images of very superficial structures in the patient, but they usually are not apparent on images of deeper-lying structures.

System resolution also is degraded by scattered radiation. This is discussed in Chapter 18, Section B. The method for combining component resolutions to determine system resolution also is discussed in Appendix G.

C. PERFORMANCE CHARACTERISTICS OF CONVERGING, DIVERGING, AND PINHOLE COLLIMATORS

Equations for collimator resolution, R_c, and efficiency, g, for converging, diverging and pinhole collimators are as follows:

CONVERGING COLLIMATOR

$$R_c \approx [d(l'_e + b)/l'_e][1/\cos\theta][1 - (l'_e/2)/(f + l'_e)] \tag{16-10}$$

$$g \approx K^2(d/l'_e)^2[d^2/(d + t)^2][f^2/(f - b)^2] \tag{16-11}$$

$$l'_e \approx (l - 2\mu^{-1})/\cos\theta \tag{16-12}$$

DIVERGING COLLIMATOR

$$R_c \approx [d(l'_e + b)/l'_e][1/\cos\theta][1+(l'_e/2f)] \tag{16-13}$$

$$g \approx K^2(d/l'e)^2[d^2/(d + t)^2][f + l)/(f + l + b)] \tag{16-14}$$

PINHOLE COLLIMATOR

$$R_c \approx d_e(l + b)/l \tag{16-15}$$

$$g \approx d_e \cos^3\theta/16b^2 \tag{16-16}$$

$$d_e = \sqrt{d[d + 2\mu^{-1}\tan(\alpha/2)]} \tag{16-17}$$

The parameters in these equations are as shown in Figure 16-17. For the pinhole collimator, d_e is the "effective" pinhole diameter, accounting for penetration of the edges of the pinhole aperture. The equations for collimator resolution R_c refer to the equivalent FWHM of the point- or

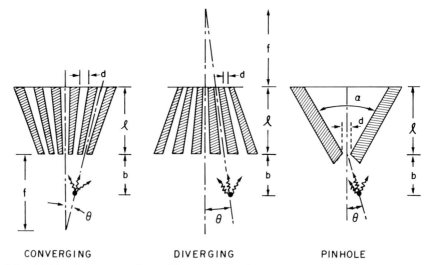

CONVERGING   DIVERGING   PINHOLE

Fig. 16-17. Parameters for collimator resolution, R (FWHM), and efficiency, g (transmitted/emitted photons), for Equations (16-17). Adapted with permission from Medical Physics Data Book, Padikal TN, Fivozinsky SP (eds). Washington DC, National Bureau of Standards, 1982, pp. 48–55.

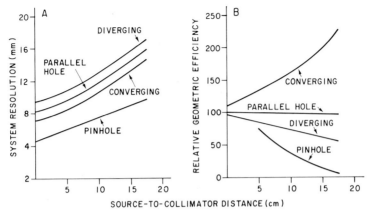

Fig. 16-18.   Performance characteristics (left, system resolution; right, point-source geometric efficiency in air) versus source-to-collimator distance for four different types of Anger camera collimators. [From Rollo FD, Harris CC: Factors affecting image formation, in Rollo FD (ed): Nuclear Medicine Physics, Instrumentation, and Agents. St. Louis, C.V. Mosby Co., 1977. Modified from Moyer RA: J Nucl. Med. *15:*59, 1974].

line-source spread function, corrected for magnification or minification of the image by the collimator (Equations 15-3, 15-5, and 15-6). Thus, if the collimator projects a profile with a 2 cm FWHM measured on the detector and the image magnification factor is ×2, the equivalent FWHM in the imaged plane is 1 cm.

The equations above may be compared with Equations 16-6 and 16-7 for parallel-hole collimator. They are similar except for the presence of additional terms involving collimator focal lengths f and, for off-axis sources, the angle θ between the source, the focal point (or pinhole), and the central axis of the collimator (Figure 16-7). The equations illustrate that for converging and diverging collimators, resolution is best at the center ($\theta = 0$, $\cos \theta = 1$).

The performance characteristics of different types of collimators are compared in Figure 16-18 which shows *system* resolution and efficiency vs. distance, including effects of camera intrinsic resolution as well as collimator magnification. Figure 16-18 illustrates that resolution always is best with the source as close as possible to the collimator. Changes in collimator efficiency with distance depend on whether the radiation source is a point source or a uniform sheet source. For a point source (Figure 16-18, right), collimator efficiency increases with increasing source-to-collimator distance with the converging collimator. Maximum efficiency is obtained at the collimator convergence point (~35 cm), where γ rays are transmitted through all of the collimator holes, and then decreases beyond that point. Point-source collimator efficiency decreases with distance for the diverging and pinhole collimators, more severely for the latter. For an extended, large-area sheet source, sufficiently large to cover the entire field of view of the collimator, efficiency does not change with source-to-collimator distance for all of these collimators. Again, for sources embedded within a patient, attenuation effects also must be accounted for.

Figure 16-18 illustrates that the converging collimator offers the best combination of resolution and efficiency at typical imaging distances (5–10 cm); however, the field of view is also somewhat limited at these distances (Equation 15-6, Example 15-2), and for this reason converging collimators are most useful with cameras having relatively large area detectors. Diverging collimators offer a larger imaging area (Example 15-1) but at the cost of both resolution and efficiency. Pinhole collimators offer very good resolution and reasonable efficiency at close distances but lose efficiency very rapidly with distance; they also have a quite limited field of view because of magnification effects at typical imaging distances (Equation 15-3). Generally they are used for imaging smaller organs that can be positioned close to the collimator, e.g., thyroid and heart. They also are useful with high-energy γ-ray emitters because they do not suffer from septal penetration problems.

Differences between the resolution and field of view obtained at different source-to-collimator distances with parallel-hole, converging, diverging, and pinhole collimators are further illustrated by Figure 16-19.

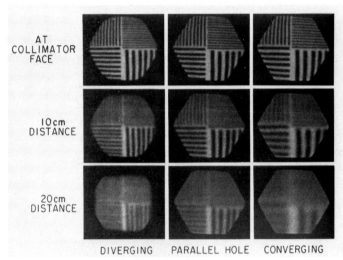

Fig. 16-19.   Bar pattern images demonstrating changing field size and resolution obtained vs. distance for three collimator types.

It should also be noted that the distortions caused by changing magnification with depth for different structures inside the body sometimes make images obtained with the converging, diverging, and pinhole collimators difficult to interpret (see Figure 15-8).

REFERENCES

1. Anger HO: Radioisotope cameras, in Hine GJ (ed): Instrumentation in Nuclear Medicine (vol 1). New York, Academic Press, 1967, chap 19
2. Strand S-E, Larsson I: Image artifacts at high photon fluence rates in single-crystal NaI(Tl) scintillation cameras. J Nucl Med 19:407–413, 1978
3. Hine GJ, Erickson JJ: Advances in scintigraphic instruments, in Hine GJ, Sorenson JA (eds): Instrumentation in Nuclear Medicine (vol 2). New York, Academic Press, 1974, chap 1
4. Hine GJ, Paras D, Warr CP: Recent advances in gamma-camera imaging. Proc SPIE 152:121–126, 1978

Additional discussions of Anger camera performance characteristics and collimator design are discussed in the following:

Hine GJ, Paras P, Warr CP: Measurement of the Performance Parameters of Gamma Cameras, Part I. Rockville, MD., U.S. Dept. H.E.W., Publ. No. (FDA)78-8049, 1977

Richardson RL: Anger scintillation camera, in Rollo FD (ed): Nuclear Medicine Physics, Instrumentation, and Agents. St. Louis, C.V. Mosby Co., 1977, chap 6

17

Radionuclide Imaging: Other Techniques and Instruments

Although the Anger camera dominates the field of nuclear medicine imaging, numerous other imaging systems also have been designed. In this chapter, we describe the basic principles and performance characteristics of those instruments that have achieved practical acceptance or that appear to offer promise for the future. The discussion of each instrument will be necessarily brief, and additional details may be found in the references listed at the end of the chapter.

A. THE RECTILINEAR SCANNER

1. Basic Principles

The rectilinear scanner, first developed during the early 1950s, was the first practical γ-ray imaging device used in nuclear medicine. At one time scanners enjoyed widespread usage, but their popularity has decreased steadily as that of the Anger camera has grown. Few, if any, scanners are sold today, but older models still are in use in some institutions.

The principle of rectilinear scanning is straightforward (Figure 17-1). A NaI(Tl) detector, suitably collimated (Section A.2), is made to scan back and forth over the area of interest on the patient, incrementing a short distance between scan passes. Linear scan speeds of up to several hundred cm/min are used, and the typical increment between scan lines is 3–4 mm. The γ-ray detector is sodium iodide, most frequently 5 cm thick

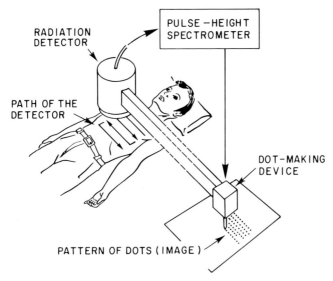

RADIATION
DETECTOR

PULSE-HEIGHT
SPECTROMETER

PATH OF THE
DETECTOR

DOT-MAKING
DEVICE

PATTERN OF DOTS (IMAGE)

Fig. 17-1. Principles of rectilinear scanning. The dot-making device is activated when a signal is received from the pulse-height spectrometer, indicating a γ-ray event detected in the selected energy window. Coupling between the detector and dot-making device may be electrical or mechanical.

× 12.5 cm in diameter, although diameters between 7.5 cm and 20 cm have been used. Signals from the NaI(Tl) detector are amplified, shaped, and analyzed using conventional circuitry (Chapter 5). Typically, a 20 percent energy window, centered on the photopeak, is used to reject scattered γ rays.

Connected to the detector by electrical or mechanical means is a *dot-making device*, which follows the motion of the scanning detector. The dot-making device prints dots on film, paper, or other image-recording medium when pulses are received by it from the pulse-height analyzer, indicating γ-ray events detected within the selected energy window. On some instruments, the number of dots printed per detected γ ray is decreased by a *dot factor*—e.g., one dot per two γ-ray events, one per four γ-ray events, etc. A dot factor is used on slower, mechanical dot printing devices so as not to exceed their maximum dot printing rates. The final image is a pattern of dots, with greatest dot densities occurring in those regions where the highest radiation intensities were recorded during the scan. On those instruments employing direct mechanical coupling between the detector and the dot-making device (i.e., attached to opposite ends of a rigid mechanical bar) the image size bears a 1:1 relationship to the size of the scanned object; however, most scanners employ electrical coupling techniques (e.g., servo motors) so that the image can be reduced in size. For example, with some scanners, it is possible to record two whole-body images on a single 35 × 43 cm (14 × 17 inch) sheet of film.

The most popular image recording technique is *photoscanning*. A small light source, generating a relatively narrow light beam (typically 1–3 mm diameter), scans over a sheet of x-ray film inside a light-tight enclosure. When a pulse is received from the pulse-height analyzer, the light beam is turned on momentarily, projecting a small spot of light onto the film. When the scan is completed, the film is developed, and a pattern of blackened dots appears that outlines the distribution of radioactivity within the scanned area. Figure 18-12 is an example of a photoscan image.

Another image-recording technique employs a persistence oscilloscope. The oscilloscope beam follows the motion of the scanning detector across the CRT face and is turned on momentarily when γ rays are recorded. A very long persistence time is used so that the dots—and thus the image—remain on the CRT face essentially permanently, or until erased to record a new image. Another older method for image recording employed a mechanical stylus traveling over an ordinary sheet of paper; as γ-ray events were recorded, the stylus was activated to imprint a dot on the paper through a carbon ribbon positioned in front of the stylus.

Most modern scanners are provided with photoscan and persistence oscilloscope imaging capabilities. Of the two, photoscanning provides images of the most satisfactory appearance, and generally these are used for diagnostic interpretations. The persistence oscilloscope permits the image to be viewed during the scan procedure, so that positioning errors or instrument malfunctions can be detected quickly.

2. Focused Collimators for Scanning

The purpose of the collimator on a scanner is to restrict the field of view of the detector to a small, well-localized region in front of it. Early scanners used lead collimators with a single, narrow hole (Figure 17-2A). These provide very low geometric efficiency. For example, achieving collimator resolution of about 1 cm requires a collimator hole diameter of less than 1 cm. Only a very small portion of the detector area is exposed to radiation, and the collimator efficiency and recorded counting rate are therefore very low. Only by increasing the collimator hole diameter and severely sacrificing resolution could larger-diameter detectors be used efficiently with single-hole collimators.

Multihole focused collimators permit large-diameter detectors (7–20 cm) to be used while still maintaining reasonable collimator resolution (≲1 cm). Multiple, tapered holes converge to a common point in front of

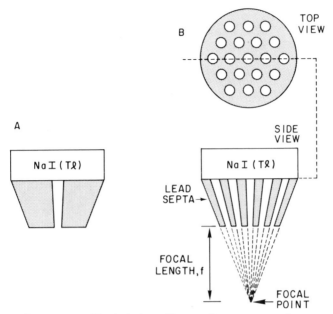

Fig. 17-2. (A) Single-hole collimator for a scanner detector. (B) Multihole focused collimator permits the use of larger diameter detectors with collimator resolution comparable to that of a single-hole collimator.

the collimator, called the collimator *focal point* (Figure 17-2B). The distance from the collimator face to the focal point (typically 7–12 cm) is the collimator *focal length f*. The holes are arranged in a hexagonal pattern and are separated from each other by lead *septa* of sufficient thickness to prevent γ rays from crossing from one hole to another. Design considerations for septal thickness and hole length and diameter are similar to those described for Anger camera collimators (Chapter 16, Section B).

The response characteristics of focused collimators are quite different from those of Anger camera collimators. Figure 17-3 shows typical point or line spread functions recorded when a focused collimator is passed over a point or line source of radiation at different distances from the collimator. The maximum radiation intensity (maximum profile height) is obtained when the source is at the collimator focal point. The narrowest profile (smallest FWHM) is recorded when the source is scanned in the collimator focal plane. Broader profiles (and hence poorer resolution) are obtained at other distances Focused collimators thus provide a *tomographic* imaging effect (Chapter 19) because the image of

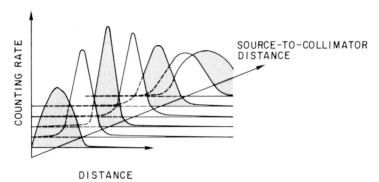

Fig. 17-3. Point or line spread functions versus distance from a focused collimator. (Compare to Figure 16-15.)

the source distribution at the depth of the collimator focal plane in the
patient is brought into sharpest focus, while images of source distributions in planes above and below the focal plane are somewhat blurred.
This can be used to advantage in situations where the depth of a specific
structure to be imaged is known accurately. Generally, however, this is
not the case, and it is better to image with good resolution over as great
a range of depths as possible. Strong tomographic effects are generally
undesirable in routine imaging.

The range of depths over which good image resolution is achieved is
called the collimator *depth of field* λ. This is defined as the distance over
which collimator resolution (FWHM) is not worse than two times the
resolution at the focal point depth. Depth of field *increases* (i.e., tomographic effect *decreases*) with increasing collimator focal length f and
decreasing detector diameter d. Thus

$$\lambda \propto f/d \qquad (17\text{-}1)$$

Large-diameter detectors with short focal length collimators provide
the strongest tomographic effects (smallest λ). Scanners with 20 cm
diameter NaI(Tl) detectors were commercially available at one time.
They provided very high efficiencies and counting rates because of the
large area of detector surface available; however, they also provided
strong tomographic effects, and eventually disappeared from the market
as a result. Depth of field also is smaller for high-resolution collimators
(see Table 17-1).

Focused collimator efficiency g is defined in terms of the total
number of γ rays passing through the collimator holes during a scan of a

Table 17-1
Performance Characteristics for Commercially
Manufactured Focused Collimators for 12.5 cm
Diameter Detectors 8.9 cm Focal Length

Collimator Type	Suggested Maximum Energy (keV)	Resolution at Focus (mm)	Depth of Field λ (cm)	Geometric Efficiency g
Low energy, high resolution	180	7	1.8	1×10^{-4}
Low energy, medium resolution	180	10	2.6	2×10^{-4}
Low energy, high sensitivity	180	15	3.9	4.1×10^{-4}
Medium energy	370	10	2.6	1.5×10^{-4}
High energy	550	10	2.6	0.75×10^{-4}

Adapted with permission from Hine GJ, Erickson JJ: Advances in scintigraphic instruments, in Hine GJ, Sorenson JA (eds): Instrumentation in Nuclear Medicine (vol 2). New York, Academic Press, 1974, Table IA.

point source; this is, essentially, the total area under a point or line spread function (Figure 17-3). Efficiency also can be defined in terms of the number of γ rays passing through the collimator from a uniform sheet source of activity with a stationary source and detector. Collimator efficiency increases as the square of collimator resolution R_c (FWHM at the focal point distance), as it does for Anger camera collimators:

$$g \propto R_c^2 \qquad (17\text{-}2)$$

Also, as with Anger camera collimators, efficiency for a source in air does not depend on source-to-collimator distance. As the source moves away from the focal point, the point or line spread functions are not so high (i.e., the maximum counting decreases), but they are wider, so that the total area under them remains constant.

Table 17-1 summarizes performance characteristics for a selection of collimators provided by one manufacturer. Collimator efficiency g refers to the fraction of γ rays transmitted by the collimator from a uniform sheet source having an area larger than the collimator field of view and of activity emitting one γ ray per cm^2. As with Anger camera systems a selection of low- and medium-energy collimators with different combinations of efficiency and resolution are available. Note also that the values given for geometric efficiency, g, refer to a source in air, and do not include attenuation by the patient.

3. Contrast-Enhancement Techniques

Rectilinear scanners with photoscan image recording provide options for enhancing the contrast of the final image by changing the brightness of the light source as the average counting rate changes during the scanning procedure. Thus areas of increased activity and counting rate are represented on the final image not only by greater dot density but with darker dots, resulting in greater overall contrast (difference in film density) between areas of low and high activity.

Average counting rate is monitored during the scan by a ratemeter or a digital counting circuit. A signal indicating average counting rate (e.g., ratemeter output signal) is sent to the light source circuits (Figure 17-4), where it is used to adjust light source intensity. Electronic circuits are used to establish the exact relationship.

Figure 17-4 shows a typical relationship between counting rate and light source intensity. In low-counting-rate areas, the light source is very dim, and no dots are recorded. Then, above some threshhold counting rate (40 percent in the Figure 17-4 example), the light source intensity increases rapidly with counting rate, reaching maximum intensity at a relative counting rate of 100 percent. The range of counting rates between the values providing minimum and maximum light source intensity, expressed as a percentage of the counting rate giving maximum intensity,

PRINCIPLES OF CONTRAST ENHANCEMENT

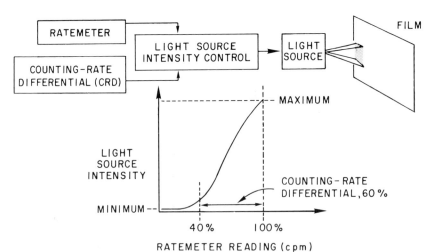

Fig. 17-4.   Principles of contrast enhancement in photoscanning.

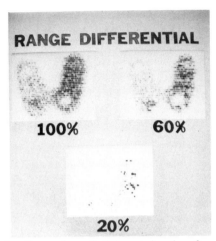

Fig. 17-5. Examples of different levels of contrast enhancement on scan images of a thyroid phantom. Range differential = CRD.

is called the *counting-rate differential* (CRD). In the example shown in Figure 17-4, the CRD is 60 percent. This is a parameter selected by the operator in the scan setup procedure. The operator positions the scanner detector over the area of desired maximum density on the photoscan image. A button is depressed to identify the counting rate recorded at that point as the "100 percent" value. Then a second button is depressed to select the CRD value. These two operations "set" the light source electronics to provide the desired amount of contrast enhancement.

Contrast enhancement must be used with caution. The smaller the CRD value, the narrower the range of counting rates displayed between minimum and maximum film densities and the greater the contrast enhancement for those areas of the image falling within this counting rate range; however, areas with counting rates below the threshold counting rate produce no image at all. Structures producing counting rates below the threshold established by the CRD values essentially are "erased" from the image. Structures producing counting rates above the identified "100 percent" value essentially are "solid black," with no useful contrast range. Figure 17-5 demonstrates the effects of varying levels of contrast enhancement on images of a thyroid phantom. Generally, contrast enhancement is most effective when one is looking for "hot spots" in the distribution, e.g., bone scanning or with various "tumor scanning" agents. Contrast enhancement is less useful when searching for "cold spots," e.g., lung scanning and liver scanning, because it enhances

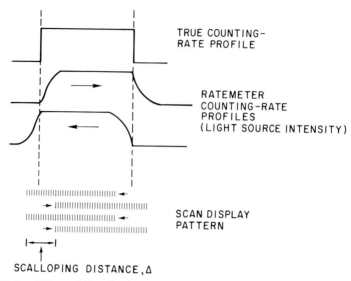

SCALLOPING DISTANCE, Δ

Fig. 17-6. Effect of "scalloping" on a photoscan image employing a ratemeter for light source intensity control.

equally the cold spot contrast and the random noise in the image surrounding the cold spot.

Contrast enhancement schemes employing a ratemeter to control light source itensity also are subject to an artefact known as *scalloping*. Because a ratemeter reading lags behind the actual change in counting rate presented to it (by about two ratemeter time constants τ), the change in light source intensity and thus image density occurring at the edge of an active structure or organ is delayed and shifted in the direction of the scan travel. On the next line, the shift is in the opposite direction. This causes a staggered density structure from one line to the next at the edges of sharp boundaries of activity and counting rate. The total shift distance between lines, Δ, is given approximately by (Figure 17-6).

$$\Delta(\text{cm}) \sim 4S\tau \qquad (17\text{-}3)$$

where S is the scan speed in cm/sec and τ is the ratemeter time constant in seconds.

Example 17-1.

What is the amount of scalloping Δ in a scan performed with a scan speed of 600 cm/min and a ratemeter time constant of 0.1 sec?

Answer.
The scan speed is 600 cm/min ÷ 60 sec/min = 10 cm/sec. Thus from Equation 17-3

$$\Delta \sim 4 \times 10 \text{ cm/sec} \times 0.1 \text{ sec}$$

$$\sim 4 \text{ cm}$$

Scalloping can be decreased by reducing the scan speed (but at the expense of longer scan time) or by shortening the ratemeter time constant (but at the expense of greater statistical fluctuations in ratemeter output; Figure 5-14, Equation 6-42). Scalloping can be a significant artefact on photoscan images if inappropriate combinations of scan speed and ratemeter time constant are employed.

4. Performance Characteristics

In comparison to Anger cameras, rectilinear scanners are less expensive, have thicker crystals and are thus more efficient for higher-energy γ-ray emitters (≤200 keV), and do not suffer from inherent imaging artefacts such as image nonuniformities, nonlinearities, or intrinsic resolution limits. With a dual-head whole-body scanner, one can obtain two opposing views of the entire body simultaneously (anterior and posterior, or two lateral views) (Figure 17-7). Rectilinear scanners provide the best resolution at some depth inside the patient, whereas the Anger camera provides sharpest images of superficial structures closest to the collimator; however, overall resolution is not greatly different for the two instruments.

The rectilinear scanner cannot compare to the Anger camera for dynamic, rapid-sequence imaging. The mechanical scanning motions require at least about a minute even for small organs, such as a single kidney or the thyroid, and larger organs require at least several minutes. Scanners are also far less flexible for unusual views, e.g., superior views of the head, oblique views, etc. These factors, and the constantly expanding variety of ^{99m}Tc-labeled compounds that are imaged very well with an Anger camera, have led to the decreasing popularity of the rectilinear scanner and probably will lead to its ultimate disappearance in the future.

B. MULTICRYSTAL SCANNERS

In multicrystal scanners, rows of detectors are positioned across the width of the patient, and images are obtained with a single linear pass of the detectors along the length of the patient.

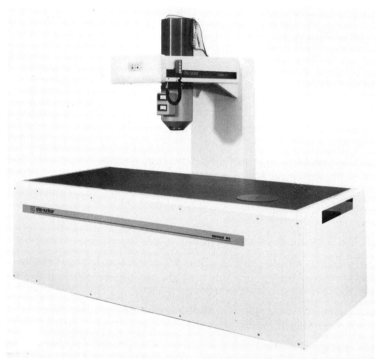

Fig. 17-7. Detector and patient support table for dual-head rectilinear whole-body scanner. Second detector is located below the patient support table. Operator console with pulse-height analyze controls, photoscanner, assembly, etc., is not shown. [Courtesy Ohio Nuclear, Solon, Ohio]

A version designed by Anger employs 64 NaI(Tl) detectors 3.2 cm diameter × 3.8 cm thick. The detectors are arranged in four rows of 16 across the 76 cm width of a scanning bed that passes over them. Each detector has its own electronics and single-hole collimator. The four rows of detectors are offset from each other so that 64 separate scan paths are traced in a single linear scan. Images are recorded on film from a CRT display. Each event recorded by a detector causes a flash of light to appear on the CRT face at a location corresponding to the position of that detector in the array. The image is recorded on a sheet of film traveling in front of the CRT display in synchronization with the scan motion.

A design used in one multicrystal scanner (Figure 17-8) employs two banks of ten NaI(Tl) detectors, one bank above and one below the patient. Each crystal is 6 cm wide and has its own electronics and focused collimator. As the detector arrays travel from patient head to foot, they execute a reciprocating side-to-side motion, so that each detector scans a

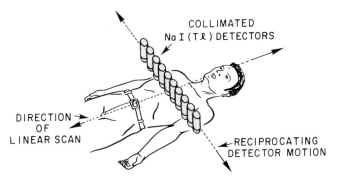

Fig. 17-8. Design principles of a multicrystal scanner. The detector bank executes a reciprocating side-to-side motion as it scans linearly from head to foot. A second bank of detectors (not shown) is positioned below the patient.

6 cm wide strip along the length of the patient. Scan data are recorded and stored digitally, permitting display and recording of images with varying levels of contrast enhancement, background subtraction, etc., at a later time.

Multicrystal scanners are used primarily for whole-body scanning. In terms of detector surface area and image quality, they are comparable to the scanning Anger camera systems Chapter 15, Section B.5). The multicrystal scanners have somewhat greater detection efficiencies for high-energy γ rays because they employ three to four times greater detector thicknesses than the Anger camera. Nevertheless, they have found only limited clinical use and will probably be reserved for research applications and for larger institutions that can afford the luxury of a specialized whole-body scanning instrument.

C. MULTICRYSTAL CAMERAS

A logical design for a γ-ray camera is a multicrystal array of small detector elements covering a large imaging area. The only such instrument to have enjoyed clinical acceptance is one based on a design first described by Bender and Blau in the early 1960s. It has been marketed commercially as the "Autofluoroscope" and later as "System 70."

The detector of this instrument consists of 294 NaI(Tl) crystals, each 0.8 cm on a side and 3.8 cm thick (Figure 17-9). They are arranged in an array of 14 × 21 elements. Lead shielding is used between the crystals to minimize intercrystal γ-ray scattering, so that the center-to-center separation between elements is 1.1 cm. The collimator is either a multihole type with one collimator hole per detector element or a pinhole type.

Individual detector crystals are coupled to PM tubes by a complicated light-piping scheme (Figure 17-10). Instead of individual PM tubes for each crystal, there is one for each row and one for each column in the array, reducing the number of PM tubes required from 294 to 35. When a γ-ray event is detected, its location in the array is determined from the two and column locations of the two PM tubes receiving light from that event.

The System 70 multicrystal camera is used for both dynamic and static imaging. Data storage and image display and analysis are under the control of a computer incorporated into the basic system. For dynamic imaging, intrinsic resolution is limited by the interdetector spacing (1.1 cm), and the imaged area is limited by the array size, 15.2 cm × 22.9 cm. For static imaging, resolution is improved by using a multihole collimator with long narrow holes. The resolution of this collimator is only a few millimeters at the face of the collimator, which is smaller than the interdetector spacing. To "fill in" the image, the detector array executes a barely noticeable rectilinear scanning motion, with each detector element scanning over a 1.1 cm × 1.1 cm area. In this way, static images are obtained with finer resolution than the interdetector spacing would otherwise allow. The detector also is programmed to image and display two adjacent 15.2 cm × 22.9 cm areas, so that a 30.5 cm × 22.9 cm area can be covered for static imaging.

The principle advantage of the multicrystal camera over an Anger camera is a higher counting-rate capability. Because the 35 PM tubes

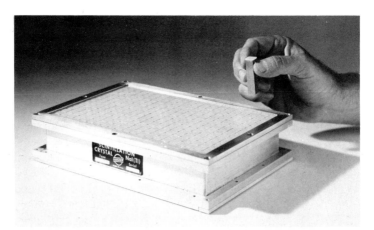

Fig. 17-9.   Detector array for a multicrystal camera. A single detector element is shown to illustrate crystal size. [Courtesy Harshaw Chemical Co., Crystal and Electronics Dept., Solon, Ohio]

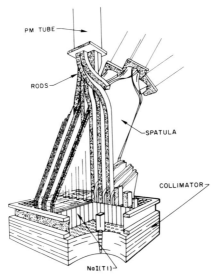

Fig. 17-10. Multihole collimator detector crystal array and light pipe array for multicrystal camera, the Baird-Atomic System 70, "Spatulas" and "rods" are optical light piping from rows and columns of detector array to PM tubes. [From ref. 1: Grenier RP, Bender MA, Jones RH: A computerized multi-crystal scintillation gamma camera, in Hine GJ, Sorenson JA (eds): Instrumentation in Nuclear Medicine (vol 2). New York, Academic Press, p. 108. 1974. With permission of the author and Academic Press.]

operate virtually independently of one another, the problem of pulse pileup (Chapter 16, Section A.6) from events recorded simultaneously in different crystals is minimized. The maximum counting rate of multicrystal camera is about 250 kcps, versus about 100 kcps for an Anger camera, and pulse pileup image artefacts are minimal. Another advantage is its greater detection efficiency for high-energy γ rays ($\gtrsim 200$ keV), resulting from its use of thicker NaI(Tl) crystals than the Anger camera.

The multicrystal camera has been used primarily for fast dynamic imaging studies, which require very high counting rates to obtain satisfactory images in short imaging times (e.g., first-pass cardiac flow studies), taking advantage of the high counting-rate capabilities of the instrument. For routine clinical imaging, its limited detector area is a serious disadvantage in comparison to the Anger camera. Also, because of light losses in its complex light-piping scheme, the multicrystal camera has substantially poorer energy resolution than the Anger camera (FWHM $\sim$ 50 percent for ^{99m}Tc, versus 12–13 percent with the Anger camera), resulting in less effective elimination of scattered radiation by pulse-height analysis and thus degraded image contrast.

In a more recent version of this camera, the individual detector crystals have been replaced with a single NaI(Tl) crystal, 20.3 × 20.3 × 2.54 cm thick, which is slotted to create an equivalent array of 20 × 20 individual detector elements. The detector is viewed by an array of 115 PM tubes that is coupled directly to the back face of the detector for coding of event location. Events are localized according to the relative amounts of light detected by different PM tubes, similar to the position coding system in the Anger camera (Chapter 15, Section B.2). This camera, known as "Scinticor", currently is undergoing clinical evaluations. The claimed advantages of this camera relative to the System 70 are a two-fold improvement in energy resolution and a four-fold improvment in counting rate capability.[2]

D. FLUORESCENCE SCANNING

All of the imaging techniques discussed thus far obtain images of radioactivity distributed internally within the body. *Fluorescence scanning* is a technique for imaging *stable* elements within the body. The basic principles of fluorescence scanning are illustrated in Figure 17-11. Gamma- or x-ray photons from a collimated *excitation source* are directed on the tissue volume of interest. The excitation source is typically a sealed source containing 1–20 Ci of ^{241}Am, a long-lived ($T_{1/2} = 463$ years) emitter of α particles and 60 keV γ rays. The α particles from the ^{241}Am

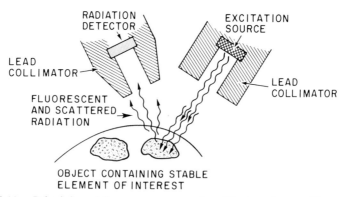

Fig. 17-11. Principles of fluorescence scanning. Photons from collimated excitation source cause fluorescence emission of characteristic x rays by photoelectric interaction with atoms of the element of interest, which are recorded by a collimated radiation detector. Scattered excitation photons are rejected by pulse-height analysis.

source do not escape from the source housing. Heavily filtered x-ray beams also have been employed. Some of the γ or x rays from the excitation source interact via the photoelectric effect with atoms of the element of interest, resulting in the emission of characteristic x rays of that element (27–33 keV for iodine). These x rays are detected by a collimated radiation detector positioned over the tissue volume of interest.

The excitation source and radiation detector are scanned in rectilinear fashion over an area of interest to obtain an image. Because of the need to separate the x rays from the relatively intense flux of scattered radiation from the excitation source ($E \sim 50$ keV for scattered photons from ^{241}Am), fluorescence scanning requires a detector with superior energy resolution, e.g., a semiconductor detector.

Only iodine in the thyroid gland occurs in natural concentrations sufficiently high to be imaged by fluorescence scanning. Poor penetration of body tissues by the relatively low-energy x rays of most elements limits the application of fluorescence scanning to relatively superficial organs such as the thyroid gland, although attempts also have been made to monitor the flow of iodinated contrast agents through the heart. Scan times of about 10 min are needed to obtain images of the thyroid gland with spatial resolution of about 1 cm.

REFERENCES

1. Grenier RP, Bender MA, Jones RH: A computerized multi-crystal scintillation gamma camera, in Hine GJ, Sorenson JA (eds): Instrumentation in Nuclear Medicine (vol 2). New York, Academic Press, 1974, Chap 3
2. Heyda BW, Croteau FR, Govaert JA: A third-generation digital camera. SPIE 454:478–484, 1984.

Additional descriptions of radionuclide imaging instruments other than the Anger camera may be found in the following:

Hine GJ, Erickson JJ: Advances in scintigraphic instruments, in Hine GJ, Sorenson JA (eds): Instrumentation in Nuclear Medicine (vol 2). New York, Academic Press, 1974, Chap 1

Graham LS, Perez-Mendez V: Special imaging devices, in Rollo ED (ed): Nuclear Medicine Physics, Instrumentation, and Agents. St. Louis, C.V. Mosby Co., 1977, Chap 7

Johnson RF: Operation and quality control of the rectilinear scanner, in Rollo FD (ed): Nuclear Medicine Physics, Instrumentation, and Agents. St. Louis, C.V. Mosby Co., 1977, Chap 9

18

Image Quality in Nuclear Medicine

The quality of nuclear medicine images is limited by several factors. Some of these factors, relating to performance limitations of the Anger camera, already have been discussed in Chapter 16. There has been steady improvement in the quality of nuclear medicine images since the introduction of imaging techniques in the 1950s. This has led to progressive improvement in the ability of the nuclear medicine physician to make diagnostic interpretations from them. Part of this has been due to improved instrumentation and part to the development of improved radiopharmaceuticals.

There are two methods for characterizating or evaluating image quality. The first is by means of physical factors that can be measured or calculated for the image or imaging system. Three such factors used to characterize nuclear medicine image quality are (1) *spatial resolution* (detail or sharpness), (2) *contrast* (difference in image density or intensity between areas of the imaged object containing different concentrations of radioactivity), and (3) *noise* (statistical noise due to random fluctuations in radioactive decay, or structured noise, e.g., due to instrument artefacts). Although they describe three different aspects of image quality, these three factors cannot be treated as completely independent parameters because improvements in one of them are frequently obtained at the expense or deterioration of one or more of the others. For example, improved collimator resolution usually involves a tradeoff of decreased collimator efficiency (Chapter 16, Section B) and hence decreased counting rates and increased image statistical noise.

The second method of characterizing or evaluating image quality involves measurement of the ability of observers to detect objects on images obtained with different imaging systems or under different imaging conditions. Although related to the physical measures of image quality described above, the relationships are not well-established due to the complexity of the human visual system and other complicating factors, e.g., observer experience. Hence, the two measures though related are somewhat independent.

In this chapter, we discuss the physical measures of image quality and the tradeoffs between them as they apply to nuclear medicine imaging. We also discuss basic methods for evaluating image quality by observer detection studies. Finally, we discuss basic techniques for quality control of imaging instruments, an essential ingredient to the maintenance of high standards of image quality. Because of its predominant role in nuclear medicine, the discussions will focus on imaging with the Anger camera.

A. SPATIAL RESOLUTION

1. Factors Affecting Spatial Resolution

Spatial resolution refers to the sharpness or detail of the image, or to the ability of the imaging instrument to provide such sharpness or detail. The sample images presented in Chapters 15–17 have demonstrated already that nuclear medicine images have rather limited spatial resolution. A number of factors contribute to the lack of sharpness in these images.

Collimator resolution (Chapter 16, Section B; Chapter 17, Section A.2) is perhaps the principal limiting factor. Because collimator hole diameters must be relatively large (to obtain reasonable collimator efficiencies) there is blurring of the image by an amount at least as great as the hole diameters (Equation 16-6). Collimator resolution also depends on source-to-detector distance (Figures 16-13, 16-15, 16-16, 16-17, and 16-18).

A second factor with camera-type imaging instruments is *intrinsic* resolution. With the Anger camera, this limitation arises primarily because of statistical variations in the distribution of light photons among the PM tubes (Chapter 16, Section A.4). Intrinsic resolution is a function of γ-ray energy with the Anger camera, becoming poorer with decreasing γ-ray energy (Figure 16-6). With multicrystal cameras, intrinsic resolution is limited by the finite size of the detector elements in the multicrystal array (Chapter 17, Section C).

Image sharpness also can be affected by patient motion. Figure 18-1

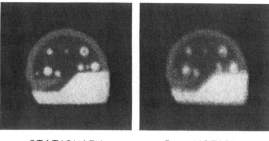

STATIONARY   5mm MOTION

Fig. 18-1. Images of a brain phantom obtained with phantom stationary (left) and with 5 mm motion (right) during the imaging procedure, demonstrating motion blurring effects.

shows images of a brain phantom obtained with and without motion. Respiratory and cardiac motion can be especially troublesome because of the lengthy imaging times required in nuclear medicine and the relatively great excursions in distance (2–3 cm) that are possible in these instances. Gated-imaging techniques (Chapter 21, Section A.3) have been employed to minimize motion blurring, especially in cardiac studies. Breath-holding techniques have been employed to minimize blurring due to respiratory motion.

Image spatial resolution also can be affected by the display or image-recording system. The image can be blurred if too large a light spot is used—e.g., defocussed dots on a CRT display or too large a light source on a photoscanner apparatus. Also, single-emulsion films generally produce sharper images than double-emulsion types.

2. Methods for Evaluating Spatial Resolution

Image spatial resolution may be evaluated by subjective or objective means. A subjective evaluation may be obtained by visual inspection of images of "organ phantoms" that are meant to simulate clinical images e.g., the brain phantom in Figure 18-1. Although they attempt to project "what the clinician wants to see," organ phantoms are not useful for quantitative comparisons of different imaging systems or techniques. Also, because of the subjective nature of the evaluation, different observers might give different interpretations of relative image quality.

Additional types of phantoms used for spatial resolution testing are shown in Figure 18-2. *Bar phantoms* are constructed of lead strips, generally encased in a plastic holder. Lead strips having widths equal to the spaces between them are used in different parts of the phantom. For example, a "5 mm bar pattern" consists of 5 mm wide strips separated edge-to-edge by 5 mm spaces. The bar phantom is placed over the detector (with or without collimator) and irradiated with a uniform

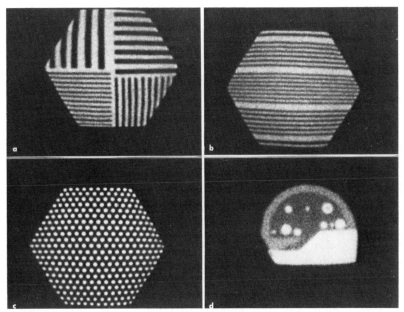

Fig. 18-2. Various types of phantoms used for evaluation of spatial resolution. (A) Four-quadrant bar phantom. (B) Parallel-line bar phantom. (C) Orthogonal hole phantom. (D) Brain phantom with simulated lesions.

radiation field, e.g., a point source of radioactivity at several meters distance or a sheet source of radioactivity placed directly behind the phantom. Spatial resolution is expressed in terms of the smallest bar pattern visible on the image. There is again a certain amount of subjectivity to the evaluation, but not so much as with organ phantoms. Similar evaluations may be made with *orthogonal hole* patterns.

To properly evaluate spatial resolution with bar phantoms, one must ensure that the thickness of lead strips used is sufficient so that they are virtually opaque to the γ rays being imaged. Otherwise, poor visualization may be due to poor contrast of the test image rather than poor spatial resolution of the imaging device. For ^{99m}Tc (140 keV) and similar low-energy γ-ray emitters, tenth-value thicknesses in lead are about 1 mm or less, whereas for ^{131}I (364 keV), annihilation photons (511 keV), etc., they are on the order of 1 cm (Table 9-4). Most commercially available bar phantoms are designed for ^{99m}Tc and are not suitable for higher-energy γ-ray emitters.

A still more quantitative approach to evaluating spatial resolution is through the *point spread function* (PSF) or *line spread function* (LSF). These are counting-rate profiles recorded across the images of point or line sources of radioactivity. A line source may be prepared using a length of thin polyethylene tubing filled with ^{99m}Tc solution. Alternatively, one can use two sheets of lead to form a narrow slit, which then is illuminated by a uniform radiation field to simulate a line source. Examples of LSFs are shown in Figure 16-15 for the Anger camera and Figure 17-3 for the rectilinear scanner.

Counting-rate profiles for a LSF may be obtained using an Anger camera-computer system (Chapter 21). Although the complete LSF is needed to fully characterize spatial resolution, a partial specification is provided by the full width at half-maximum (FWHM) of the LSF (Figure 16-12). The FWHM is not a complete specification because LSFs of different shapes can have the same FWHM; however, it is useful for general comparisons of imaging capabilities. For instruments providing magnified or minified images (e.g., with converging, pinhole, or diverging collimators on the Anger camera) the FWHM should be corrected for magnification or minification effects (Equations 15-5 and 15-6), so that spatial resolution is specified for the source plane or imaged plane. The method for combining FWHMs of different components (e.g., intrinsic and collimator resolutions) to obtain overall system resolution is discussed in Chapter 16, Section B.4 and in Appendix G.

To measure LSFs or PSFs and FWHMs accurately, the diameter of the test source should be much smaller than the resolution capability of the imaging instrument, e.g., source diameter $\lesssim \frac{1}{4}$ FWHM. Also, there should be five or more data points recorded between the FWHM points of the PSF or LSF. This may be difficult to achieve with some camera-computer systems.

Roughly speaking, the FWHM of the PSF or LSF of an imaging instrument is about 1.4–2 times the width of the smallest resolvable bar pattern (Figure 18-3). Thus, an instrument having a FWHM of 1 cm should be able to resolve 5–7 mm bar patterns.

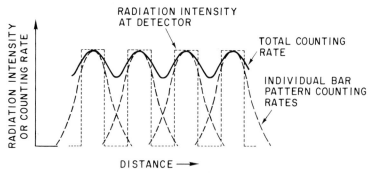

Fig. 18-3. Counting-rate profiles obtained on a bar pattern phantom with an imaging system having FWHM resolution approximately 1.6 times the width of individual bars and spaces.

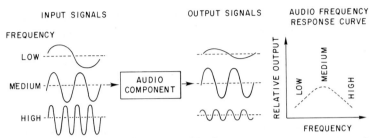

Fig. 18-4. Basic principles for generating frequency response curves for an audio system.

The most detailed specification of spatial resolution is provided by the *modulation transfer function* (MTF). The MTF is the imaging analog of the frequency response curve used for evaluating audio equipment. In audio equipment evaluations, pure tones of various frequencies are fed to the input of the amplifier or other component to be tested, and the relative amplitude of the output signal is recorded. A graph of relative output amplitude versus frequency is the frequency response curve for that component (Figure 18-4). A system with a "flat" curve from lowest to highest frequencies provides the most faithful sound reproduction.

By analogy, one could evaluate the "fidelity" of an imaging system by replacing the audio tone with a sinusoidally varying activity distribution (Figure 18-5). Instead of varying in time (cycles per second), the

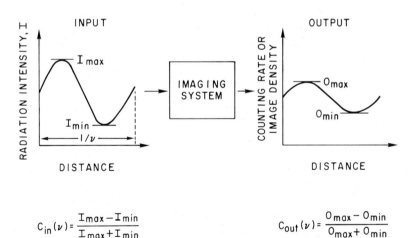

Fig. 18-5. Basic principles for determining the modulation transfer function of an imaging instrument. Input contrast is measured in terms of object radioactivity or emission rate. Output contrast is measured in terms of counting rate, image density, etc. Spatial frequency is v.

activity distribution varies with distance (cycles/cm or cycles/mm). This is called the *spatial frequency* v of the test pattern. The contrast, or *modulation*, of the test pattern is defined by

$$C_{in} = (I_{max} - I_{min})/(I_{max} + I_{min}) \qquad (18\text{-}1)$$

where I_{max} and I_{min} are the maximum and minimum radiation intensities emitted by the test pattern. C_{in} ranges from zero ($I_{max} = I_{min}$, no contrast) to unity ($I_{min} = 0$, maximum contrast). Similarly, output contrast C_{out} is defined in terms of the modulation of output image (e.g., image density or counting rate recorded from the test pattern) (Figure 18-5). The ratio of output to input contrast is the modulation transfer function for the spatial frequency v of the test pattern,

$$MTF\ (v) = C_{out}\ (v)/C_{in}\ (v) \qquad (18\text{-}2)$$

The usefulness of the MTF (or frequency response curve) derives from the fact that any image (or audio signal) can be described as a summation of sine waves of different frequencies. For audio signals, the sound "pitch" is determined by its basic sine wave frequency, while superimposed higher frequencies create the unique sound "quality" of the instrument or human voice producing it. An audio system with a "flat" frequency response curve over a wide frequency range generates an output that matches faithfully the sound of the instrument or voice producing it. Inexpensive audio systems generally reproduce the "midrange" audio frequencies accurately, but demonstrate poor response at low and high frequencies. Thus, they have poor bass response (low frequencies) and poor sound "quality" (high frequencies).

For an imaging system a flat MTF curve with a value near unity produces an image that is a faithful reproduction of the imaged object. Good low-frequency response is needed to outline the coarse details of the image and is important for the presentation and detection of relatively large but low-contrast lesions. Good high-frequency response is necessary to portray fine details and sharp edges. This is of obvious importance for small objects, but also sometimes for larger objects because of the importance of edges and sharp borders for detection of low-contrast objects and for accurate assessment of their size and shape.

Figure 18-6 demonstrates some typical MTF curves for an Anger camera collimator. The MTF curves have values near unity for low frequencies but decrease rapidly to zero at higher frequencies. Thus, the images of a radionuclide distribution obtained with this collimator show the coarser details of the distribution faithfully but not the fine details. Edge sharpness, which is a function of the high-frequency MTF values,

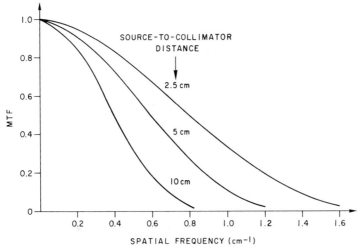

Fig. 18-6. MTF curves for a typical parallel-hole collimator for different source-to-collimator distances. [Data from ref. 1: Ehrhardt JC, Oberly LW, Cuevas JM: Imaging ability of collimators in nuclear medicine. Rockville, Md., U.S. Dept. H.E.W., Publ. No. (FDA)79-8077, p. 39, 1978. With permission.]

also is lost. This type of performance is characteristic of virtually all nuclear medicine imaging systems. Note also that the MTF curve at higher frequencies decreases more rapidly with increasing source-to-collimator distance.

The MTF curve characterizes completely and in a quantitative way the spatial resolution of an imaging system for both coarse and fine details. Images of bar patterns and similar test objects are quantitative only for specifying the limiting resolution of the imaging system, e.g., the minimum resolvable bar pattern spacing. Bar pattern images and MTF curves can be related semiquantitatively by noting that the spatial frequency of a bar pattern having bar widths and spaces of x cm is one cycle per $2x$ cm. Thus a 5 mm bar pattern has a basic spatial frequency of one cycle per cm (one bar and one space per cm). Roughly speaking, bar patterns are no longer visible when the MTF for their basic spatial frequency drops below a value of about 0.1. MTF curves thus can be used to estimate approximately the minimum resolvable bar pattern for an imaging system.

In practice, MTFs are not determined using sinusoidal activity distributions, as illustrated in Figure 18-5. Instead, they are obtained by mathematical analysis of the LSF or PSF. The methods used in this analysis are beyond the scope of this text and are described in references listed at the end of this chapter.†

MTF curves can be obtained for different components of an imaging system. For example, one can obtain a MTF for the intrinsic resolution of the Anger camera detector, $MTF_i(v)$, and another for the collimator, $MTF_c(v)$ (Figure 18-6). The system MTF is then given by

$$MTF_s(v) = MTF_i(v) \times MTF_c(v) \tag{18-4}$$

In general, system MTF is the product of the MTF values of the system components.

When two systems having MTF curves of the same general shape are compared, one can predict confidently that the system with the higher MTF values will have the superior resolution; however, the situation is more complicated when comparing two systems having MTF curves of different shapes. For example, Figure 18-7 shows MTF curves for two collimators, one of which would be better for visualizing large low-contrast structures, the other for fine details (high frequencies). To gain an impression of comparative image quality in this situation, one would probably have to evaluate organ phantoms or actual patient images obtained with these collimators.

B. CONTRAST

Image contrast refers to differences in density (or intensity) in parts of the image corresponding to different concentrations of activity in the patient. A mathematical definition of contrast was given in Equation 18-1. Part of the image contrast problem is related to the choice of the imaging radiopharmaceutical. In general, it is desirable to use an agent having the highest lesion-to-background uptake or concentration ratio. Although this is an important part of the nuclear medicine imaging problem, it is beyond the scope of this text. Instead we will concentrate on instrumentation and other physical factors affecting contrast.

Film contrast is one factor in image contrast. As discussed in Chapter 15, Section B.4, transparency film provides greater image contrast than

---

† The equation for obtaining the MTF from the LSF is

$$MTF(v) = \int_{-\alpha}^{\alpha} A(\varepsilon) \cos(2\pi v\varepsilon) \, d\varepsilon \bigg/ \int_{-\alpha}^{\alpha} A(\varepsilon) \, d\varepsilon \tag{18-3}$$

where $A(\varepsilon)$ is the amplitude of the LSF at a distance ε from the origin of the LSF coordinate system. The limits of the integration, $\pm\alpha$, are several times the FWHM of the LSF.

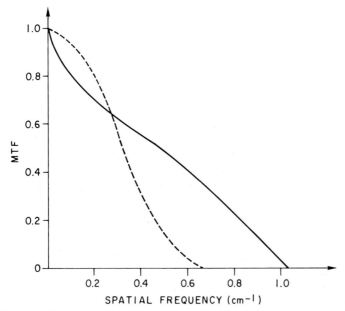

Fig. 18-7. MTF curves for two different collimators. One has better low-frequency resolution (coarse details, dashed line), while the other is better for fine details (solid line). [Data from ref. 1: Ehrhardt JC, Oberly LW, Cuevas JM: Imaging ability of collimators in nuclear medicine. Rockville, Md., U.S. Dept. H.E.W., Publ. No. (FDA)79-8077, p. 20, 1978. With permission.]

Polaroid film, and there are different grades of contrast available in different types of transparency film. It should be noted, however, that a high-contrast film will enhance not only the desired image contrast but also contrast and structure due to noise—e.g., Anger camera image nonuniformities and random noise (Section C).

The presence of *background activity* also affects contrast. For example, suppose that in the absence of background activity a certain object (e.g., a lesion) in the image has contrast

$$C_l = (R_l - R_o)/(R_l + R_o) \qquad (18\text{-}5)$$

where R_l is the counting rate recorded over the lesion and R_o is the counting rate recorded adjacent to it (Figure 18-8). Suppose that the lesion is then surrounded by radioactivity, so that a uniform background counting rate R_b is added to the image. Then the lesion contrast is

$$C_l = [(R_l + R_b) - (R_o + R_b)]/[(R_l + R_b) + (R_o + R_b)] \qquad (18\text{-}6)$$

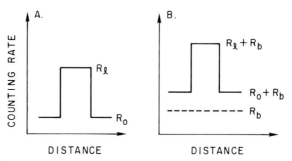

Fig. 18-8. Effect on image contrast of adding a uniform background counting rate R_b.

$$= (R_l - R_o)/(R_l + R_o + 2R_b) \qquad (18\text{-}7)$$

Contrast is decreased by the additional factor $2R_b$ in the denominator.

Example 18-1.

Suppose that $R_l = 2R_o$ and that $R_b = R_o$. Calculate the image contrast with and without the added background.

Answer.

Using Equation 18-5 for the contrast without background,

$$C_l = (2R_o - R_o)/(2R_o + R_o)$$

$$= \tfrac{1}{3}$$

When background is added, according to Equation 18-7

$$C_l = (2R_o - R_o)/(2R_o + R_o + 2R_o)$$

$$= \tfrac{1}{5}$$

Example 18-1 illustrates that background counting rates—e.g., due to activity underlying or overlying the lesion of interest—can reduce image contrast substantially. Figure 18-9 demonstrates the effect on images of a brain phantom.

Scattered radiation and *septal penetration* are additional causes of contrast degradation. Both have the effect of adding a background counting rate to the image in the vicinity of radiation sources. Mathematically, their effect on contrast is similar to that described by Equation 18-7 for the addition of background radiation. Pulse-height analysis is used to help decrease the amount of scattered radiation recorded in the image;

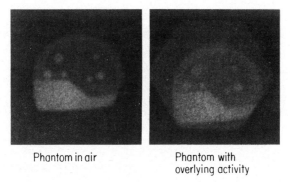

Phantom in air   Phantom with
                        overlying activity

Fig. 18-9.   Effect of adding overlying activity on contrast of
brain phantom images.

however, NaI(Tl) systems cannot reject all scatter, and rejection becomes
especially difficult for γ-ray energies below about 200 keV, as illustrated
by Figure 11-8. Using a narrower analyzer window for scatter rejection
also decreases the recorded counting rate and increases the statistical
noise in the image (Section C.2). It has been determined experimentally
that the best tradeoff between noise and scatter rejection for imaging
systems using NaI(Tl) detectors is obtained with a 20 percent energy
window centered on the γ-ray energy of interest.[2]

Some investigators have suggested the use of "offset" windows
centered above the photopeak (e.g., lower level at −5 percent, upper
level at +15 percent of the photopeak center) to further decrease the
amount of scattered radiation recorded; however, this technique must be
used with caution on the Anger camera because of the possible introduction of image nonuniformities with offset windows (Chapter 16, Section
A.2). There also has been an interest in applying semiconductor detectors
to nuclear medicine imaging to take advantage of their superior energy
resolution for discrimination against scattered radiation by pulse-height
analysis (Figure 11-14).

Figure 18-10 demonstrates the effect of scattered radiation on the
contrast of images of a brain phantom. With a very wide analyzer
window, there is virtually no rejection of scattered radiation and a
noticeable loss of image contrast.

Decreased contrast results in poorer visibility of both large low-
contrast objects as well as fine details in the image. Figure 18-11, for
example, illustrates the effects of scattered radiation (or septal penetration, which has similar effects) on the line-spread function and MTF of an
imaging system. The addition of long "tails" to the LSF results first in the
suppression of the MTF curve at low frequencies. This is reflected in

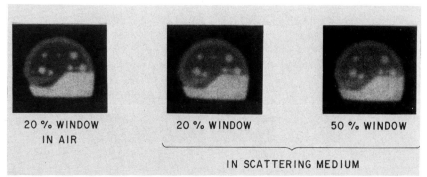

20 % WINDOW   20 % WINDOW   50 % WINDOW
IN AIR

IN SCATTERING MEDIUM

Fig. 18-10. Effect of scatter and pulse-height analysis on contrast of brain phantom images.

poorer contrast of large objects which makes large low-contrast objects more difficult to detect and define. There also is a suppression of the high-frequency portion of the MTF curve that has the effect of shifting the limiting frequency for detection of high-contrast objects, e.g., bar patterns, to lower frequencies. Thus, the contrast-degrading effects of scatter and septal penetration decrease the visibility of all structures in the image, particularly those that are near the borderline of detectability. Background radiation, e.g., from over- and underlying activity, has similar effects. These effects are apparent in Figures 18-9 and 18-10, both of which demonstrate a perceptible loss of image sharpness as well as overall image contrast when overlying activity or scattered radiation are present.

Image contrast is improved in emission computed tomography (ECT, Chapters 19 and 20) because ECT permits imaging of an isolated slice from the activity distribution with a minimum of superpositioning of activities in different structures. ECT may offer significant improvements for perception of low-contrast lesions.

C. NOISE

1. Types of Noise

Image noise may be either random or structured. *Random noise* refers to the mottled appearance of nuclear medicine images caused by random statistical variations in counting rate (Chapter 6). This is a very important factor in nuclear medicine imaging and is discussed in detail in Section C.2.

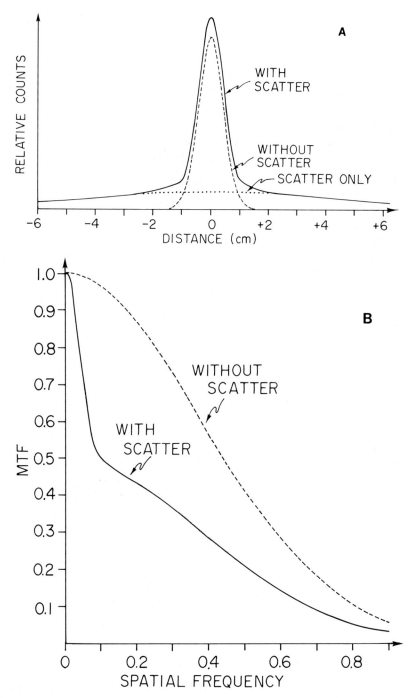

Fig. 18-11. Demonstration of effects of scatter and/or septal penetration on line spread function (A) and MTF (B) of an imaging system. The long "tails" on the LSF have the effect of suppressing the MTF curve at both low and high spatial frequencies.

375

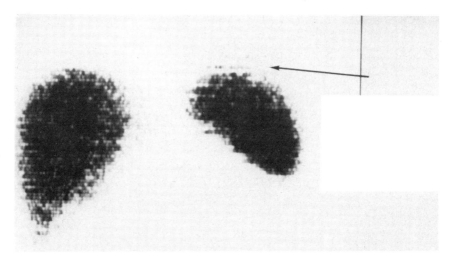

Fig. 18-12. Example of respiratory motion artefacts (arrow) in rectilinear scanning.

Structured noise refers to nonrandom variations in counting rate superimposed on and interfering with perception of the object structures of interest. Some types of structured noise arise from the radionuclide distribution itself. For example, uptake in the ribs may be superimposed over the image of the heart in studies to detect myocardial infarction with ^{99m}Tc-labeled pyrophosphates. Bowel uptake presents a type of structured noise in studies to detect inflammation or abscess with ^{67}Ga. Another example in scanning is object motion, especially respiratory motion for structures near the diaphragm (Figure 18-12).

Structured noise also can be caused by imaging system artefacts. Nonuniformities in Anger camera images (Figure 16-3 and 16-5) and scalloping in rectilinear scanning (Figure 17-6) are examples. In rectilinear scanning, raster lines themselves are a type of structured noise. Some computer displays consist of a well-defined matrix of display points, which superimposes an undesirable noise structure on the image structures of interest. Proper display techniques can offer marked improvements in computer display image quality (Figure 21-4).

2. Random Noise

Random noise, also called statistical noise or mottle, is related directly to the number of counts recorded, or the *information density* of the image. Information density is defined as the number of counts recorded per unit area of the image, e.g., cts/cm^2. Information density changes over the area of the image, depending on the local counting rate recorded in each area. For Anger camera imaging, the information density in an area of the image where the counting rate recorded per unit area is R(cts/sec/cm^2) is given by

$$\text{ID (cts/cm}^2) = Rt \qquad (18\text{-}8)$$

where t is the imaging time. For rectilinear scanning, the local information density is given by

$$\text{ID (cts/cm}^2) = R/S\Delta \qquad (18\text{-}9)$$

where R(cps) is the counting rate, S(cm/sec) is the scan speed, and Δ(cm) is the spacing between scan lines. Information density can be increased in camera imaging by increasing the counting rate (e.g., by using more activity or more efficient collimator) or imaging time and in scanning by increasing the counting rate or by decreasing the scan speed or line spacing.

Information density has important effects on the minimum detectable size and contrast of lesions in nuclear medicine imaging. Suppose it is desired to detect a lesion of cross-sectional area A in a part of the image where the information density is ID(cts/cm^2). The number of counts recorded, N, in an area A in that part of the image is given by

$$N = A \times \text{ID} \qquad (18\text{-}10)$$

The standard deviation in counts recorded in an area A is

$$\sigma = \sqrt{A \times \text{ID}} \qquad (18\text{-}11)$$

or

$$V_n(\%) = (1/\sqrt{A \times \text{ID}}) \times 100\% \qquad (18\text{-}12)$$

where V_n is the percentage standard deviation in counts, or "noise contrast."

Thus, in order to detect a lesion of size A, one would have to distinguish it from random noise fluctuations in the image of magnitude given by Equations 18-11 and 18-12. Usually, a lesion contrast of three to five times the noise contrast, V_n, is required for visual detection. Taking a value of 4 for this requirement, one therefore has a required minimum lesion contrast C_{min} expressed as a percentage difference in counts recorded between the lesion and its surroundings, given by

$$C_{min} \approx (4/\sqrt{A \times \text{ID}}) \times 100\% \qquad (18\text{-}13)$$

Note that the lesion contrast requirement increases as lesion size A decreases.

Example 18-2.
Estimate the minimum detectable lesion contrast in an area of the image where the information density is 400 cts/cm^2, for lesions of 1 cm^2 and 4 cm^2 cross-sectional area.

Answer.
From Equation 18-13, for the 1 cm^2 lesion

$$C_{min} = [4/\sqrt{1 \times 400}] \times 100\%$$
$$= (4/20) \times 100\%$$
$$= 20\%$$

For the 4 cm^2 lesion

$$C_{min} = [4/\sqrt{4 \times 400}] \times 100\%$$
$$= (4/40) \times 100\%$$
$$= 10\%$$

Example 18-12 illustrates that for small, low-contrast lesions, random noise may be the detection-limiting factor. Figure 18-13 illustrates this further for images of a liver phantom. Although spatial resolution and contrast are the same for all of the images shown, there are marked

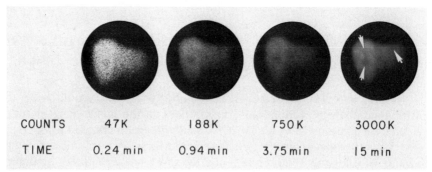

| COUNTS | 47K | 188K | 750K | 3000K |
| TIME | 0.24 min | 0.94 min | 3.75 min | 15 min |

Fig. 18-13. Example of effects of information density on perceptibility of low-contrast lesions in a liver phantom. There are two lesions in the right lobe. One very small lesion in the left lobe is seen only with the highest information density.

differences in lesion perceptibility because of differences in information density and noise.

Information densities in nuclear medicine are typically in the range 100–3000 cts/cm². This is well below the levels encountered in radiography and photography, in which information densities (x-ray or visible light photons detected to form the image) are on the order of 10^6 events/mm^2. In nuclear medicine, information densities are limited by the relatively low radiation source intensities and by inefficient utilization of the emitted radiation, especially with absorptive collimation. Information density can be increased by using a collimator with larger hole diameters or shorter holes and thus greater collimator efficiency (Equation 16-7); however, this results in a loss of spatial resolution (Equation 16-6), which already is quite limited in nuclear medicine imaging. Practical limitations on imaging time, acceptable spatial resolution, and the amount of activity that can be administered safely to patients are serious impediments to substantial further improvement in nuclear medicine information densities and are the reason why photographic or radiographic image quality will be very difficult to ever achieve in nuclear medicine.

Limited information density is a serious impediment to "high-resolution" imaging in nuclear medicine. As shown by Example 18-2, detection of very small objects requires greater contrast or longer imaging time. This applies to comparisons of images or imaging systems having the *same* spatial resolution. "High-resolution" collimators provide better image contrast and improved visibility even for smaller numbers of counts in the image (Figure 18-14); however, they also have lower sensitivity and thus provide lower counting rates than "low-resolution" collimators. For visibility of very fine details, e.g., comparable to that seen in radiography, the sensitivity of the required collimators would be prohibitively low and the imaging times impractical. The same tradeoffs between contrast and statistical noise exist in radiography; however, as noted above the photon flux levels in x-ray imaging are much higher, permitting the detection of much smaller details.

D. EVALUATION OF DETECTION AND OBSERVER PERFORMANCE

The physical measures of image quality discussed above are helpful for comparing different imaging systems, as well as for preparing purchase specifications, establishing quality control parameters, etc. They also can in some cases provide useful estimates of minimum detectable object size and contrast, e.g., as in Example 18-2. In most cases, however, these estimates are determined more accurately by detection

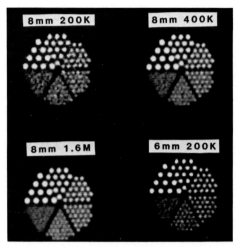

Fig. 18-14. Demonstration of effects of improved resolution on contrast and detectability of small objects. Improved spatial resolution results in improved contrast, lower right, providing improved visibility in spite of fewer counts in comparison to the other images. Decreased sensitivity of "high-resolution" collimators ultimately sets practical limits for "high-resolution imaging" in nuclear medicine. Reproduced with permission from Muehllehner G: Effect of resolution improvement on required count density in ECT imaging: a computer simulation. Phys Med Biol 30 (2):163–173, 1985

experiments using human observers. Two types of experiments commonly are used for nuclear medicine imaging, *contrast-detail (C-D)* studies, and *receiver operating characteristic (ROC)* studies.

1. Contrast-Detail (C-D) Studies

A contrast-detail study is performed using images of a phantom having a set of objects of varying sizes and contrasts. An example is the Rollo phantom, shown in Figure 18-15. The phantom consists of solid spheres of four different diameters immersed in four different thicknesses of a radioactive solution of uniform concentration. Images of this phantom thus contain "cold" lesions of different sizes and contrasts (Figure 18-15, right).

To perform a contrast-detail study with this or a similar phantom, a set of images are obtained using the different imaging systems or techniques to be evaluated. An observer then is given the images, usually without identification and in random order to avoid possible bias, and asked to indicate the smallest-diameter of sphere that is visible at each level of contrast. "Borderline" visibility may be indicated by selecting a diameter "between" two of the diameters actually present in the image. The results then are presented on a contrast-detail diagram as illustrated by Figure 18-16.

A contrast-detail study can be helpful for comparing detectability of both large low-contrast lesions as well as small high-contrast lesions. For example, in Figure 18-16, system A would be preferred for the former and system B for the latter. Because of the subjective nature of the C-D studies, the use of multiple observers is recommended. Also, because observers may change their detection threshhold from the study to the next or as they gain familiarity with the images, it usually is helpful to repeat the readings for verification of results.

Contrast-detail studies have a number of disadvantages. Because they are subjective, they are susceptible to bias and other sources of difference in the observer's detection threshholds. They also are lacking in clinical realism. Most importantly, perhaps, they do not test for the

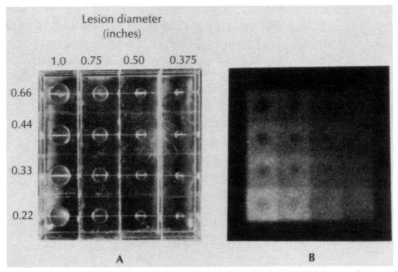

Fig. 18-15. Example of a phantom, the Rollo phantom, which can be used to obtain images for a contrast-detail study. Left: phantom, right: example image. (Reproduced from ref. 2: Rollo FD, Harris CC: Factors affecting image formation, in Rollo FD (ed): Nuclear Medicine Physics, Instrumentation, and Agents. St. Louis, C.V. Mosby Co., 1977, p. 397. With permission.)

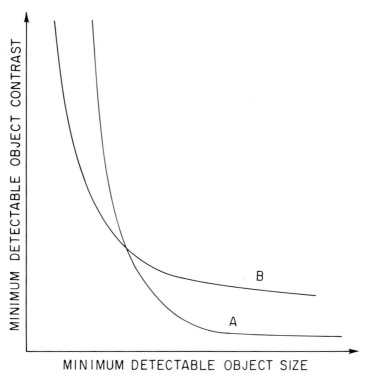

Fig. 18-16.   Hypothetical results of a contrast-detail study comparing two imaging systems, A and B. System A provides better detectability for large low-contrast objects, suggesting perhaps better lesion-to-noise contrast ratio, whereas System B is better for small high-contrast lesions, suggesting perhaps better spatial resolution.

possibility of false positives, i.e., the detection of objects that actually are not present in the image. This is particularly important for noisy images in which noise not only can mask the presence of real objects, but also can create apparent structures that masquerade as real objects.

2. Receiver Operating Characteristic (ROC) Studies

Deficiencies of the contrast-detail method are overcome by the ROC method. For an ROC study, a set of images is obtained with the different imaging systems or techniques to be tested. Phantoms containing simulated lesions can be used, but it also is possible to use actual clinical images. In the simplest approach, each image contains either one or no lesions. The former are called "positive" images and the latter are called "negative" images. The images are given to the observer who is asked to indicate whether the lesion is present or absent in each image, as well as where it is and his or her confidence that it actually is present. Usually the confidence levels are numbered and about four different levels are permitted, e.g., 1 = certainly present, 2 = probably present, 3 = probably not present, and 4 = certainly not present. Then, for each confidence level, the following parameters are calculated:

True positive fraction (TPF) = fraction of positive images correctly identified as positive by the observer.

False positive fraction (FPF) = fraction of negative images incorrectly identified as positive by the observer.

The TPF also is sometimes called the *sensitivy* and $(1 - FPF)$ the *specificity* of the test or the observer. Two other parameters that sometimes are calculated are the *true-negative fraction*, TNF = $(1 - FPF)$, and the *false-negative fraction*, FNF = $(1 - TPF)$.

The ROC curve then is obtained by plotting TPF vs. FPF for progressively relaxed degrees of confidence, i.e., highest confidence = level 1 only, then confidence levels $1 + 2$, confidence levels $1 + 2 + 3$, etc. An example of data and the resulting ROC curve are shown in Figure 18-17. The ROC curve should lie above the ascending 45° diagonal which would represent "guessing", i.e., equal probability of true and false positive detection. The farther the curve lies above the 45° line and the greater the area under the curve, the better the performance of the imaging system and/or observer.

An ROC curve shows not only the true-positive detection rate for an observer and/or an imaging system or technique, but also its relationship to the false-positive detection rate. Thus, it is relatively immune to the sources of observer bias that can occur in contrast-detail studies. It also is applicable to other types of detection questions, i.e., presence or absence of disease, as opposed to simple detection of lesions.

Several difficulties may be encountered in ROC studies. These include verification of absolute truth for images obtained from actual clinical studies, possible presence of multiple lesions on a single image, and statistical comparisons of the results for different observers and sets of images. These issues are dealt with in the references provided at the end of the chapter.

E. QUALITY CONTROL TESTING OF THE ANGER CAMERA

Quality control procedures are used to ensure that nuclear medicine imaging devices are providing images of optimal quality. Accreditation standards of the Joint Commission on the Accreditation of Hospitals

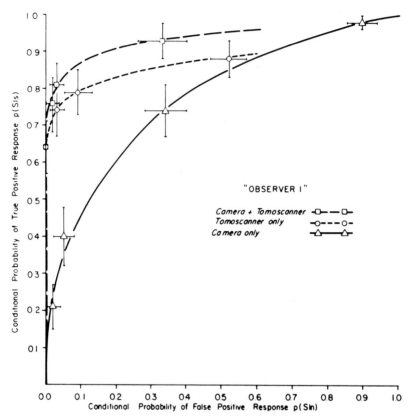

Fig. 18-17. Example of ROC data from an experiment comparing lesion detect-
ability using Anger camera and tomoscanner images. p(S|s) is the true positive
fraction and p(S|n) is the false positive fraction. Reproduced with permission from
Turner DA, et al, Brain scanning with the Anger multiplane tomographic scanner as
a second examination. Evaluation by ROC method. Radiology *121*: 115–124, 1976.

(JCAH) as well as guidelines of the Nuclear Regulatory Commission
(NRC) require that all nuclear medicine laboratories establish routine
quality control procedures.

Quality control of imaging instruments usually is based on visual
evaluation of images of test objects or test patterns. The evaluation may
be augmented by a quantitative analysis of these images using a computer
when such capabilities are available. Although uniform standards have
not as yet been established, generally accepted procedures have been
recommended by various governmental, scientific, and professional or-
ganizations. In this section, we discuss procedures recommended for
quality control of the Anger camera. Additional details may be found in
the references listed at the end of the chapter.

1. Quality Control Testing Methods

Quality control of Anger cameras consists of obtaining images and other data to evaluate *image uniformity*, *spatial resolution*, and *linearity*. In addition, these images permit one to evaluate imaging system *sensitivity*, the presence of *artefacts*, and the performance of *accessory devices*, such as multiformat cameras, computer interfaces, display systems, etc. Two variables in quality control testing are the *radionuclide* used and testing of *intrinsic versus extrinsic* performance.

Quality control tests usually are performed with either a ^{99m}Tc or a ^{57}Co radiation source. The advantages of ^{99m}Tc include its ready availability in most laboratories, and that it tests system performance for the radionuclide most commonly used for clinical imaging. Disadvantages include the need for daily replenishment of source activity, possible contamination during source loading and handling, and difficulty in monitoring source activity on a daily basis due to residual activity in the source from previous uses. The latter is important when it is desired to monitor changes in system sensitivity, e.g., cpm/μCi.

Advantages of ^{57}Co sources include ease of use and handling, and its relatively long half-life (270 days). Its principal emissions are reasonably close in energy to those of ^{99m}Tc (122–136 keV vs. 140 keV). On the other hand, ^{57}Co sources are relatively expensive, require long-term storage facilities, and do not test the camera under the exact conditions used clinically. Also, they sometimes are contaminated with ^{56}Co and ^{58}Co, which emit high-energy (400–700 keV) γ rays that can degrade image quality. The presence and amount of contaminating radionuclides can be determined by spectroscopic methods, as described in Chapter 11. The contamination problem can be overcome by allowing these relatively short-lived radionuclides ($T_{1/2} \lesssim 75d$) to decay for several months before using the source. It should be noted that when a ^{57}Co source is used, the same percentage PHA window setting should be used as is used for clinical imaging with ^{99m}Tc, typically 20%.

A second variable in the method of performing quality control tests is testing of intrinsic vs. extrinsic system performance. *Intrinsic* testing is performed with the collimator removed and with the detector exposed directly to the source, whereas *extrinsic* testing is performed with a collimator attached to the detector. The two methods of testing are illustrated in Figure 18-18. Intrinsic testing usually is performed with a small-volume source of radioactivity, e.g., a syringe, placed at a distance from the detector exceeding at least five times the detector diameter. To avoid the edge-packing artefact, a mask is placed over the edges of the detector. This is important because without the mask as much as 50% of the counts may be recorded in the edge-packing area. Extrinsic testing is performed with a sheet source of activity sufficiently large to cover the

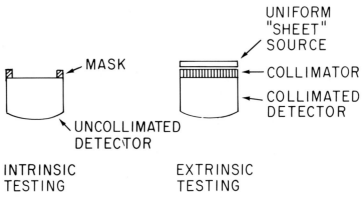

Fig. 18-18. Methods for intrinsic (left) vs. extrinsic (right) testing of Anger camera performance. Intrinsic testing is performed with a small-volume source placed at a distance of greater than five times the detector diameter from the detector, with collimator removed and a lead mask over outer borders of the detector to eliminate edgepacking artifacts. Extrinsic testing is performed with a sheet source in direct contact of the collimated detector. Various lead bar or hole phantoms are placed between the source and detector to evaluate spatial resolution, linearity, etc.

entire detector and placed in direct contact with the collimated detector. Sheet sources of [57]Co usually consist of the radioactivity embedded in a ceramic matrix, whereas ^{99m}Tc sheet sources commonly consist of a plastic container that can be filled with radioactive solution. The solution sources must be mixed uniformly before using.

As with the choice of radiation source material, there are advantages and disadvantages to each of these methods. Intrinsic testing can be performed with considerably less activity, typically a few hundred μCi($\sim$10MBq) versus several mCi ($\sim$100MBq), and small-volume sources are relatively easy to handle in comparison to the sheet sources required for extrinsic testing. However, intrinsic testing does not test the performance of the collimator and is somewhat more time-consuming in that the collimator must be removed and a mask installed to perform the tests. Extrinsic testing is somewhat more convenient but is susceptible to nonuniformities in the source distribution itself, due either to manufacturing defects for [57]Co sources or to inadequate mixing of ^{99m}Tc sources.

Sheet sources also are more expensive to construct and more difficult to handle and store than point sources.

The choice of radiation source and of intrinsic vs. extrinsic testing is an option of the individual user with advantages and disadvantages as noted above. Of more importance is the careful design, execution, and recording of results of the selected testing procedures. The following sections describe the types of testing recommended.

2. Recommended Types and Frequencies of Tests

Table 18-1 summarizes the recommended types and frequencies of quality control tests for the Anger camera. The results of all studies should be evaluated as they are obtained and then recorded and filed in a permanent and easily accessible location to permit day-to-day evaluation and comparison of results. In addition to filing images, other pertinent data including the number of counts in the images, elapsed time, source activity, system gain, and CRT intensity settings should be recorded.

DAILY TESTS

Daily testing should begin with adjustment of dot size and shape (focus and astigmatism) on the CRT, and cleaning of the CRT face and the lenses and rollers in the recording camera. Collimators, cables, and other components also should be inspected visually for any signs of damage.

Table 18-1
Recommended Types and Frequencies of Quality
Control Tests for an Anger Camera

Frequency	Test
Daily	1. Adjust size and sharpness of dots on CRTs.
	2. Clean lens, rollers, etc., on cameras.
	3. Inspect collimators, cables and other components for signs of mechanical damage.
	4. Obtain flood-field uniformity image.
	5. Calculate system sensitivity.
Weekly	1. Obtain resolution-phantom image.
	2. Obtain linearity-phantom image.
	3. Test performance of accessory devices (multiformat cameras, whole-body scanning tables, computer systems and interfaces, etc.).
Semiannual	1. Evaluate energy resolution.
	2. Evaluate counting-rate capability.
	3. Evaluate multiple-window energy registration.

Uniformity is tested by obtaining a flood-field image with a point or sheet source. Prior to obtaining this image, the pulse-height analyzer should be adjusted using the same source. Source activity should be such that the counting rate does not exceed about 20Kcps to avoid pileup artefacts. The flood-field image should contain about 10^4 cts/cm^2, i.e., about 0.5-2 million counts, depending on detector size. The preset number of counts and image orientation should be the same from day-to-day. The image should be obtained with uniformity and linearity correction circuits "on" and with the camera in the "normal" count-rate mode.

The images are evaluated by visual inspection and compared to reference images for nonuniformities and artefacts immediately after they are obtained, i.e., *before they are filed*. As a rule of thumb, image nonuniformities can be detected visually on Polaroid film if they exceed about 10%, and on transparency film if they exceed about 6–7%, due to the somewhat higher contrast of the latter (see Figure 15-9). Nonuniformities due to the collimator or camera detector and electronics can be distinguished from those in display devices by performing an image rotation of 90° on the camera and repeating the study. If the nonuniformity pattern does not rotate with the image, it can be assumed to reside in the display device, e.g. in the CRT phosphor.

Sensitivity can be evaluated by recording the amount of time needed to record the preset number of counts in the flood-field image. This requires that the activity in the source be known accurately, i.e., by correcting for ^{57}Co decay or by carefully measuring the activity used in a ^{99m}Tc source. The latter may be difficult to establish, due to residual activity from previous use. When intrinsic testing is used, it also is important to maintain a constant source-to-detector distance for accurate evaluation of sensitivity.

WEEKLY TESTS

Weekly testing should include an evaluation of image *spatial resolution* and *linearity*. Usually both of these parameters can be tested with the same phantom. Commonly used phantoms include various bar patterns and hole patterns, examples of which are illustrated in Figure 18-2. Of these phantoms, those having a single pattern of bars or holes extending across the entire image seem to be the most useful. The four-quadrant bar phantom, for example, requires multiple images to evaluate resolution and linearity in all areas of image. Again, the images are evaluated visually and compared with reference images before filing.

Weekly testing also should include evaluation of various *accessory* devices, such as multiformat cameras. Images of the resolution/linearity phantom should be recorded in all commonly used multiformat camera modes. For Anger cameras with whole-body imaging capabilities, an image of the resolution/linearity phantom also should be obtained in this mode to evaluate for the presence of "strip" artefacts and other scanning problems.

OTHER TESTS

Less frequent (e.g. semiannual) testing is recommended for evaluating *energy resolution, counting-rate capability*, and, for cameras with multiple window capabilities, *energy-window registration*. These tests are more complicated and time-consuming than the daily and weekly tests described above. Details are described in the references listed at the end of the chapter.

Computers can be helpful for the performance and evaluation of quality control studies, principally by providing quantitative values for the measured parameters. For example, nonuniformities can be quantified as illustrated in Figure 18-19. Camera-computer systems also require periodic quality control testing, e.g., to test for nonuniformities due to ADC nonlinearities. Generally, the tests performed parallel those described for the Anger camera. Hasegawa[3] has described a protocol whereby the camera-computer system is used with an orthogonal-hole

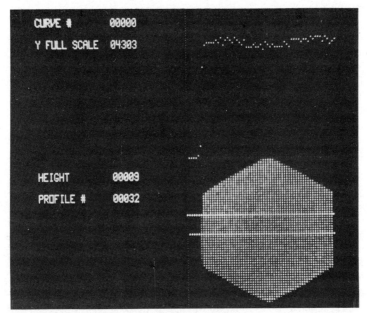

Fig. 18-19.   Profile slice (top) obtained on an Anger camera-computer system to evaluate uniformity of a flood-field image (bottom).

phantom to calculate automatically the spatial resolution, uniformity, linearity, and sensitivity of the camera-computer system.

3. Acceptance Testing

Regardless of the specific methods and phantoms used, a useful starting point for a quality control program is to have a well-documented set of acceptance tests available for comparison. A recommended set of acceptance tests for the Anger camera has been prepared by the AAPM.[4] Acceptance testing should be performed under the direction of a physicist or engineer when the imaging system is first installed to verify that performance specifications are met. Usually, these tests are much more complicated than those that are used in routine quality control; however, some of the recommended acceptance tests closely parallel those of a quality control program. Thus, they provide a baseline set of performance standards that can serve as the basis for detecting subtle, long-term changes in system performance. Also, the quantitative results of the acceptance tests can be helpful for evaluating problems discovered during the performance of quality control tests.

REFERENCES

1. Ehrhardt JC, Oberly LW, Cuevas JM: Imaging ability of collimators in nuclear medicine. Rockville, Md., U.S. Dept. H.E.W., Publ. No. (FDA)79-8077, 1978
2. Rollo FD, Harris CC: Factors affecting image formation, in Rollo FD (ed): Nuclear Medicine Physics, Instrumentation, and Agents. St. Louis, C.V. Mosby Co., 1977, Chap 8, 10, 11
3. Hasegawa BH, Kirch DL, McFree LT, et al: Quality control of scintillation cameras using a minicomputer. J Nucl Med 22:1075, 1981
4. Scintillation Camera Acceptance Testing and Performance Evaluation. AAPM Report No. 6. Chicago, Ill., Amer Assoc Phys Med, 1980

Additional discussion of nuclear medicine image quality and quality assurance procedures may be found in the following:
Graham LS: Quality assurance of Anger cameras, in Rao DV, Chandra R, Graham MC (eds): Physics of Nuclear Medicine, Recent Advances, New York, American Institute of Physics, 1984, pp. 68–83
Paras P: Quality assurance in nuclear medicine, in Medical Radionuclide Imaging, Proceedings (vol 1). Vienna, IAEA, 1977, pp 3–41
A comprehensive discussion of methods for evaluating detection and observer performance is found in:
Swets JA, Pickett RM: Evaluation of Diagnostic Systems: Methods from Signal Detection Theory. New York, Academic Press, 1982

19

Nuclear Medicine Tomography: Principles

A basic problem in conventional radionuclide imaging is that the images obtained are two-dimensional projections of three-dimensional source distributions. Images of structures at one depth in the patient thus are obscured by images of overlying and underlying structures. One solution is to obtain images from different projections around the patient, e.g., posterior, anterior, lateral, and oblique views. The person interpreting the images then must sort out the structures from the different views mentally to decide the true three-dimensional nature of the distribution. This approach is only partially successful; it is very difficult to apply it to complex distributions with many overlapping structures. Also, deep-lying organs often have overlying structures from all projection angles.

An alternative approach is *tomographic imaging*. Tomographic images are two-dimensional representations of structures lying within a selected plane or depth in a three-dimensional object. The classical approach to tomographic imaging, first developed in diagnostic radiology and later extended to nuclear medicine, involves using geometric techniques to blur the image of objects not in the plane of interest while leaving objects in the selected plane in focus. Modern tomographic techniques such as positron emission tomography (PET), single-photon emission computed tomography (SPECT), x-ray computed tomography (x-ray CT), and magnetic resonance imaging (MRI), use quantitative "projection" data obtained with detection systems placed or rotated around the object and mathematical algorithms to "reconstruct" images of selected planes within the object from these data. The mathematical method underlying this approach was first published by Radon in 1917, but it was not until the 1950s and 1960s that work in radioastronomy and chemistry resulted in practical applications. The development of x-ray CT in the early 1970s initiated application of the principles of image reconstruction in medical imaging.

In this chapter, we describe the basic principles of tomographic imaging, emphasizing modern reconstruction imaging techniques. Tomographic systems and devices are discussed in Chapter 20.

A. FOCAL-PLANE TOMOGRAPHY

Focal-plane tomography (also called ''blurring tomography'') was the first widely used method for producing tomographic medical images. Figure 19-1 illustrates the concept for x-ray imaging. As the source (x-ray tube) and image receptor (film) move in opposite directions, a focal plane is defined by those points (B) for which the projected images remain stationary throughout the motion. Points in other planes are translated into blurred images (A' to A''). The result is a tomographic image in which objects in plane B remain in focus whereas objects in other plans are blurred. The thickness of tissue that remains relatively in focus depends on the range of angles swept by the tomographic motion. Larger tomographic angles produce thinner sections.

In essence, focal-plane tomography involves acquiring images from different projection angles and then shifting and superimposing these images to bring different planes into focus. In the example above, the shifting is accomplished by mechanical motion. It also can be accomplished by acquiring separate projection images and then shifting and superimposing, e.g., using digitized images and computer systems (Chapter 21). One such approach that has been used in nuclear medicine is so-called ''pinhole tomography,'' in which a collimator with multiple pinholes is used to acquire different pinhole projection images that are shifted and superimposed to bring different planes into focus. Another is the ''rotating slant-hole collimator.'' The principles of these devices are discussed further in Chapter 20, Section A.

Another simple form of focal-plane tomography is achieved by the use of focused collimators for rectilinear scanning (Chapter 17, Section A.2). Usually, however, the intention in rectilinear scanning is to obtain a simple two-dimensional projection image over an extended range of depths within the patient. Hence, strongly focused collimators (shallow depth-of-field, Equation 17-1) generally are not used, and the tomographic effect, though available, is ignored.

A further example of nuclear medicine tomography achieved by a combination of focused collimation and image projection shifting is the Anger tomoscanner. This also is described in Chapter 20, Section A.

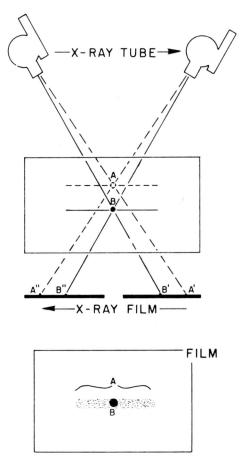

Fig. 19-1. Principles of focal-plane tomography. The x-ray tube and film moving in opposite directions produce a tomographic image with points in plane B in focus while points lying in other planes such as A are blurred. Note that the resultant image is a superpositioning of in-focus (B) and out-of-focus (A) information.

There are two fundamental problems with focal-plane tomographic approaches for nuclear medicine. The first is that the images produced contain blurred structures and counts from superimposed out-of-focus planes. This tends to obscure details in the in-focus plane and contributes to increased statistical noise. For example, if the total number of counts collected for the tomographic image is 500,000 and the focal plane contributes only 25,000 of these counts, the final image is dominated by statistical noise from the 475,000 counts from out-of-focus planes. The signal-to-noise ratio thus may be very poor, even when off-plane structures are properly blurred.

A second problem is that the projection images for focal-plane tomography are collected only from a limited range of angles around the patient. For this reason, focal-plane tomography often is referred to as *limited-angle tomography*. As discussed in Section B.2, a severe limitation in reconstructing a quantitatively accurate image is imposed unless the range of angular projections extends at least over 180°. Limited-angle tomography thus cannot be used reliably for quantitative applications in nuclear medicine.

Focal-plane tomography also can be performed mathematically with computers, with the result that the distinction between focal-plane tomography and true "computed" tomography itself becomes blurred. However, there are fundamental differences related to the limitations summarized above that will become clear in the discussion on reconstruction tomography in the next section.

B. COMPUTED (RECONSTRUCTION) TOMOGRAPHY

Computed tomography (CT) techniques differ from focal-plane and other geometric approaches because they are based on rigorous mathematical algorithms and because they collect and process data only from the tissue section of interest. Individual tomographic planes, or "slices," are physically distinct and nonoverlapping. They thus provide an intrinsically better signal-to-noise ratio as well as a more accurate representation of the actual activity distribution, which is of importance for quantitative nuclear medicine studies. The tomographic planes usually are oriented perpendicular to the long axis of the body; however, other orientations of the planes also can be obtained. In contrast to x-ray CT, which uses transmitted radiation, nuclear medicine uses emitted radiation; hence, nuclear medicine techniques generally are referred to as *emission computed tomography*, or ECT. Two specific types of ECT, *single-photon emission computed tomography*, or SPECT, which uses ordinary γ-ray emitters, and *positron emission tomography*, or PET, which uses positron emitters, will be discussed after the general principles are described.

1. Principles of Image Reconstruction From Projections

The input data for computed reconstruction tomography consist of a set of standard two-dimensional projection images (e.g., scintigrams) taken at many angles about the body. It is possible to generate or "reconstruct" the original two-dimensional activity distribution in the plane if a sufficient number of scan projection profiles are acquired over an adequate range of projection angles.

Consider the scan profiles for the simple case of a point source of activity within an object (Figure 19-2). Each profile maps the location of the point source in the direction parallel to the scan profile; however, the source could lie at any point along the line perpendicular to that profile. For a point source, this ambiguity is easily resolved by inspection of profiles from other angles, but with distributed sources this judgment becomes ambiguous and complex. Since the depth of the activity is unknown, a first approximation for the source distribution can be obtained by projecting the data from each scan profile back across the entire image grid (Figure 19-2C, D). That is, equal values are assigned to all points in the object plane contributing to the scan profile. This operation is known as *backprojection*. If the backprojections of all the scan profiles then are added together, an approximation of the original object distribution results (Figure 19-2C, D). The complete operation, using simple addition of uncorrected scan profiles, is called *linear superposition of backprojections* (LSBP).

Increasing the number of views with LSBP improves the tomographic effect (Figure 19-2D); however, even with an infinite number of views, the final image still is blurred. The point spread function describing this blurring is proportional to $1/r$, where r is the distance from the point source (Figure 19-2E). Mathematically, it can be shown that the relationship between the true image and the LSBP image is given by:

$$\text{LSBP image} = \text{True image} * (1/r) \tag{19-1}$$

where $*$ is the operation of convolution (Appendix G).

To reconstruct the true image from the LSBP image, the $1/r$ blurring factor must be eliminated. To understand how this is accomplished, it is helpful to introduce the concept of the *Fourier transform*. The Fourier transform of a function is essentially a change of coordinates, in which the function $f(x,y)$ is described not in terms of its amplitude at individual spatial coordinates, (x,y), but as a summation of sine and cosine functions of different spatial frequencies, v_x and v_y, in the x and y directions. This general concept was introduced in Chapter 18 (Section A.2) to describe the modulation transfer function (MTF), which describes the spatial resolution of an imaging system in terms of its ability to resolve different spatial frequency patterns. The Fourier transform, $F(v_x,v_y)$, of a function, $f(x,y)$, is the representation of that function in "frequency space," as opposed to "real space." It is obtained by integrating the product of the original function with sine and cosine functions and usually is expressed symbolically as

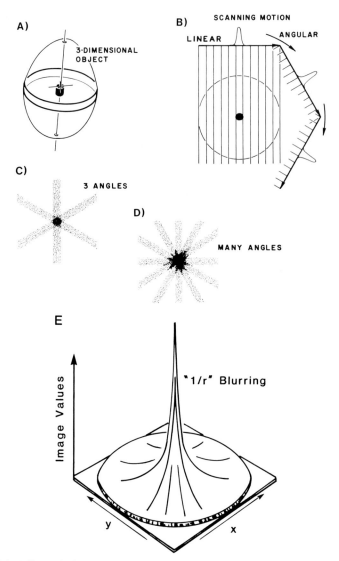

Fig. 19-2. Steps in backprojection process. (A) Unknown source distribution. For simplicity, the object in this example contains only a single point source. (B) Profile scans obtained at various angles around the object. (C) Backprojection and superpositioning of profiles obtained at three angles produces an approximation of the original object distribution. Approximation improves as the number of angles increases (D); however, even with an infinite number of projections (E), there is residual blurring. Blurring is described by a "1/r" function. (Reprinted from ref. 1: Phelps ME, Hoffman EJ, Gado M, et al: Computerized transaxial reconstruction, in DeBlanc H, Sorenson J (eds): Non Invasive Brain Imaging, Computed Tomography and Radionuclides. Society of Nuclear Medicine, 1975, pp 111–146. With permission.)

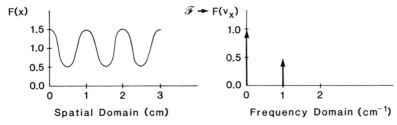

Fig. 19-3. (Left) Function consisting of a cosine function with maximum amplitude 0.5 units superimposed on a constant level of amplitude 1.0 units. (Right) Fourier transform ($\mathscr{F}$) of this function showing frequencies and amplitudes of the spatial frequency components. Distance in the spatial domain is measured in centimeters while spatial frequency in the frequency domain is in units of cm^{-1}. (ie, cycles per cm).

symbolically as

$$F(\nu_x, \nu_y) = \mathscr{F}\,[f(x,y)] \tag{19-2}$$

A simple example of a function and its Fourier transform is shown in Figure 19-3. The function consists of a constant level of 1.0 unit of amplitude with a superimposed cosine function of frequency 1 cm^{-1} and amplitude of 0.5 units. The Fourier transform of this function is represented by two amplitudes, one with a value of 1.0 at spatial frequency 0 cm^{-1} and the second with a value of 0.5 at spatial frequency 1 cm^{-1}.

Other examples of Fourier transforms are the MTF curves illustrated in Figures 18-6 and 18-7. The modulation transfer function is, in fact, simply the Fourier transform of the line spread function (LSF) of the imaging system or device. Unlike the simple example in Figure 19-3, however, the LSF for most imaging systems contains many different spatial frequency components, and its Fourier transform therefore contains a spectrum of spatial frequency components.

Returning now to Equation 19-1, and taking the Fourier transform ($\mathscr{F}$) of both sides, one obtains:

$$\mathscr{F}(\text{LSBP image}) = \mathscr{F}(\text{true image}) \times \mathscr{F}(1/r) \tag{19-3}$$

This relatively simple expression results because the complicated convolution operation in the spatial domain is equivalent to a simple multiplication of Fourier transforms in the frequency domain (Appendix G). The true image can be retrieved from this equation simply by dividing by the Fourier transform of the function, 1/r:

$$\mathscr{F}(\text{true image}) = \mathscr{F}(\text{LSBP image})/[\mathscr{F}(1/r)] \tag{19-4}$$

It can be shown that the Fourier transform of the function (1/r) is simply:

$$\mathscr{F}(1/r) = 1/\nu \qquad (19\text{-}5)$$

where ν = spatial frequency. Thus

$$\mathscr{F}(\text{true image}) = \mathscr{F}(\text{LSBP image}) \times \nu \qquad (19\text{-}6)$$

Taking the inverse Fourier transform of each side of this equation, one finally obtains:

$$\text{True image} = \text{LSBP image} * g \qquad (19\text{-}7)$$

where g now is the function in the spatial domain whose Fourier transform is equal to ν in the frequency domain.

The function g is a correction "filter" that can be convolved with the scan profiles to eliminate the 1/r blurring effect. Alternatively, the correction filter could be applied by taking the Fourier transforms of the scan profiles and multiplying each frequency component by a factor proportional to the spatial frequency. The approaches are entirely equivalent, and both are used in practice. The correction filter has a simple ramp shape in the frequency domain and a somewhat more complicated shape in the spatial domain (Figure 19-4). Because of its shape in the frequency domain, this filter is sometimes referred to as a *ramp filter*. From its shape in the frequency domain, it can be seen that correction for

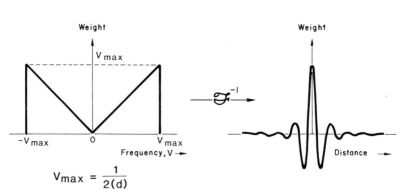

Fig. 19-4.   Ramp filter to correct for 1/r blur in the frequency domain (left) and corresponding spatial domain filter (right). The ramp filter is the Fourier transform ($\mathscr{F}$) of the spatial domain filter. (Reprinted from ref. 1: Phelps ME, Hoffman EJ, Gado M, et al: Computerized transaxial reconstruction in DeBlanc H, Sorenson J (eds): Non Invasive Brain Imaging Computed Tomography and Radionuclides. Society of Nuclear Medicine, 1975, pp 111–146. With permission.)

the 1/r blurring is achieved by giving increasing weight to higher spatial frequencies in the Fourier transform of the LSBP image. This can be understood intuitively by recognizing that blurring is a process that suppresses high spatial frequency information; hence, the correction for the specific blurring effect of LSBP is achieved by the reverse process of selectively amplifying these frequencies. In practice, filter functions are used that have somewhat rounded shapes in the frequency domain to avoid artefacts resulting from oscillations caused by sharp spatial frequency cutoff and to avoid excessive enhancement of high-frequency noise in the image.

The entire reconstruction process, including the filtering process, is known as *linear superposition of filtered backprojections* (LSFBP). Figure 19-5 reviews the basic principles.

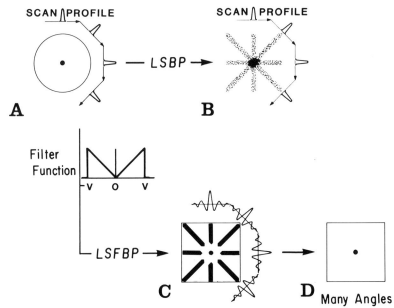

Fig. 19-5. Illustration of linear superposition of backprojections (LSBP) and filtered back projections (LSFBP). Linear superposition of back projections (LSBP) produces an approximation of the actual activity distribution with 1/r blurring as shown in Figure 19-2. Applying the ramp filter to the scan profiles results in filtered scan profiles (C), which, when backprojected, eliminate the 1/r blurring. As the number of scan profiles increases, extraneous information included in (C) disappears and the original object distribution is reproduced (D). (Reprinted from ref. 1: Phelps ME, Hoffman EJ, Gado M, et al: Computerized transaxial reconstruction, in DeBlanc H, Sorenson J (eds): Non Invasive Brain Imaging, Computerized Tomography and Radionuclides. Society of Nuclear Medicine, 1975, pp 111–145. With permission.)

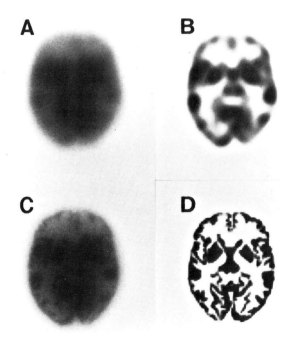

Fig. 19-6. Computer simulation illustrating effects of 1/r and detector blurring. (A) Image reconstruction with LSBP with a 12 mm FWHM detector resolution. (B) Image reconstruction from same data as (A), but with LSFBP to remove 1/r blurring. (C) Image reconstructed by LSBP but with 1-mm FWHM detector resolution. (D) Image reconstructed with same data as (C) but with LSFBP to remove 1/r blurring. (Reprinted from ref. 2: Phelps ME, Huang SC, Hoffman EJ, et al: An analysis of signal amplification using small detectors in positron emission tomography. J Comput Assist Tomogr 6:551–565, 1982. With permission.)

Although LSFBP and the equivalent Fourier filtering technique remove the 1/r blurring created by the backprojection process, they do not remove blurring that occurs in the data collection process itself caused by spatial resolution limitations of the imaging device. Figure 19-6 shows a computer simulation illustrating the relative effects of 1/r and detector blurring. The image in Figure 19-6A was reconstructed using the LSBP technique with simulated data from a 12-mm FWHM detector and contains both 1/r and detector blurring. Figure 19-6B illustrates the removal of the 1/r blur by LSFBP reconstruction to the limit set by the 12-mm detector resolution. Figure 19-6C is a LSBP reconstruction for 1 mm FWHM detector resolution. Note the appearance of detail even though the image contains 1/r blurring. Figure 19-6D, showing the same data reconstructed by LSFBP, has both sources of blurring removed, at least to the limit of a 1 mm detector resolution. Although the image in Figure 19-6C appears to be a reasonable tomographic image, the actual contrast between structures is very low because of the 1/r blurring, as can be seen by comparison to Figure 19-6D. If a realistic level of statistical noise was added to the data, it would remove most of the perceived structure in Figure 19-6C. In Figure 19-6D, image contrast is high and the reconstructed image data are quantitatively accurate.

The LSFBP and equivalent Fourier-filtering techniques described above are the most commonly used reconstruction methods for ECT at this time. Algebraic methods based on solving simultaneous equations with the scan projection profiles as input data also have been used and were in fact the methods used on the original EMI CT scanners. These methods are called algebraic reconstruction techniques (ART), simultaneous iterative reconstruction techniques (SIRT), and similar names. They are described in references listed at the end of the chapter.

2. Sampling Requirements

Scan profiles are not continuous functions but collections of discrete point-by-point samples of the scan projection profile. The distance between these points is the *linear sampling distance*. In addition, scan profiles are obtained only at a finite number of *angular sampling intervals* around the object. The choice of linear and angular sampling intervals and the maximum frequency of the correction filter (the cutoff frequency), in conjunction with the detector resolution, determine the reconstruction image resolution.

The *sampling theorem*[3] states that to recover spatial frequencies in a signal up to a maximum frequency, v_{max}, requires a linear sampling distance d given by:

$$d \leq 1/(2v_{max}) \tag{19-8}$$

This means that the highest spatial frequency component to be recovered from the data must be sampled at least two points per cycle. Coarser sampling does not allow higher spatial frequencies to be recovered accurately and leads to image artefacts known as *aliasing*. The linear sampling distance sets a resolution limit for any imaging system. This limit (v_{max} in Equation 19-8) is known as the *Nyquist frequency*. This sampling requirement put in terms of the FWHM detector resolution requires $d \leq FWHM/3$.

In ECT, image resolution also depends on detector resolution and on the cutoff frequency used for the reconstruction filter. Figure 19-7

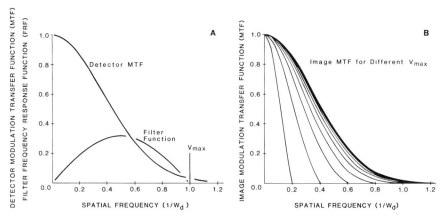

Fig. 19-7.   (A) Detector modulation transfer function (MTF) and reconstruction filter function with a cutoff frequency ν_{max}. Spatial frequencies are expressed in units of $(1/W_d)$, where W_d is the FWHM of the detector line spread function. (B) MTF for image reconstructed with different cutoff frequencies, starting at $\nu_{max} = 0.2$ and increasing in increments of 0.2 units. As cutoff frequency is increased, image MTF approaches a limit determined by the detector.

illustrates the tradeoffs between these variables. If the filter cutoff frequency is low compared with the detector resolution, then the reconstruction filter determines the tomographic image resolution. As the filter cutoff frequency is increased, tomographic image resolution initially increases in proportion to the cutoff frequency. However, as the cutoff frequency is further increased, improvements in image resolution become disproportionately smaller and eventually reach the limit determined by the detector resolution. Beyond this point, no improvement in image resolution can be achieved unless the detector resolution is increased. Once the limiting resolution determined by detector resolution and filter cutoff frequency have been established, the linear sampling distance should be selected to properly recover this resolution.

The angular sampling interval (angle between projections) should provide sampling around the periphery at approximately the same intervals as the linear sampling distance. Thus, if projections are acquired around a field of view of diameter D and the linear sampling distance across each projection is d, the number of angular views should be approximately the length of $180°$ arc over which projections are taken divided by the sampling distance:

$$\text{number of angular views} = \pi D/2d \qquad (19\text{-}9)$$

Figure 19-8 illustrates the effect of angular sampling interval in emission tomography.

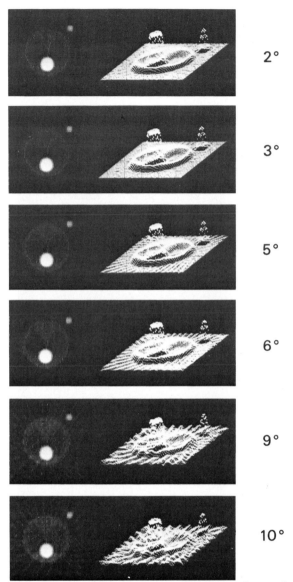

	2°
	3°
	5°
	6°
	9°
	10°

Fig. 19-8. Effects of angular sampling interval on emission computed tomography. As the angles between views increases (and the number of views decreases), artefacts are created as a consequence of angular undersampling. In this example, the artefacts are insignificant for angular separations of 5° or less. (Reprinted from ref. 4: Budinger TF: Physical attributes of single-photon tomography. J Nucl Med 21:579–592, 1980. With permission.)

It also is necessary that data be collected over a full 180° arc. If an arc of less than 180° is used, the data set is insufficient to correctly reconstruct the tomographic distribution of activity. Figure 19-9 demonstrates that projections missing from the full 180° arc cause data to flare out past the true object and produce geometric distortions perpendicular to the direction of the missing projections. This was a problem for a number of unsuccessful tomographic techniques developed in nuclear medicine that were classified as "limited-angle tomography" (7-pinhole, rotating slant-hole tomography). These techniques collected data from an arc considerably less than 180° and therefore yielded distortions in the resultant images similar to those illustrated Figure 19-9. Such distortions are not easy to "read out" of the images because they are variable in shape and magnitude depending upon where the objects are in the field of view.

C. QUANTITATIVE ASPECTS OF EMISSION CT

1. Spatial Resolution

Spatial resolution in SPECT and PET is characterized by line spread functions and MTFs, as for other imaging systems (Chapter 18, Section A.2). Because of their three-dimensional characteristics, ECT devices have two components of spatial resolution, *in-plane*, measured within the imaged plane, and *axial*, measured perpendicular to the imaged plane.

In-plane spatial resolution is affected by the intrinsic resolution of the imaging device (detector and positioning electronics for a gamma camera, or size and spacing of individual detector elements in a multicrystal device), collimator resolution, sampling interval (linear and angular), reconstruction filter function, scattered radiation, image display matrix, and in the case of PET, accidental coincidence events. Most manufacturers specify image resolution for the finest possible sampling, a high value of v_{max} for the filter function, and the finest possible image display matrix. In SPECT, it is not uncommon for manufacturers to specify image resolution for a high-resolution collimator, but to specify sensitivity for a high-sensitivity (low-resolution) collimator. In most imaging applications, the high-sensitivity collimator usually is used because of the demanding statistical requirements of ECT; hence, the spatial resolution achieved in practice often is less than quoted performance levels.

Axial resolution depends on slice thickness, which is determined by the detector resolution in the axial direction. Axial resolution is not affected by linear or angular sampling, reconstruction filter, or display matrix. The effect of decreasing axial resolution, i.e., increasing slice thickness, is to increase the amount of averaging or blurring of structures

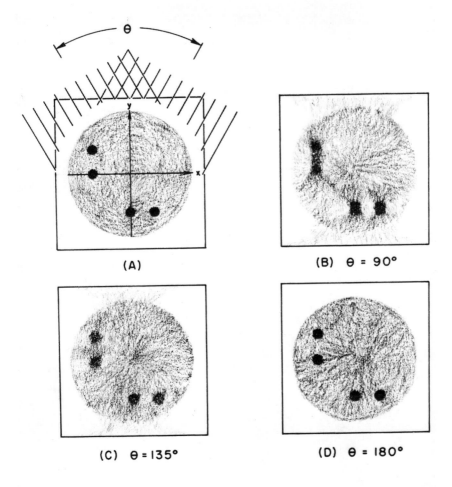

(A)

(B) Θ = 90°

(C) Θ = 135°

(D) Θ = 180°

Fig. 19-9. Effects of angular sampling range. (A) Definition of angular sampling range, and images obtained by sampling over (B) 90°, (C) 135°, and (D) 180° ranges. Note that sampling over an interval of less than 180° distorts the shapes of the objects and adds artefactual data to the image. (Reprinted from ref 1: Phelps ME, Hoffman EJ, Gado M, et al: Computerized transaxial reconstruction, in DeBlanc H, Sorenson J (eds): Non Invasive Brain Imaging, Computed Tomography and Radionuclides. Society of Nuclear Medicine, 1975. pp 111–146. With permission.)

along the axial direction. It also results in increased sensitivity by increasing the thickness of tissue defining the plane of interest. In addition, for both PET and SPECT, increased slice thickness usually implies an increase in the thickness of exposed detector area per slice. Thus, sensitivity usually increases as the square of the axial resolution. An exception to this occurs in SPECT with a fixed gamma camera and collimator when axial resolution is decreased simply by summing image planes. In this case sensitivity is increased in direct proportion to axial resolution.

The uniformity of resolution across the field of view is another important characteristic of an ECT device. Reconstruction algorithms are based on the assumption that each data point within a scan profile reflects the sum of activity within a well-defined column of tissue through the body. Nonuniform resolution with depth impairs the validity of this assumption and produces artefacts in the reconstructed image. In PET and SPECT these errors tend to cause blurring effects rather than sharp high-spatial-frequency artefacts.

Patient motion also degrades spatial resolution (Chapter 18, Section A.1). While it usually is possible to monitor for significant motion during a study, some types of motion (diaphragmatic and cardiac) cannot be controlled. In these situations, gating the acquisition will improve image resolution. Short scan times also minimize the effects of both voluntary and involuntary motion.

2. Partial-Volume Effects

A tomographic system has a characteristic "resolution volume" determined by the combination of its in-plane and axial resolutions. This volume has an approximately cylindrical shape of height = 2 × FWHM axial resolution and diameter = 2 × FWHM in-plane resolution. The images produced by an ECT system reflect the amount of activity within these individual volume elements. For a source of this size or larger, the response reflects both the amount and concentration of activity. Smaller objects only partially occupy the characteristic volume. In this case, the system response reflects the amount but not the concentration of activity within the object. If the concentration of radioactivity within an object is held constant, the apparent concentration in the image decreases as object size decreases. This effect is illustrated in Figure 19-10, in which objects of identical concentration are seen to decrease in intensity with decreasing size. Total counts are conserved for the smaller objects; however, they are distributed over an area larger than the physical

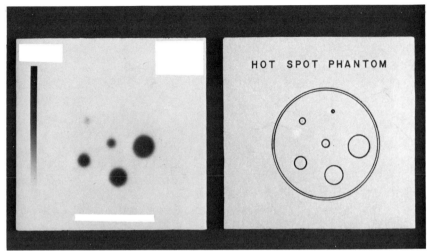

Fig. 19-10.   Illustration of partial volume effect with PET. Test object shown on the right is a 21 cm diameter water-filled cylinder containing six smaller cylinders of 6.35, 9.53, 15.9, 22.2, 31.8, and 38.1 mm. Although each of the cylinders has the same concentration of positron emitting isotope, the intensity and therefore the apparent concentrations in the cylinders appears to decrease as cylinder size decreases. Imaging system resolution is 11.6 mm. (Reprinted from ref. 5: Hoffman EJ, Huang SC, Phelps ME: Quantitation of positron emission computed tomography: 1. Effect of object size. J Comput Assist Tomogr 3:299–308, 1979. With permission.)

dimensions of the object and thus appear to represent larger objects of less than their actual activity concentrations.

This *partial-volume effect* is important for both qualitative and quantitative interpretation of ECT data. Although they may be visible in the image, small objects near the resolution limits of the device appear to contain smaller concentrations of radioactivity than they actually do. The ratio of the apparent concentration to true concentration is called the *recovery coefficient* (RC). The RC for a three-dimensional object is a product of the RCs in each dimension. Figure 19-11 illustrates RC vs. object size (in units of in-plane FWHM) for several different image resolutions of a PET device. In principle, if an ECT system has a known and uniform spatial resolution and if the size of the object is known, a "recovery coefficient correction factor" can be applied to correct for the partial-volume underestimation of concentrations for small objects. While this approach works well in phantom studies in which object sizes are well characterized, the sizes of in vivo objects usually are too poorly defined for this method to be useful.

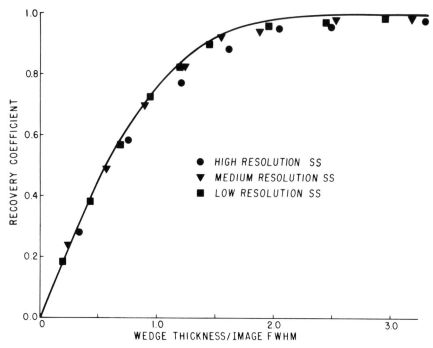

Fig. 19-11.   Recovery coefficient, RC, vs. object size (in units of size/FWHM) for a PET system. Objects were wedges of varying widths that were much thicker than the axial resolution of the tomogram. The smooth line is a theoretical RC response for a system with a Gaussian-shaped LSF. Data points were measured with a PET system operated in high-resolution (circles), medium-resolution (triangles), or low-resolution (squares) modes. (Reprinted from ref. 5: Hoffman EJ, Huang SC, Phelps ME: Quantitation in positron emission computed tomography: 1. Effect of object size. J Comput Assist Tomogr 3:299–308, 1979. With permission.)

3. Effects of Photon Attenuation

The attenuation of a monochromatic photon beam is described by:

$$I = I_0 e^{-\mu x} \tag{19-10}$$

where I_0 is the incident intensity, I is the transmitted intensity, x is the path length through the absorber, and μ is the linear attenuation coefficient of the absorber for the energy of incident radiation (Chapter 9, Section B.1). Because body tissues absorb or scatter a significant amount of radiation, it is necessary to apply attenuation corrections to avoid image distortions in ECT.

The magnitude of attenuation effects in SPECT is illustrated in Figures 19-12 and 19-13. In Figure 19-12, projection data acquired with a gamma camera from a water-filled cylinder containing a uniform concentration of activity are shown for 511 keV annihilation photons ($\mu = 0.1$ cm^{-1}) and 140 keV ^{99m}Tc photons ($\mu = 0.15$ cm^{-1}). Also illustrated is the profile for $\mu = 0$, i.e, no attenuation. For thicker sections of the cylinder, the effect of attenuation is pronounced and in fact is the dominant factor in the measured profile values. Figure 19-13 illustrates SPECT images and measured count densities for uniform cylinders of activity with various

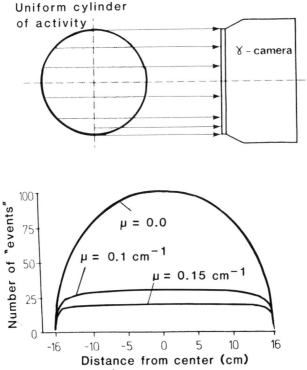

Fig. 19-12. Scan profiles of detected events across a uniform cylinder of activity, for different values of linear attenuation coefficient. $\mu = 0.1$ cm^{-1} (511 keV annihilation photons), $\mu = 0.15$ cm^{-1} (140 keV ^{99m}Tc photons), and $\mu = 0$ (no attenuation). Note that under actual measurement conditions, most photons are eliminated by attenuation. (Reprinted from ref. 6: Larsson SA: Gamma camera emission tomography: Development and properties of a multi-sectional emission computed tomography system. Acta Radiol (Suppl 363), 1980. With permission.)

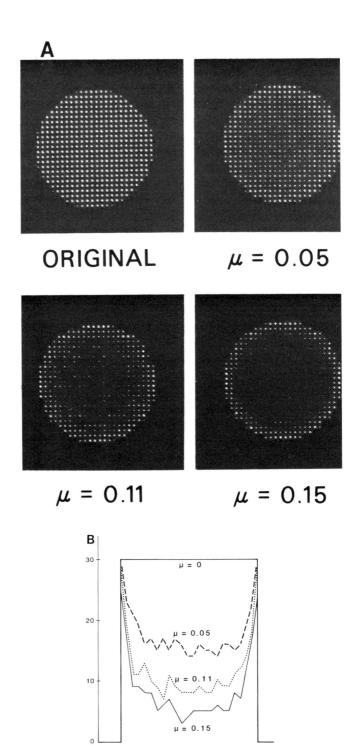

A

ORIGINAL $\mu = 0.05$

$\mu = 0.11$ $\mu = 0.15$

B

410

attenuation values. As the attenuation coefficient μ increases, the resultant images and image count profiles reveal progressively greater suppression of counts at the center of the image.

Several methods have been used for attenuation correction in SPECT. Most are based on the assumption that the linear attenuation coefficient at a given energy is constant for all body tissues. In the most common approach, an initial image produced without correction provides an estimate of x, the average attenuation path length through tissue. The corrected image then is determined from Equation 19-10 using the average attenuation path length for each pixel and a constant value for the attenuation coefficient, μ.

Other approaches include using the arithmetic $[(I_1 + I_2)/2]$ or geometric $\sqrt{I_1 \times I_2}$ mean of scan profiles obtained at 180° angles to each other and correcting the scan profiles for attenuation before image reconstruction. The rationale for using the geometric mean is as follows. Consider the source of activity shown in Figure 19-14. The attenuation of photons directed toward detector 1 is given by

$$I_1 = I_{01} \, e^{-\mu a} \tag{19-11}$$

and for those directed toward detector 2 by

$$I_2 = I_{02} \, e^{-\mu b} \tag{19-12}$$

where a and b are the source depths. Note that $b = D - a$. Taking the product and then the square root of Equations 19-11 and 19-12, one obtains

$$\sqrt{(I_1 \times I_2)} = \sqrt{(I_{01} \times I_{02})} \, e^{-\mu D/2} \tag{19-13}$$

Thus, the geometric mean of counts from opposed detectors depends on total tissue thickness, D, but not on source depths, a and b. This result is exact only for a point or a plane source, but corrections can be applied as approximations for simple extended sources, e.g., uniform volume sources.[8] The geometric mean also depends on the unattenuated counts,

←

Fig. 19-13. SPECT images (A) and reconstructed count profiles (B) for a uniform cylinder of activity for various values of linear attenuation coefficients μ. (Reprinted from ref. 7: Budinger TF, Gullberg GT: Transverse section reconstruction of gamma-ray emitting radionuclides in patients, in Ter-Pogossian MM, Phelps ME, Brownell GL, Cox JR, Davis DO, Evens RG (eds): Reconstruction Tomography in Diagnostic Radiology and Nuclear Medicine. Baltimore, University Park Press, 1977, pp 315–342. With permission.)

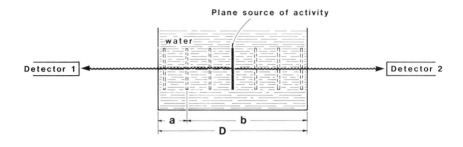

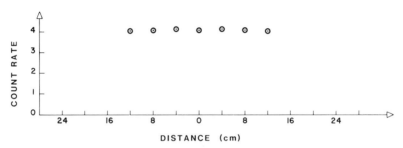

Fig. 19-14. (Top) Plane source of activity at different depths in an attenuating medium. For ordinary γ-ray emitters, effects of attenuation and distance can be compensated for by using the geometric or arithmetic mean and a correction for total tissue thickness, D. For positron emitters, the coincidence count rate (bottom) also depends only on total thickness, D, and not on specific location, a and b. See text for equations. (Reprinted from ref. 9: Phelps ME, Hoffman EJ, Mullani NA, et al: Application annihilation coincidence detection to transverse reconstruction tomography. J Nucl Med 16:210–224, 1975. With permission.)

I_{01} and I_{02}, which may change with a and b because of distance effects; however, for systems using parallel-hole collimators, e.g., SPECT gamma camera systems, unattenuated counts do not change with distance (Chapter 16, Section B.3, Figure 16-14).

The analysis and equations above are accurate for a single point source of activity. When multiple sources are present, the situation is more complicated, as shown by the following example.

Example 19-1.

Derive the equation for the geometric mean of counts from two point sources located along a line between two detectors and show why it cannot be described only in terms of the unattenuated counts, I_0, and I_{02}, and μ and D (distance between the detectors) as can be done for a single point source (Equation 19-13).

Answer:

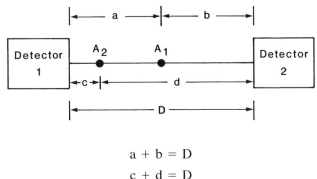

$$a + b = D$$
$$c + d = D$$

I_1 = measured counts
from detector 1 = $I_{02}e^{-\mu c} + I_{01}e^{-\mu a}$

I_2 = measured counts
from detector 2 = $I_{01}e^{-\mu b} + I_{02}e^{-\mu d}$

geometric mean = $\sqrt{I_1 \times I_2}$

$$= \sqrt{(I_{02}^2 e^{-\mu(c+d)} + I_{01}^2 e^{-\mu(a+b)} + I_{01}I_{02}e^{-\mu(c+b)} + I_{01}I_{02}e^{-\mu(a+d)}}$$

$$= \sqrt{(I_{02}^2 + I_{01}^2)e^{-\mu D} + I_{01}I_{02}e^{-\mu(c+b)} + I_{01}I_{02}e^{-\mu(a+d)}}$$

Only the first term in the last expression depends only on I_{01}, I_{02}, μ, and D. The other two terms contain exponential terms $[e^{-\mu(c+b)}$ and $e^{-\mu(a+d)}]$ that depend upon the relative locations of the two sources between the detectors. Therefore, attenuation effects depend upon the source distribution, and the simple correction scheme for point sources and line sources must be modified for more complicated source distributions.[8]

Equations similar to Equations (19-11)–(19-13) can be written for the arithmetic mean, although in this case the effects of source depth are not eliminated completely, even for point sources. Figure 19-15 and Table 19-1 show line spread functions for a single gamma camera detector and for the arithmetic and geometric means of counts from opposed detectors for a point source of ^{99m}Tc in air (left) and at different depths in a water phantom (right). From this it can be seen that attenuation has much stronger effects than distance. The combined effects of distance and

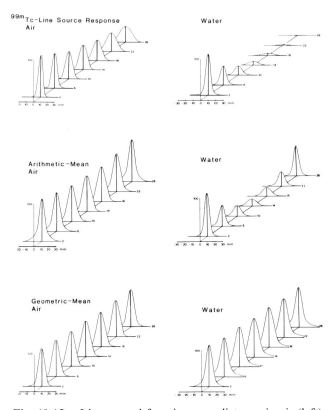

Fig. 19-15. Line spread functions vs. distance in air (left) and in water (right) for high-resolution parallel-hole collimator on Anger camera. The line source was a 100 mm long plastic tube with an internal diameter of 2.5 mm. The tube was mounted inside a tank (methacrylate) measuring 410 mm in length, 310 mm in width, 300 mm in thickness. Measurements were made either with the tank empty (in air) or filled with water. (Top): single detector only; (middle): arithmetic mean of opposing detector profiles; (bottom): geometric mean of opposed detector profiles. (Reprinted from ref. 6: Larsson SA: Gamma camera emission tomography: Development and properties of a multi-sectional emission computed tomography system. Acta Radiol Suppl 363. 1980. With permission.)

Table 19-1
Numerical data for Figure 19-15

Distance from Collimator (cm)	AIR Relative* Maximum Response (%)	Resolution FWHM (mm)	Distance from Collimator (cm)	WATER Relative* Maximum Response (%)	Resolution FWHM (mm)
		^{99m}Tc line source response			
2	100	7.4	2	100	7.5
6	84	8.6	6	47	9.4
10	66	10.0	10	23	11.2
14	58	12.5	14	10	13.9
18	49	14.7	18	8.1	16.3
22	44	17.2	22	1.9	19.1
26	38	20.0	26	0.8	21.6
		Arithmetic Mean			
2–28	100	8.5	2–28	100	7.8
6–24	93	10.6	6–24	50	8.6
10–20	84	12.3	10–20	25	11.5
14–16	84	13.2	14–16	17	14.3
18–12	82	12.7	18–12	21	13.0
22–8	90	11.2	22–8	34	10.4
26–4	99	9.8	26–4	71	8.1
		Geometric Mean			
2–28	100	9.4	2–28	100	9.9
6–24	98	10.8	6–24	93	11.7
10–20	94	12.4	10–20	95	13.3
14–16	94	13.2	14–16	93	14.3
18–12	93	12.7	18–12	95	14.1
22–8	97	11.7	22–8	93	13.2
26–4	100	10.4	26–4	96	11.9

Adapted from ref 6: Larsson SA: Gamma camera emission tomography: Development and properties of a multi-sectional emission computed tomography system. Acta Radiol (Suppl 363), 1980.
* Valve at peak of line spread function.

415

attenuation result in a 100-fold range in counts recorded with a single detector (Figure 19-15, top right). With the arithmetic mean (Figure 19-15, middle) the range is reduced to a factor of five, and with the geometric mean (Figure 19-15, bottom), they are virtually eliminated, although there still is a small reduction in relative counts when the source is at the deepest location in the phantom.

To correct for attenuation using the geometric or arithmetic mean an estimate for tissue thickness, D is required. This generally is accomplished by estimating body thickness from a preliminary uncorrected image reconstruction or by assuming a standard body size and shape. SPECT attenuation correction methods that use a constant value for linear attenuation coefficients for body tissues work reasonably well for relatively uniform and symmetric body sections, e.g., the head and abdomen, but are less successful in the thorax because of the variable shapes and attenuation characteristics of internal structures. Methods for incorporating variable attenuation coefficients and accurately measured internal path lengths (e.g., from transmission scans) have been implemented in SPECT[7], but generally are not convenient for routine use. Accurate attenuation correction remains a significant problem for SPECT and is one of the major limitations for quantitative applications of the technique as well as a significant source of image artefacts and distortions. Similar distortions also can occur in PET. An example of the effects of attenuation on ECT is shown in Figure 19-16.

Although physical attenuation processes are similar for PET systems, the coincidence detection methodology (Chapter 20, Section D.1) facilitates a more effective solution to the problem. Positron annihilation results in the emission of two oppositely directed 511 keV photons from the site of the annihilation event (Chapter 2, Figure 2-7). Coincidence detection requires that both 511 keV photons reach the opposing detectors simultaneously (see Figure 20-8). The probability that an individual photon will escape the body is given by (I/I_0) from Equation 19-10. Therefore, the probability that two 511 keV photons with respective path lengths of a and b will escape from the body is given by:

$$\text{Probability} = e^{-\mu a}\, e^{-\mu b} = e^{-\mu(a+b)} = e^{-\mu D} \qquad (19\text{-}14)$$

where D is the total path length (body thickness) as shown in Figure 19-14.

For coincidence detection of annihilation photons, the attenuation factor thus is independent of the position, a and b, of the positron source between the detectors and depends only on the total tissue thickness, D. Furthermore, Equation 19-14 is accurate for both thin (point or plane) and for multiple or extended (volume) sources of positron emitter. This is

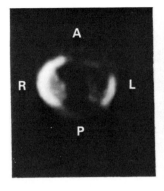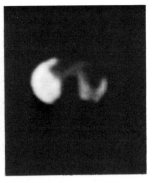

NO
ATTENUATION
CORRECTION

TRANSMISSION
ATTENUATION
CORRECTION

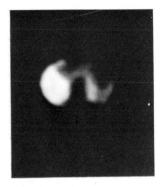

GEOMETRIC
ATTENUATION
CORRECTION

Fig. 19-16. Tomographic images of an abdomen obtained with a PET system and ^{13}N-labeled ammonia. Left: Image reconstructed with no attenuation correction. Right: Image reconstructed with attenuation correction based on direct measurement of tissue attenuation by transmission technique. Bottom: Image reconstructed using assumed elliptical body shape fitted to uncorrected image and constant value of $\mu = 0.09$ cm^{-1}. ^{13}NH$_3$ distributions in the liver, pancreas, spleen, and left kidney are represented accurately in attenuation corrected images. In the uncorrected image, activity appears to be most intense at the periphery, where attenuation is least. (Reprinted from ref. 10 Phelps ME, Hoffman EJ, Mullani NA, et al: Some performance and design characteristics of PETT III, in Ter-Pogossian MM, Phelps ME, Brownell GL, Cox JR, Davis DO, Evens RG (eds): Reconstruction Tomography in Diagnostic Radiology and Nuclear Medicine. Baltimore, University Park Press, 1977, pp 371–392. With permission.)

Table 19-2

Average pathlength linear attenuation coefficients (μl)
measured in PET.

	Level	μ (cm^{-1}) S.D. (% S.D.)
Head	4 cm above orbital meatal line	0.088 ± 0.003 (3.4)
Abdomen	4 cm below tip of xiphoid	0.089 ± 0.007 (7.9)
Chest	4th intercostal space	0.067 ± 0.018 (27)

Reprinted from ref. 10: Phelps ME, Hoffman EJ, Mullani NA, et al. Some performance and design and characteristics of PETT III, in Ter Pogossian MM, Phelps ME, Brownell GL, Cox JR, Davis DO, Evens RG (eds): Reconstruction Tomography in Diagnostic Radiology and Nuclear Medicine. Baltimore, University Park Press, 1977, pp 371–392. With permission.

unique to coincidence detection with PET and permits more accurate correction for attenuation than in SPECT.

There are two methods of attenuation correction in PET: calculated approximation and direct measurement approaches. The calculated correction method assumes a constant linear attenuation coefficient and utilizes values of D obtained from the object itself or geometric approximations of its outline, e.g., using an ellipse as a border for a head section. In either case, the boundary is chosen from initial images reconstructed without attenuation correction. Equation 19-14 then is applied on a point-by-point basis to the projection profiles and the image is reconstructed from the corrected profiles. While this approach also suffers from inaccuracies based upon variations in μ as do the similar methods in SPECT, the thickness D can be measured with reasonable accuracy, and the values of μ vary much less for annihilation photons than they do for the lower-energy photons commonly used for SPECT (Table 19-2). In addition, the value of μ is the average value along all the attenuation path lengths across the object from all the projections around the object. For example, in the worst-case situation of the chest, the average pathlength value of μ has a measured standard deviation of about 27 percent. This is much smaller than the point-to-point variation in the attenuation coefficient of lung tissue of 0.032 cm^{-1} to muscle of 0.088 cm^{-1} (i.e., a variation of 275 percent).

In the direct measurement method, attenuation profiles are measured with an external ring source of positron activity placed between the patient and the detectors of the PET system. Measurements are obtained with (I) and without (I$_0$) the patient in place, and the ratio of the two measurements provides a correction factor that can be applied on a point-by-point basis to the emission projection profiles. The corrected data then are used to reconstruct the final image. This method requires two additional scans to acquire the transmission data; however, the attenuation correction is very accurate. In contrast, the calculation method introduces errors as a result of small inaccuracies in defining the body contour.

The transmission correction method adds error mainly because of statistical noise in the transmission data. These errors are propagated into the final emission data through the correction process. Additional errors can occur if the amounts of scattered radiation in the transmission and emission data are significantly different. These errors usually are small in a properly designed PET system. An intermediate approach is to use a rapid transmission scan, reconstruct a tissue density image from the transmission data to define the outside boundaries and major internal structures of varying attenuation, e.g., lungs vs. bone or soft tissue, and calculate average path length attenuation corrections from these data by assigning known values of μ to the various types of tissues along the attenuation path. This approach has the favorable properties of both the calculated and transmission correction methods while minimizing the errors of each. Figure 19-16 illustrates the impact of attenuation correction on a set of images.

4. Image Noise

Image noise usually is analyzed in terms of signal-to-noise ratio (S/N) rather than absolute noise levels, because the significance of the noise depends on its magnitude in comparison to the signal levels of interest. Often the noise level is expressed as $(S/N)^{-1} \times 100$ percent, because this expression describes the noise level relative to the signal. For example, if a radioactive sample provides 100 counts, the noise (standard deviation) is 10 counts (Chapter 6, Section B.1). The signal-to-noise ratio is (100/10) = 10, and the noise level is 10 percent.

To analyze the signal-to-noise characteristics of a tomographic image, consider Figure 19-17. Images A and B are composed of an array of square picture elements, or pixels (Chapter 21, Section A), each characterized by a total number of counts, N_p. From the discussion above, it would be expected that the noise in a given pixel to be simply the square root of the pixel counts, $\sqrt{N_p}$; however, this is the case only when the data for individual pixels are independent of other pixels in the image. This applies to standard planar imaging but not the ECT, because the reconstructed value for each pixel is influenced by the values in other pixels crossed by the same sampling lines (Figure 19-17B). In the backprojection process, counts for each pixel are distributed among all of the pixels along the sampling line and then removed from the inappropriate pixels by the reconstruction filter. This process, however, produces noise from these arithmetic operations (Chapter 6, Section C) that is propogated among all of the pixels along the sampling line in the sampling and backprojection processes. The noise propagation effect is greater for longer path lengths through the body and also increases as the number of pixels along the line increases, i.e, as spatial resolution is increased. This increase occurs because the number of arithmetic operations, and therefore the magnitude of error propagation, increases. The propagation of noise requires the accumulation of a large number of image counts for ECT.

The signal-to-noise ratio, S/N, for a reconstructed image of a uniform distribution of activity is given by[11]:

$$\text{Signal/Noise} = \sqrt{12\ N/\pi^2(D/d)^3} \tag{19-15}$$

where D is the object diameter (e.g., the diameter of a body section), d is the linear sampling distance, and N is the total number of counts in the recontructed image. Noise is expressed as a standard deviation of recorded signal counts, N, in the above relationship. Equation 19-15 assumes the use of a ramp filter and a linear sampling distance d given by Equation 19-8.

The signal-to-noise ratio increases as the total counts increases and decreases as the number of resolution elements (D/d) increases. For a given signal-to-noise ratio, improvement of spatial resolution by a factor of 2 (i.e., d changes to $d/2$) requires the total number of counts to increase by a factor of 8 to keep the signal-to-noise ratio constant per resolution element.

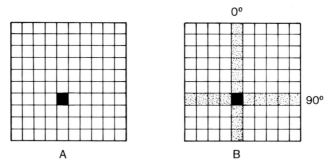

Fig. 19-17.   In standard planar imaging (A), noise in a given pixel is determined only by the number of counts in that pixel. In ECT (B), the number of counts in a pixel is calculated from measurements made through many other pixels. Noise is thus determined by the number of counts in all measurements crossing the pixel, as exemplified by 0° and 90° projections.

From Equation 19-15, it can be shown that for ECT, the image signal-to-noise ratio, in terms of reconstructed counts per resolution element (N_r) and the total number of resolution elements (R) is given by:

$$\text{Signal/Noise} = \sqrt{(N_r)}/^4\sqrt{R} \qquad (19\text{-}16)$$

Therefore, the "intuitive" signal-to-noise ratio of $\sqrt{N_r}$ that would be obtained by analogy to planar imaging is reduced by a factor of $^4\sqrt{R}$ in ECT. It is assumed that for both ECT and planar imaging that all image noise originates from statistical noise in the counting data. While this is not strictly correct, it facilitates a numerical description of noise and its impact on the image signal-to-noise ratio for both ECT and planar imaging. In addition, if measured image noise is greater than predicted from equations 19-15 and 19-16, then it is apparent that other sources of noise are significant.

Example 19-2.
   Given two square images of uniform activity, one planar and one ECT as in Figure 19-17, each 20 × 20 cm with 1 × 1 cm pixel size, and each containing 1 million counts, what is the average percentage of noise per pixel in each image?

Answer:
   (A):   planar image
      percentage of noise = (noise/signal) × 100%
      total number of pixels = 20 × 20 = 400
      counts per pixel = $10^6/400$ = 2500
      percentage of noise = $\sqrt{(2500)}/(2500)$ × 100% = 2%

   (B):   ECT image
      resolution element and pixel size are the same in this case (each is a 1 cm × 1 cm square)
      percentage of noise = (noise/signal) × 100%
      From Equation 19-15:

$$(N/S) \times 100\% = [1/\sqrt{12 \ N/\pi^2(D/d)^3}] \times 100\%$$

$$= [1/\sqrt{12 \times 10^6/\pi^2(20/1)^3}] \times 100\% = 8.1\%$$

Example 19-3.
   Given the same image data described in Example 19-2, what is the average percentage of noise for a 3 × 3 pixel region of interest on each image?

Answer:

(A)   planar image:

percentage of noise = (noise/signal) × 100%

3 × 3 ROI has 9 pixels each with 2500 counts

percentage of noise = $[\sqrt{9 \times 2500}/9 \times 2500)] \times 100\%$
$$= 0.67\%$$

(B)   ECT image:

percentage of noise = (noise/signal) × 100%

3 × 3 ROI has 9 pixels and 9 resolution elements, therefore the total number of resolution elements in the image is 400/9. Thus, from Equation 19-16

$$\text{noise/signal} \times 100\% = {}^{4}\sqrt{(400/9)}/\sqrt{(9 \times 2500)} \times 100\% = 1.7\%$$

Example 19-4.

Assume that the 1 million count ECT image in Examples 19-2 and 19-3 was acquired in 1 minute. If the linear sampling distance d is decreased to 0.5 cm in order to double the resolution, how much time and how many counts would be necessary to obtain an image with a signal-to-noise ratio per pixel equal to that of the original?

Answer:

From Equation 19-15

$$\text{original (signal/noise)} = \sqrt{(12 \times 10^{6})/\pi^{2}(20/1)^{3}} = 12.33$$

Therefore, if N is the number of counts in the new image and $d = 0.5$ cm,

$$\sqrt{(12 \times N)/\pi^{2}(20/0.5)^{3}} = 12.33$$

Solving for N:

$$N = 8 \text{ million counts in 8 minutes}$$

REFERENCES

1.   Phelps ME, Hoffman EJ, Gado M, et al: Computerized transaxial reconstruction, in DeBlanc H, Sorenson J (eds): Non Invasive Brain Imaging, Computed Tomography and Radionuclides. Society of Nuclear Medicine, Inc., 1975, pp 111–146

2. Phelps ME, Huang SC, Hoffman EJ, et al: An analysis of signal amplification using small detectors in positron emission tomography. J Comput Assist Tomogr 6:551–565, 1982
3. Oppenheim AV, Wilsky AS: Signals and Systems. Englewood Cliffs, NJ Prentice-Hall, Inc., 1983, Chapter 8.
4. Budinger TF: Physical attributes of single-photon tomography. J Nucl Med 21:579–592, 1980
5. Hoffman EJ, Huang SC, Phelps ME: Quantitation in positron emission computed tomography: 1. Effect of object size. Comput Assist Tomogr 3:299–308, 1979
6. Larsson SA: Gamma camera emission tomography: Development and properties of a multi-sectional emission computed tomography system. Acta Radiol (Suppl 363), 1980
7. Budinger TF, Gullberg GT: Transverse section recontruction of gamma-ray emitting radionuclides in patients, in Ter-Pogossian MM, Phelps ME, Brownell GL, Cox JR, Davis DO, Evens RG (eds): Reconstruction Tomography in Diagnostic Radiology and Nuclear Medicine. Baltimore, University Park Press, 1977, pp 315–342
8. Sorenson JA. Quantitative measurement of radioactivity in vivo by whole-body counting, in Hine GJ, Sorenson JA (eds): Instrumentation of Nuclear Medicine, vol 2. New York, Academic Press, 1974
9. Phelps ME, Hoffman EJ, Mullani NA, et al: Application annihilation coincidence detection to transverse reconstruction tomography. J Nucl Med 16:210–224, 1975
10. Phelps ME, Hoffman EJ, Mullani NA, et al: Some performance and design characteristics of PETT III, in Ter-Pogossian MM, Phelps ME, Brownell GL, Cox JR, Davis DO, Evens RG (eds): Recontruction Tomography in Diagnostic Radiology and Nuclear Medicine. Baltimore, University Park Press, 1977, pp 371–392
11. Hoffman EJ, Phelps ME: Positron emission tomography: principles and quantitation, in Phelps ME, Mazziotta JC, Schelbert HR (eds): Positron Emission Tomography and Autoradiography: Principles and Applications for the Brain and Heart. New York, Raven Press, 1986, pp 237–286

Additional descriptions of tomographic imaging techniques may be found in Budinger.[4]

20
Nuclear Medicine Tomography: Systems and Devices

As discussed in Chapter 19, tomography is performed in nuclear medicine using two basic approaches: focal-plane techniques and computed reconstruction techniques. The reconstruction techniques in turn can be categorized as those based on ordinary γ-ray emitters (SPECT) and those based on annihilation photons from positron emitters (PET). In this chapter we describe systems and devices for performing each of these types of tomography and some practical problems associated with them.

A. FOCAL-PLANE SYSTEMS

Focal-plane tomography is performed by obtaining images from different projection angles and then shifting and superimposing these images to bring a selected plane into focus while blurring the images of off-plane structures. Focal-plane tomography as performed in nuclear medicine often is called *collimator tomography* because the systems used achieve the tomographic effect by collimator projection techniques. It also is referred to as *longitudinal*, as opposed to *transaxial*, tomography, because the tomographic planes are oriented parallel to the collimator face. A simple example of collimator tomography, discussed in Chapter 19, Section A, is the focused collimator used for rectilinear scanning.

A variety of other devices are included in this category, most of

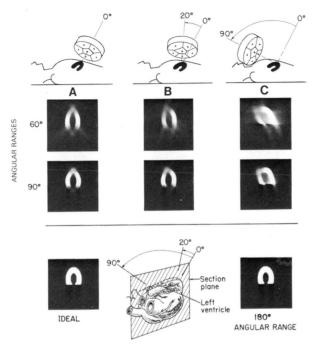

Fig. 20-1. Illustration of the 7-pinhole collimator tomography technique and simulated images of the myocardium with the collimator aligned (A) along the ventricular axis, (B) 20° off axis, and (C) 90° off axis, for angular sampling ranges of 60° or 90°. The ideal image is shown at the lower left and simulated results for 180° angular sampling at the lower right. Image distortion increases as the acquisition deviates from the ventricular axis, and distortions are more marked for a more limited angular sampling range. (Reprinted from ref. 1: Budinger TF: Physical attributes of single-photon tomography. J Nucl Med 21:579–592, 1980. With permission.)

which are primarily of historical interest. Examples include multiple-pinhole arrays (Figure 20-1) and rotating slant-hole collimators (Chapter 15, Section B.3). These collimator devices produce different views of the object either with the collimator held stationary (multiple-pinhole collimators) or with the collimator moved to different positions (rotating slant-hole collimator). The different views then are shifted and superimposed (i.e., backprojected) to geometrically reconstruct tomographic images at different depths. The unprocessed views obtained with multiple-pinhole collimators may be physically separated, as with the 7-pinhole collimator (Figure 20-1), or overlapping. The latter is referred to as *coded aperture* tomography. The overlapping of images in the coded-aperture technique requires an additional processing step to "decode" the projections before image reconstruction. A rotating slant-hole collimator is simply a collimator with parallel holes directed obliquely rather than perpendicular to the collimator face. Rotating the collimator is equivalent to moving the gamma camera head to another position around the patient.

A more complex device based on a combination of detector motion and focused collimators is the *Anger tomoscanner*. Although no longer manufactured, a number of these instruments still are in use. The device is a rectilinear scanner with two detector heads, one above and one below the patient table. The detectors are small (7-PM tube) Anger cameras, each 21.6 cm in diameter and fitted with a focused collimator of 8.9-cm focal length.

The method of obtaining images with the tomoscanner is illustrated in Figure 20-2. A point source between the collimator and the collimator focal point projects an image onto the detector, magnified in size by the converging collimator effect (Equation 15-5) but otherwise similar to a conventional Anger camera image. As the detector scans across the source, the image moves across the detector in a direction opposite to the scanning motion. A point source beyond the focal point also projects a point-source image, but moving in the same direction as the scanning motion. A point source in the collimator focal plane is not seen at all until it is close to the focal point, where it projects a much magnified image covering the entire detector.

Images from different depths are brought into focus for recording by moving the image on the CRT display or by moving the image-recording medium (i.e., the film) in front of the display in synchronization with the motion of sources at the chosen depth. Sources not at the chosen depth do not remain stationary when this is done, resulting in motion blurring of off-plane structures. The displayed image also is magnified or minified to compensate for collimator effects on displayed image size. The tomoscanner produces 12 images simultaneously (six planes for each detector at approximately 2.5 cm intervals), as illustrated in Figure 20-3. (It should be noted that in later versions of the tomoscanner, the image motions, magnifications, minifications, and superpositioning steps were performed by computers operating on digitized images; however, the optical principles described above still are valid descriptions for the image formation process.)

The Anger tomoscanner was perhaps the most successful example of a focal-plane tomography device in nuclear medicine, and was in fact capable of providing improved detectability of lesions in careful clinical

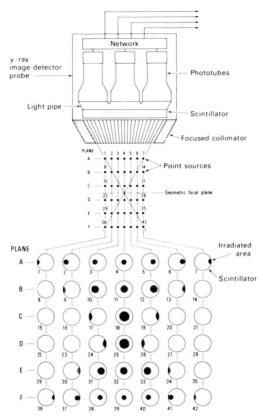

Fig. 20-2. Principles of the Anger tomoscanner. Darkened areas are projections of the radiation field from sources at different distances and at different positions in front of the collimated detector. Sources at different depths produce images of different sizes and with different relative motions on the detector crystal. Different planes are brought into focus by different relative motions and magnifications or minifications of the image on the display device. (Reprinted from ref. 2: Anger HO: Tomography and other depth-discrimination techniques, in Hine GJ, Sorenson JA (eds): Instrumentation in Nuclear Medicine, vol 2. New York, Academic Press, 1974. With permission.)

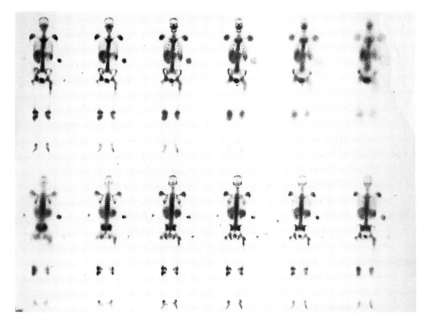

Fig. 20-3. Whole-body bone scan recorded by an Anger tomoscanner. The top
and bottom row of images were recorded by the anterior and posterior detectors,
respectively. The most anterior image is on the upper left while the most posterior
image is on the lower right.

comparisons to conventional planar imaging (see Figure 18-17). However,
along with other focal-plane devices, it did not enjoy long-standing
success. Each of these devices suffers from the fact that the angle over
which projections are collected is insufficient to meet the 180° sampling
requirement for accurate reconstruction of the image (Chapter 19, Section
B.2). The term *limited-angle tomography* often is applied to these
techniques. In addition to producing characteristic angular undersampling
artefacts (see Figures 19-8 and 19-9), their effective depth resolution
produced distortions dependent of object shape and subject orientation.
Thus, while limited-angle approaches may provide usable results in some
regions, e.g., 7-pinhole imaging of the left ventricle of the heart, where
there is some degree of symmetry along the ventricular axis, in most
applications significant image distortions occur. Even when imaging the
myocardium along the ventricular axis, small positioning errors distort
the anatomy and large positioning errors may invalidate the results
completely (Figure 20-1).

   An additional limitation, discussed in Chapter 19, Section A, is that
blurred images and noise from activity above and below the focal plane
obscure the structures of interest in the focal plane. For these reasons,

focal-plane tomography has largely been replaced in clinical settings with rotating gamma camera SPECT devices.

B. GAMMA CAMERA SPECT SYSTEMS

1. Data Acquisition

Most nuclear medicine tomography is performed with Anger camera systems having 1 to 3 detector heads mounted on a gantry to allow rotation around the patient for 180° to 360° angular sampling. These systems typically have an on-line computer and display system and permit the user to choose the display grid and reconstruction filter (e.g., cutoff frequency, shape of filter, etc.). The gamma camera and computer system do not necesssarily have to come from the same manufacturer. Figure 20-4 shows an example of a single-head gamma camera SPECT device. The data acquisition process is outlined in Figure 20-5.

The gamma camera obtains a two-dimensional image at each angular position around the patient. Although 180° angular sampling is adequate

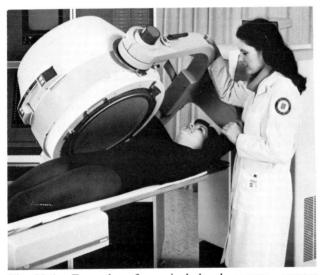

Fig. 20-4. Example of a single-head gamma camera SPECT system. A large-field-of-view detector is attached to a gantry that rotates around the long axis of the patient. Most such devices make circular orbits, although some employ elliptical orbits to maintain the closest possible distance between the body and collimator during rotation. The patient is centered at the axis of rotation of the camera. (Courtesy of Siemens, Inc.)

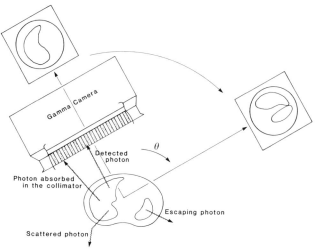

Fig. 20-5.   Gamma camera SPECT data acquisition. As the
gamma camera rotates about the patient, completing an arc
of 180°–360°, two-dimensional images are obtained at each
scanning angle. Scan profiles from these projection images
are used as input for the reconstruction algorithm to compute a tomographic image.

to satisfy angular sampling requirements for ECT, many gamma camera
SPECT studies are performed with 360° rotation to minimize errors
resulting from attenuation and loss of resolution with depth. For most
SPECT applications, the projection images are divided into matrix sizes
of 64 × 64 or 128 × 128 picture elements or *pixels* (Chapter 21, Section
A.1). A plot of the counts from one row of pixels across the image
provides a single scan-projection profile. Thus, a 64 × 64 acquisition
matrix potentially can generate 64 different slice projections, and a
complete set of angular projections can provide 64 tomographic slices. In
practice, the pixels from adjacent rows are added together to improve
counting statistics, thus providing thicker but fewer slices. Typical slice
thicknesses range from 12 to 24 mm.

   A camera with a circular field of view (FOV) completely samples a
spherically shaped volume in one complete rotation around the patient,
whereas a rectangular FOV results in complete sampling of a cylindrical
volume. Both types of camera head shapes are used for SPECT. Most
systems permit the user to define the limits of reconstruction within the
sampled volume, i.e., the number of slices and spatial extent of the
reconstructed volume. For example, a reasonable approximation for the
sampled volume for a circular FOV camera is a cube, whereas for a
rectangular FOV camera it can be approximated by an elongated box

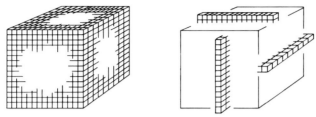

Fig. 20-6.   The sampled volume for a rotating gamma camera can be approximated by a cube of side length equal to the diameter of the camera field of view. Transverse, sagittal, or coronal views can be generated by data sorting routines and appropriately displaying different sections, as shown on the right.

(Figure 20-6). Transverse as well as sagittal and coronal images can be generated from this data set. It also is possible in most systems to generate tomographic images for oblique sections by appropriate interpolation of the data; however, these images do not have spatial resolution equal to that of the basic set of orthogonal planes. If the dimension of the cube is equal to the diameter of the FOV of the camera, then some elements in the corners of the cube are undersampled. Nevertheless, objects of interest are sampled adequately if they are centered in the cube.

2. Spatial Resolution

Spatial resolution in SPECT is limited primarily by collimator resolution and particularly by the variation to collimator resolution with depth (Figure 16-15). Usually, the arithmetic mean of opposed projections is used (Chapter 19, Section C.3). This tends to average the spatial resolution from the two projections and produce a more uniform resolution through the thickness of the patient, but the averaging also tends to degrade resolution to a value that exists at some distance from the collimator (e.g., see Figure 19-15). Typical gamma camera SPECT systems have in-plane spatial resolution in the final reconstructed image of 15–20 mm, FWHM.

3. Sensitivity and Uniformity of Response

The propagation of statistical noise that occurs in the reconstruction process requires that a large number of counts be acquired for SPECT. For example, whereas a conventional planar image of high quality usually can be obtained with about 500,000 counts, a study of similar statistical quality in SPECT requires acquisition of 5–15 million counts (Chapter 19,

Section C.4). To achieve this number of counts in a reasonable imaging time requires that the detector system be designed for high photon-collection efficiency. One approach is to use multiple detectors around the patient to collect several projections at once; however, even with three detector heads, many data collection intervals are required. This makes gamma camera SPECT unsuitable for dynamic imaging of processes that occur within periods of minutes.

Another issue relating to error propagation is that high-frequency noise and artefacts are maximally amplified by the reconstruction filter. In particular, errors and artefacts that occur at frequencies near the sampling frequency will be strongly amplified. A major source of such artefacts is gamma camera nonuniformities (Chapter 16, Section A.2). Although a variety of correction schemes have been developed to deal with this problem for planar imaging (Chapter 16, Section A.3), small differences between flood-field data acquisition and patient imaging conditions, e.g., scatter conditions, still can lead to significant artefacts in SPECT. The problem is compounded by the fact that the rotating motion of the gamma camera moves the nonuniformities around a circular path, resulting in characteristic "ring" artefacts (Figure 20-7). Also, statistical errors in the flood-field image used to correct nonuniformities are propagated and amplified in the final image. Flood-field images used for SPECT should

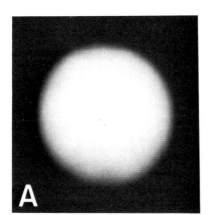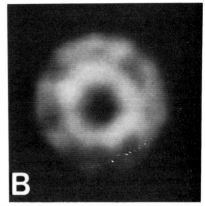

Fig. 20-7. Example of "ring" artifacts in rotating camera SPECT. The object was a uniform cylinder of ^{99m}Tc. Camera uniformity correction was not performed (B) in order to exaggerate artefacts that can occur from camera nonuniformity during circular orbit data collection and image reconstruction. (A) Image reconstruction after camera uniformity correction. (Courtesy of J. Links, Johns Hopkins Medical Institution, Baltimore, Md.)

contain at least 10 million counts to minimize this additional source of image noise.

If the phototubes in the camera are not well-shielded, the effects of the earth's magnetic field (or stray fields from nearby NMR units) can cause image distortions that lead to further artefacts. This results from small changes in PM-tube gain as the camera is rotated in different orientations in the magnetic field. This does not cause problems in conventional planar imaging because the effects are subtle; however, it can lead to significant artefacts in SPECT because of error propagation effects in the reconstruction process.

4. Effects of Scattered Radiation

In comparison with the effects of photon attenuation and camera nonuniformities, the effects of Compton scattering within the patient are of lesser magnitude. Nevertheless, Compton scattering still can have a significant impact on image quality and quantitative relationships between the reconstructed image and source activity. Several correction methods have been proposed. The simplest involves the use of an "effective" linear attenuation coefficient in the attenuation correction that is smaller than the actual value for body tissues. Typically, the value used for 140 keV ^{99m}Tc photons is 0.12 cm^{-1}, instead of the actual value of 0.15 cm^{-1}. By using the smaller value, count values reconstructed for areas near the center of thick objects are underestimated, but the error is offset by the corresponding increase in the number of scattered photons detected from these areas. This approach results in a cosmetic improvement in appearance, e.g., for cylindrical phantoms; however, it is not a good quantitative solution because some of the reconstructed counts represent scattered photons, not true source counts from the reconstructed region.

Another approach involves estimating the distribution of scattered photons from the reconstructed image, e.g., by deconvolution with an assumed scatter distribution function. This method assumes that the scatter distribution function is spatially invariant and of the same general magnitude and shape for all organ and body thicknesses, and may not produce accurate results in all cases.

Yet another method that involves minimal assumptions is to collect counts with both a photopeak window and with a "scatter window" set below the photopeak to generate an approximate image of the scatter distribution.[3] For example, the photopeak window for ^{99m}Tc might be set to 127–153 keV, while the scatter window is set to 92–125 keV. The resulting "scatter image" then is subtracted from the photopeak image to obtain the "true image" without scatter. The weighting factor applied to the scatter image for the subtraction process must be determined experimentally. Images produced by this technique are reasonably accurate for objects 2 cm or larger. This approach also increases statistical noise in the image because of error propagation in the subtraction process.

C. OTHER SPECT SYSTEMS

In addition to the multidetector gamma camera approach, a number of SPECT systems have been constructed with arrays of collimated detector elements. The most well-known of these is the Mark IV brain scanner developed by Kuhl, Edwards, and Ricci.[4] Other systems were subsequently developed that used converging collimators with square or hexagonal arrays of NaI(Tl) detector elements, with up to four such arrays around the patient.[1] Another approach under investigation uses a single cylindrical NaI(Tl) crystal that surrounds the object, and an array of PM tubes to determine the location of events detected within this crystal, similar to the positioning electronics used for a conventional Anger camera.[5] Each of these systems has a circumferential detector array to provide higher photon-collection efficiency and more rapid data acquisition, possibly for dynamic studies. To date, however, none has found widespread use, and their ultimate role in nuclear medicine remains to be determined.

D. PET SYSTEMS

1. Annihilation Coincidence Detection

The fundamental physical difference between PET and SPECT is the use of *annihilation coincidence detection*, or ACD, in the detection process in PET (Figure 20-8). ACD is based on the fact that two 511-keV photons are emitted in opposite directions following the annihilation of a positron and an ordinary electron (see Figure 2-7). Two detectors oriented at 180° to each other are used to detect those photons. A *coincidence circuit* records only those pairs of events that are detected within a narrow time interval that is determined by the resolving time of the detectors and their associated electronics (typically 5–20 nanoseconds). An energy threshhold of 100–350 keV also is used in most systems. As shown in Figure 20-8, ACD defines a volume between the detectors from which true coincidence events can originate. For this reason, ACD sometimes is referred to as an *electronic collimation* technique. Coincidence events involving scattered radiation and accidental coincidences between unrelated events also can occur. These must be dealt with as discussed in Section D.5 below.

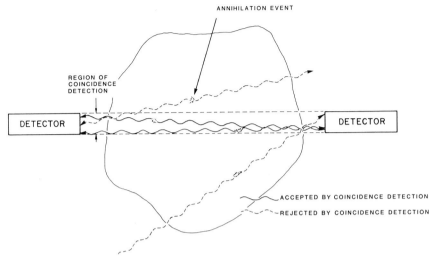

Fig. 20-8.   Principles of annihilation coincidence detection (ACD). Two events must be detected simultaneously to be recorded. Events registered in only one detector are rejected electronically. This defines a sensitive volume between the detectors for true coincidence detection; hence, the name "electronic collimation." (Reprinted from ref. 6: Phelps ME, Hoffman EJ, Mullani NA, et al: Applications of annihilation coincidence detection to transaxial reconstruction tomography. J Nucl Med 16:210–224, 1975. With permission.)

2. Spatial Resolution

Two factors place an ultimate limit on spatial resolution in ACD: the range of positrons in tissue before annihilation, and deviation from 180° in the angle between the emitted photons. The range of positrons in tissue is determined by their energy, and thus is a characteristic of the radionuclide (Chapter 2, Section G.). For most positron emitters, the maximum range in soft tissues is between 2 and 20 mm (Table 20-1); however, the effect on spatial resolution is much smaller for several reasons. First, positrons are emitted with a spectrum of energies, and only a small fraction travel the maximum range. Second, the projection data are two-dimensional, which compresses the range in the third dimension, i.e., there is no loss of resolution for positrons traveling along a line between the detectors. Thus, the resolution limit is much smaller than the maximum positron range (FWHM and FWTM, Table 20-1).

Deviation from exact 180° emission of annihilation photons results from the fact that the positron–electron pair is not completely at rest when annihilation occurs. The angular spread is represented by a Gaussian distribution with FWHM of about 0.3°. This translates into a spatial

Table 20-1
Resolution Broadening Due to Positron Range

Isotope	Max Positron Energy (MeV)	Max Positron Range (mm)	FWHM (mm)	FWTM (mm)
^{18}F	0.64	2.6	0.22	1.09
^{11}C	0.96	3.8	0.28	1.86
^{68}Ga	1.90	9.0	1.35	5.92
^{82}Rb	3.35	16.5	2.60	13.20

resolution effect of about 2.8 mm for 100 cm detector separation (i.e., whole-body tomograph) and about 1.4 mm for 50 cm detector separation (i.e., head tomograph). The combination of positron range and deviation from exact 180° angular separation results in a limiting spatial resolution of 1.5–3.0 mm for PET. The resolution also depends on detector resolution, i.e., width of individual detector elements. For most detector materials and detector shapes, the FWHM of the LSF is about 0.4–0.5 times the width of the detector elements.

The spatial resolution achieved by ACD is quite uniform with depth. Over an imaging field-of-view restricted to the center 40–50% of the detector separation, the line spread function varies by only about 10% (Figure 20-9). After image reconstruction, the variation is even less, about 5%. System resolution is a combination of detector resolution, positron range, and angular spread of photon emissions. These factors are not additive but are determined by a convolution of individual response functions (Appendix G). Combining all of these effects, modern PET systems have in-plane tomographic image resolution in the range of 4–8 mm.

3. Detector Systems

Although NaI(Tl) is satisfactory for most imaging systems used with ordinary γ-ray emitters, the 511 keV annihilation photons require detectors with greater stopping power for efficient detection in PET. Increased stopping power for photons generally is achieved with detectors of higher density and atomic number. In addition, the detectors should have a short scintillation decay time, to permit the use of narrow coincidence timing windows and minimize random or accidental coincidence events (Section D.5). Bismuth germanate (BGO) is currently the preferred detector material, even though its scintillation light yield is somewhat low and decay time somewhat long. BGO also is nonhygroscopic, which permits close packing of detector elements in arrays and favors long detector life. Other materials that have been used include BaF_2, which has a very short decay time (0.8 nsec plus a slow component with 620 nsec) needed for

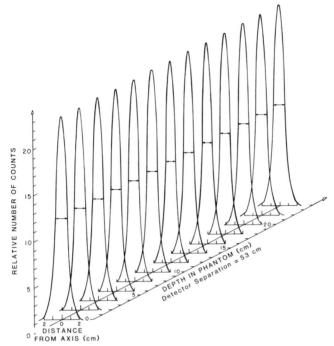

Fig. 20-9. Line spread functions vs. distance between detectors for an ACD system. The separation of detector
systems was 53 cm in this example.

"time-of-flight" techniques (Section D.9), but also has lower detection
efficiency than BGO, and gadolinium orthosilicate (GSO), which has
many of the favorable properties of BGO and BaF_2, but at present is
expensive and in limited supply. The properties of these detector materials are summarized and compared in Table 4-2.

4. Sensitivity

In ACD, each detector can be operated in coincidence with multiple
detectors on the opposite side of an array (Figure 20-10). Each detector
element therefore can define multiple sampling paths over a range of
angles, resulting in a fan-beam response for each detector. Multiple-
coincidence detection provides a dramatic increase in sensitivity in
comparison with systems having only a single sampling path per detector
point or element. For example, in comparison with gamma camera
SPECT, the multiple coincidence lines provide an increase in sensitivity
of 10–20 times. The fan-beam response also is ideally suited for data
collection for reconstruction tomography.

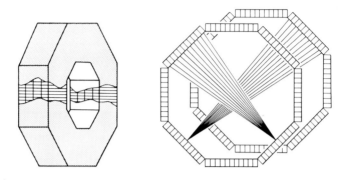

OCTAGONAL RING
PET CAMERA

Fig. 20-10.   Example of a detector geometry design configuration for an octagonal ring PET system. Each detector in
each bank of detectors is connected in coincidence with all
the detectors in the opposing bank. In addition, a ring of
detectors can be operated in coincidence with detectors of
another ring.

5. True, Scatter, and Accidental Coincidence Events

The total coincidence counting rate, R_{total}, for a pair of detectors is
given by

$$R_{total} = R_t + R_{sc} + R_a \qquad (20\text{-}1)$$

where R_t represents true coincidences for annihilation events occurring
within the volume defined by the detector pair and electronic collimation
(Figure 20-8), R_{sc} represents scatter coincidences involving annihilation
events occurring outside this volume but for which one or both of the
photons are scattered to produce a coincidence event, and R_a is the
accidental coincidence rate caused by chance detection of photons from
unrelated annihilation events within the coincidence timing window.

The true coincidence rate, R_t, for a positron-emitting source located
in an absorbing medium between a pair of coincidence detectors is given
by:

$$R_t = E \, \varepsilon^2 g \, e^{-\mu D} \qquad (20\text{-}2)$$

where E is the source emission rate (positrons/sec), ε is the intrinsic
efficiency of the two detectors (assumed to be equal), i.e., fraction of
incident photons detected, and g is the geometric efficiency of an
individual detector, i.e., fraction of emitted photons intercepted by the

detector. Note that g appears only to the first power in this equation, because if one of the photons is emitted from within the true coincidence region in a direction so as to be detected by one detector, the other automatically is emitted in the proper direction toward the other detector. D is the object thickness and μ is the linear attenuation coefficient of the absorbing medium (Equation 19-14). Modern PET systems use arrays of individual detector elements. For a circumferential array of detectors (e.g., Figure 20-10), each individual detector having surface area, A_d, arranged in a ring of radius r around the source, the geometric efficiency of an individual detector pair is given by (Equation 12-6):

$$g = A_d/4\pi r^2 \qquad (20\text{-}3)$$

Hence, the true coincidence rate for an individual detector pair in the array decreases as $1/r^2$. The number of detectors in the ring increases in proportion to radius r; thus the total geometric efficiency for a ring of detectors decreases as $1/r$, as does the total coincidence counting rate for a source located at the center of the ring.

The accidental coincidence rate, R_a, for an individual detector pair is given by

$$R_a = 2\tau R_s^2 \qquad (20\text{-}4)$$

where τ is the coincidence resolving time of the detectors and associated electronics, and R_s is the single-channel, i.e., the noncoincidence count rate, in each detector (assumed to be equal for each detector in this example). For a source with emission rate E (positrons/sec) located near the midpoint between the detector pair, the single-channel count rate is given by

$$R_s = (2E)\ \varepsilon g\ e^{-\mu D/2} \qquad (20\text{-}5)$$

The factor 2E enters this equation because each positron results in two annihilation photons. Thus, since g decreases as $1/r^2$ (Equation 20-3), the accidental coincidence rate for an individual detector pair (Equation 20-4) decreases as $1/r^4$. For a circumferential array of detectors, the total geometric efficiency decreases as $1/r$; hence, the total accidental coincidence rate for an array decreases as $1/r^2$.

Scatter coincidences can originate from within or outside the imaged plane (Figure 20-8). They arise from the same annihilation event (i.e., they are in true coincidence) and, unlike accidental coincidences, cannot be eliminated by using shorter coincidence resolving time. The scatter coincidence rate in an individual detector pair for a source having an emission rate E, located near the center of the detector array, can be expressed as

$$R_{sc} = E\,K\,\varepsilon^2\,g^2 \tag{20-6}$$

where ε is the intrinsic efficiency of each detector, and g is the geometric efficiency. K is a constant that depends in a complicated way on the detector–patient geometry, detector shielding, etc., and must be determined empirically for each tomograph design.

Equations 20-5 and 20-6 assume that the sources for accidental and scatter coincidences are near the center of the field of view; however, as shown in Figure 20-11, they can originate from sources anywhere within the volume of tissue exposed to the detectors, and even from outside this volume, as a result of penetration of shielding around the detectors and backscatter from neighboring objects and surfaces. Thus, the accidental and scatter coincidence rates are strongly dependent on the design of the PET system. Accidental coincidences also can originate from ordinary γ rays emitted by the positron-emitting radionuclide or from other

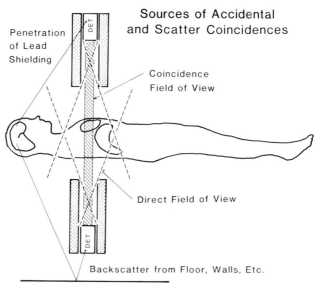

Fig. 20-11.   Sources of accidental and scatter coincidences. The coincidence field of view defines the potential locations of true coincidences. Scatter and accidental coincidences originate primarily within the direct field of view of the detectors, defined by the dashed lines. Additional accidental coincidences can result from poor shielding or backscatter and from ordinary γ rays from the administered radionuclide. (Reprinted from ref. 7: Phelps ME, Mazziotta JC, Schelbert HR (eds): Positron Emission Tomography and Autoradiography. New York, Raven Press, 1986. With permission.)

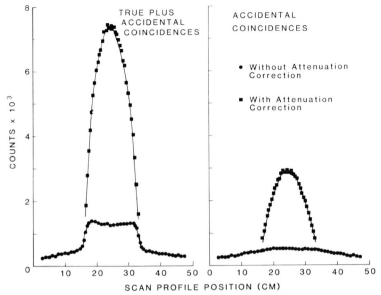

Fig. 20-12. Profiles of true and accidental coincidences for a 20-cm-diameter cylinder containing a uniform concentration of positron emitter. The profile on the left includes both true and accidental coincidences, whereas the profile on the right includes only accidental coincidences measured at the same time with a delayed timing window. (Reprinted from ref. 8: Hoffman EJ, Huang SC, Phelps ME, et al: Quantitation in positron emission computed tomography; 4. Effect accidental coincidences. J. Comput Assist Tomogr 5:391–400, 1981. With permission.)

radionuclides in the body. As shown in Figures 20-12 and 20-13, accidental and scatter coincidences produce a relatively flat background across the field of view for a distributed source of positron radioactivity.

There are two methods of correcting for accidental coincidences. The first, a direct measurement technique, requires a parallel time circuit for the coincidence detection circuit with a time delay on the signal from one detector. This delay typically is greater than ten times 2τ so that no true coincidence events will register in that branch of the circuit. Events in this branch can result only from accidental (i.e., random) overlap of detected events. The events counted in the accidental coincidence circuit are subtracted from those counted in the true coincidence circuit to provide a corrected estimate of the true coincidence counting rate. Figure 20-12 shows examples of true and accidental coincidence rates determined in this way. Typically, the corrections are performed automatically in hardware circuits.

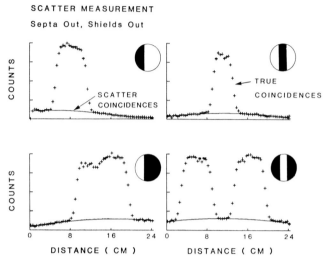

SCATTER MEASUREMENT

Septa Out, Shields Out

Fig. 20-13. Profiles of true and scatter coincidences in a 17.8-cm-diameter water-filled cylinder with three chambers: a 5-cm-wide chamber in the center with two equal-sized chambers on either side. Dark areas contain activity and white areas contain no activity. Fraction of coincidence counts attributed to scatter is the portion under the solid line in each profile. The ratio total of scatter-to-true coincidences in these data is about 0.3. (Reprinted from ref. 9: Hoffman EJ, Phelps ME, Huang SC, et al: Evaluating the performance of multiplane positron tomographs designed for brain imaging. IEEE NS-29:469–473, 1982. With permission.)

Alternatively, R_a can be estimated from Equation 20-4. This requires separate counting channels to determine single channel-counting rates. These corrections usually are performed using softward routines.

Correction for scatter coincidences is not as simple because the factor K in Equation 20-6 usually is not known accurately and is somewhat variable across the field of view. Typically, the distribution of scatter coincidences across the field of view is relatively flat (Figure 20-13); thus, one approach is to measure the coincidence rate at the edge of the field of view, where no activity is present, and extrapolate a profile back across the field of view to approximate the distribution of scatter coincidences. The approximated distribution then is subtracted from the recorded profiles. Another approach is to measure the scatter distribution for line sources in phantoms and use these measured data to deconvolve the scatter from measured patient data. This approach is difficult to apply in practice. It should be noted that in each of these cases, scatter correction must be performed before attenuation corrections and image reconstruction.

6. Deadtime

In PET systems with multiple coincidence detector pairs, (e.g., the fan-beam geometry in Figure 20-10), more than one detector pair is assigned to each coincidence circuit for economic reasons. Overlapping of coincidence events in the same circuit from neighboring detector pairs results in rejection of both events and contributes to system deadtime. These multiple coincidences (usually called "triples") can be a major source of deadtime losses in a PET system. Overlap of pulses in the single channel detector circuits also can occur and cause deadtime losses (Chapter 12, Section C). Deadtimes can be monitored and mathematical corrections applied if both the single-channel and coincidence counting rates are monitored for each coincidence circuit. If the activity is relatively constant with time and over the area of image, an average value for deadtime correction can be used. If activity is rapidly changing, deadtime corrections must be made using values appropriate for the varying range of counting rates for the scan.[7]

7. Signal-to-Noise Ratio in PET

Noise in PET has several components in addition to Poisson counting statistics of the true coincidence events. These include additional statistical fluctuations from accidental and scatter coincidences as well as noise introduced by attenuation corrections and further amplified by the reconstruction process.

The geometry of the detector system strongly influences the signal-to-noise ratio in PET. As discussed in Section D.5, the signal (i.e., true coincidence counting rate) is proportional to the square of intrinsic detector efficiency and inversely proportional to the radius of the detector ring. Scatter and accidental coincidences also increase with increasing intrinsic detector efficiency; however, increasing the intrinsic detection efficiency for 511 keV annihilation photons usually increases the signal more than the noise, because scatter and accidental coincidences often involve lower-energy photons that already are easily stopped by less efficient detectors. Detectors with high intrinsic efficiency and large photofractions for 511 keV photons thus provide higher signal-to-noise ratios than detectors with low intrinsic efficiency and small photofractions. These properties also allow the use of higher energy-discriminator settings, which further reduces noise by decreasing the detection efficiency for scatter and accidental coincidences.

For an array of detectors, signal counts from true coincidences as well as noise counts from scatter and accidental coincidences decrease with increasing radius of the array; however, as discussed in Section D.5, the noise counts decrease faster ($1/r^2$) than signal counts ($1/r$). Thus, for activity contained within one image axial slice width, the ratio of true coincidences to accidental or scatter coincidences increases with the radius of the detector ring.

$$R_t/R_a \propto r \qquad \qquad (20\text{-}7)$$

$$R_t/R_{sc} \propto r \qquad \qquad (20\text{-}8)$$

For most imaging situations, the activity extends well beyond a single axial slice width, and the scatter and accidental coincidences will also depend upon the amount of off-plane activity viewed by the detectors. As a result, the relative increase in S/N with r is greater than indicated in Equations 20-7 and 20-8 and is a complex function of system design.

Scatter and accidental coincidence profiles tend to be rather smoothly distributed over the image (Figure 20-12 and 20-13) and consist primarily of low-spatial-frequency components. The signal in a highly structured image (e.g., brain) consists of a broad range of spatial frequency components. These different frequency features of signal and noise allow the use of subtraction techniques for removing scatter and random coincidences as first-order corrections.

From the above discussion it is clear that the signal-to-noise ratio in PET is optimized by a combination of system geometry, properties of detector materials, and knowledge of the spatial frequency components of signal and noise. In general, geometric discrimination against sources of scatter and accidental coincidences is very effective. This is accomplished by using relatively large detector ring diameters (50–60 cm for head tomograph, 100 cm for body tomograph), and by limiting the detector field of view as much as possible to regions from which true coincidences are obtained (Figure 20-11). In such systems, a compromise must be made between limiting the detector view in the axial direction to reduce accidental and scatter coincidences, while allowing true coincidence events between one detector plane and the next (Figure 20-10).

Accidental coincidences also are reduced by using detectors with fast scintillation decay times, allowing shorter coincidence time windows (Equation 20-4). However, it should be noted that accidental coincidences are reduced by the first power of the coincidence time window and by the *second* power of the single-channel counting rate. Thus, reductions in the latter, e.g., by optimizing detector and shielding geometry, often can be more effective than shorter coincidence time resolution.

8. Signal Amplification Technique

The signal amplification technique (SAT[10]) in PET is a design approach for improving the image signal-to-noise ratio. As discussed in Chapter 19, CT image reconstruction is performed using filter functions that amplify the higher spatial frequency components of the projection data. Typically, to maximize spatial resolution, the cutoff frequency of the reconstruction filter is placed at or near the upper limit of the frequency response of the detector (see Figures 19-7, 20-14). Unfortunately, this approach also amplifies high-frequency noise. Indeed, the highest resolution components of detector response, which have low amplitude, are recovered at the expense of significantly amplifying high-frequency noise in the image. These points are illustrated by Figure 20-14.

In the SAT approach, the same or similar filter functions are used, but with improved detector resolution by using smaller detector elements. The use of the same filter function results in the same image noise levels, but the improved detector response results in the maximum amplification of the filter function being applied to a higher level of signal; hence, the signal-to-noise ratio is improved.

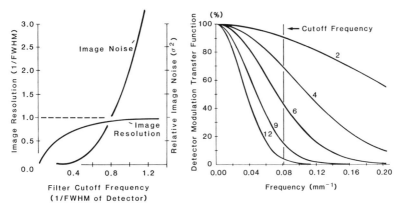

Fig. 20-14. (Left) As cutoff frequency of reconstruction filter is increased, image resolution increases non-linearly to an asymptotic value determined by detector resolution, but image noise (variance, σ^2) continually increases as a third power of cutoff frequency. Thus, raising cutoff frequency to maximize image resolution produces small increases in image resolution with large increases in image noise. A conventional cutoff frequency is usually at about 1/FWHM. (Right) MTFs of detectors with 12, 9, 6, 4 and 2 mm FWHM resolutions. Vertical line is location of a conventional cutoff frequency for a 12 mm FWHM detector resolution. (Reprinted from Ref. 10: Phelps ME, Huang SC, Hoffman EJ, et al: An analysis of signal amplification using small detectors in positron emission tomography. J Comput Assist Tomogr 6:551–565, 1982. With permission).

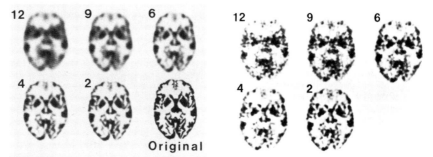

Fig. 20-15. Computer simulation of SAT on brain images. Original is digitized brain section with gray to white matter ratio of 4. Angular projection with Poisson noise were generated with different detector resolutions (in mm) shown adjacent to images. All images were reconstructed with identical filter function and 20 million (left) or 250,000 (right) image counts. Note image resolution improvement with improving intrinsic detector resolution even though cutoff frequency is not changed. In noisy images with 250,000 count (right) it appears that SAT decreases image noise. However, noise is the same in each image; it is only that signal-to-noise is increasing due to selective signal amplification in the detectors. (Reprinted from Ref. 10: Phelps ME, Huang SC, Hoffman EJ, et al: An analysis of signal amplification using small detectors in positron emission tomography. J Comput Assist Tomogr 6:551–565, 1982. With permission.)

Figure 20-14 (Right) illustrates how the amplitude of spatial frequencies between zero and a conventional cutoff frequency are progressively amplified with increasing intrinsic detector resolution. Thus, for a fixed number of image counts and cutoff frequency (i.e., the one for 12 mm detector in Fig. 20-14), the image noise is constant but spatial resolution and image signal-to-noise is increased with increasing intrinsic detector resolution (Fig. 20-15). The principle of SAT is illustrated by the example images in Figure 20-15. SAT provides improved resolution and higher signal-to-noise ratio. Alternatively, fewer counts are required for a given signal-to-noise ratio. The latter is useful for shortening study times (e.g., rapid dynamic studies) or decreasing patient dose.

Some improvements in image quality can be achieved in SPECT by improved detector resolution (e.g., see Figure 18-14); however, one cannot achieve the same improvement in signal-to-noise ratio that can be achieved by SAT in PET. The improved signal-to-noise ratio of SAT requires that intrinsic resolution be improved without loss of sensitivity, which can be accomplished in PET by using closely packed small detector elements of high stopping power. In SPECT imaging, improved resolution usually is achieved with finer resolution collimators, which reduces sensitivity by the square of the resolution (Equation 16-8). This offsets the potential gain in signal-to-noise ratio that might be achieved by SAT in SPECT.

9. Time of Flight

Time-of-flight (TOF) techniques are another potential method for improving the signal-to-noise ratio in PET imaging. Annihilation photons travel at the speed of light, i.e., about 30 cm/nsec. With sufficiently fast coincidence timing resolution, the location of the origin of the two photons can be estimated by the difference in their arrival times at the two detectors (Figure 20-16). Because the *difference* between arrival times is measured, the localization error is only half what would be predicted from directly measuring the transit time for each photon. For example, with a timing accuracy of 1 nsec the origin of the event can be determined to within about 15 cm, rather than 30 cm, the distance that light travels in 1 nsec.

In conventional PET image reconstruction, no a priori knowledge is available of the origin of the photons along the line between two detectors. Instead, the reconstruction algorithm assumes that the events are distributed uniformly along this line. This results in a propagation of statistical noise from counts in one pixel to another, as discussed in Chapter 19, Section C.4. Time-of-flight provides information about the distribution of activity along the line between the detectors, resulting in smaller noise propagation effects. Incorporation of this information places constraints on the reconstruction process and therefore provides what is known as a *constrained estimation* reconstruction. Figure 20-17 illustrates schematically how TOF reduces the propagation of image noise in the reconstruction process.

The better the TOF timing resolution, the greater the noise suppres-

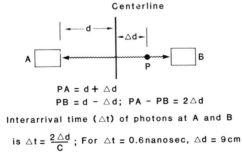

$$PA = d + \Delta d$$
$$PB = d - \Delta d; \quad PA - PB = 2\Delta d$$

Interarrival time (Δt) of photons at A and B

is $\Delta t = \dfrac{2\Delta d}{c}$; For $\Delta t = 0.6$ nanosec, $\Delta d = 9$ cm

Fig. 20-16.   Illustration of interarrival time measurements in time of flight between two coincidence detectors A and B. P is the point of annihilation and emission of the two 511 keV photons.

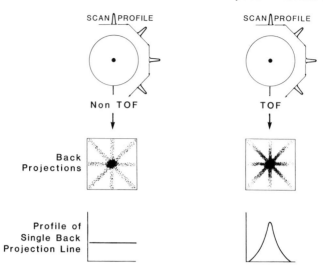

Fig. 20-17. PET reconstruction using (left) conventional (non-TOF) and (right) time-of-flight (TOF) image data. Both techniques backproject data across multiple pixels, but additional information provided by TOF limits the backprojection of data to a narrower range, thus decreasing the propagation of noise by the reconstruction algorithm.

sion and improvement in signal-to-noise ratio. It can be shown that, for a uniform cylinder of activity, the improvement in signal-to-noise ratio in the reconstructed images is equivalent to a gain in sensitivity or counts recorded, G, given by:

$$G = D/\Delta d \qquad (20\text{-}9)$$

where D is the diameter of a cylinder and Δd is the distance equivalent (FWHM) of the timing resolution. For object diameters, D, of 15 cm (head) and 30 cm (body) containing uniformly distributed activity, and Δd of 5 cm (i.e., time resolution = 0.33 nsec), G equals 3 and 6, respectively. This corresponds to an equivalent increase in counts recorded by the same factors. Since noise decreases as the square root of counts recorded, the corresponding improvements in signal-to-noise ratio are 1.7 and 2.5, respectively. These results must be modified if the activity is not uniformly distributed. For example, in a typical heart study, the activity ratio between the heart and surrounding tissue can be on the order of 4 to 1, with the heart occupying about a 10 cm diameter circle. The sensitivity gain in this case would be about 2, corresponding to the concentration of activity in the heart.

The detector material used in current TOF systems is BaF_2, and the timing resolution achieved is about 0.8 nsec (i.e., about 9 cm, see Table 4-2). This results in signal-to-noise improvements of 1.3 and 1.8 for 15 cm and 30 cm objects. The fast response of BaF_2 also results in fewer accidental coincidence events, which can be an important advantage for studies involving very high count rates, e.g., some fast dynamic studies with high activity injections. However, the slow decay time component of BaF_2 (620 nsec) limits count rate because of deadtime. On the other hand, BaF_2 provides smaller light yields and lower intrinsic detection efficiency than BGO. Thus, there are tradeoffs in performance characteristics of conventional vs. TOF systems for PET at this time. Development of improved detector systems for TOF could result in significant advantages for this technique in the future.

10. System Configurations

Modern PET systems use between 2 and 8 circumferential arrays of detectors arranged in circles, octagons, or hexagons around the patient, patterned after the designs of the first PET scanners developed by Phelps, Hoffman, and colleagues.[6,7] Each adjacent pair of detector planes pro-

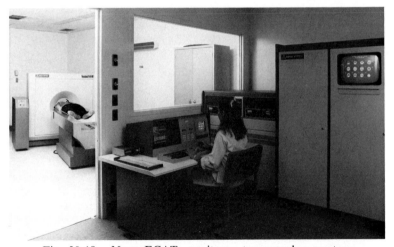

Fig. 20-18. NeuroECAT positron tomography system (CTI, Inc., Knoxville, Tenn.). This system contains three octagonal rings of BGO detectors. The technologist sets up the scanning and processing variables with the system's computer. The patient lies on a movable bed. This device was specifically designed for brain studies. (Reprinted from ref. 11: Phelps ME, Mazziotta JC, Huang SC: Study of cerebral function with positron emission tomography. J Cereb Blood Flow Metab 2:113–162, 1982. With permission.)

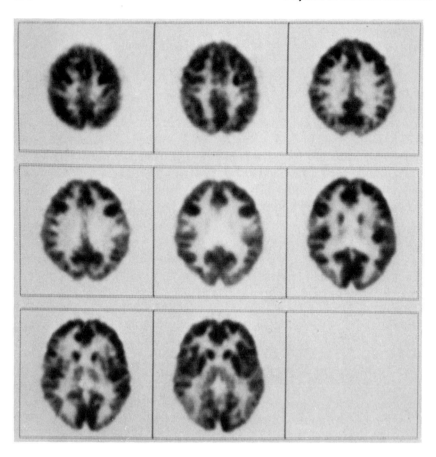

Fig. 20-19. PET transverse images of the cerebral metabolic rate for glucose using 2-deoxy-2[^{18}F]-fluoro-D-glucose and a modern positron tomograph. Gray scale is in units of μmoles/min/g of tissue with black being the highest. Anterior is at top of each image and left is left side of each image. Images proceed from left to right and top to bottom from a superior level down to the level of the basal ganglia. Note the clear delineation of cortical and subcortical structures. (Reprinted from ref. 7: Phelps ME, Mazziotta JC, Schelbert HR (eds): Positron Emission Tomography and Autoradiography. New York, Raven Press, 1986. With permission.)

vides a pair of direct coincidence planes plus a cross-plane between them; thus, the total number of coincidence planes is between 3 and 15. Physically, these systems are similar to x-ray CT and SPECT systems. An example is shown in Figure 20-18. Software for tracer kinetic modeling (Chapter 22) usually is incorporated directly into these systems. Examples of images obtained with modern PET systems are shown in Figures 20-19 and 22-18.

REFERENCES

1. Budinger TF: Physical attributes of single-photon tomography: J Nucl Med 21:579–592, 1980
2. Anger HO: Tomography and other depth-discrimination techniques, in Hine GJ, Sorenson JA (eds): Instrumentation in Nuclear Medicine, vol 2. New York, Academic Press, 1974
3. Floyd CE, Jaszczak RJ, Harris CC, et al: Monte carlo evaluation of compton scatter subtraction in single photon emission computed tomography. Med Phys 12:776–778, 1985
4. Kuhl DE, Edwards RQ, Ricci AB, et al: The Mark IV system for radionuclide computed tomography of the brain. Radiology 121:405–413, 1976
5. Logan KW, Holmes RA: The design and function of MUMPI (Missouri University multiplane imager). J Nucl Med 25:P148, 1984
6. Phelps ME, Hoffman EJ, Mullani NA, et al: Applications of annihilation coincidence detection to transaxial reconstruction tomography. J Nucl Med 16:210–224, 1975
7. Phelps ME, Mazziotta JC, Schelbert HR (eds): Positron Emission Tomography and Autoradiography: Principles and Applications in the Brain and Heart. New York, Raven Press, 1986
8. Hoffman EJ, Huang SC, Phelps ME, et al: Quantitation in positron emission computed tomography: 4. Effect of accidental coincidences. J Comput Assist Tomogr 5:391–400, 1981
9. Hoffman EJ, Phelps ME, Huang SC, et al: Evaluating the performance of multiplane positron tomographs designed for brain imaging. IEEE NS-29: 469–473, 1982
10. Phelps ME, Huang SC, Hoffman EJ, et al: An analysis of signal amplification using small detectors in positron emission tomography. J Comput Assist Tomogr 6:551–565, 1982
11. Phelps ME, Mazziotta JC, Huang SC: Study of cerebral function with positron emission tomography. J Cereb Blood Flow Metab 2:113–162, 1982

Additional information regarding position tomography may be found in the following:
Reivich M, Alavi A (eds): Position Emission Tomography, New York, Alan R. Liss, 1986
Heiss W-D, Phelps ME (eds): Positron Emission Tomography of the Brain. Springer-Verlag, New York, 1983

21
Digital Image Processing in Nuclear Medicine

Image processing refers to a variety of techniques that are used to maximize the information yield from a picture. While most such processing is performed by computers, image processing and computer processing are not necessarily synonymous terms. For example, the contrast of images formatted on x-ray film depends on factors related to film exposure and development, which also can be adjusted to optimize the display of image information. Computer-based techniques provide more flexible and powerful image-processing capabilities, and are of importance both for processing raw data, e.g., computed tomography studies such as PET and SPECT (Chapters 19 and 20), and for analyzing the resultant images, e.g., generating kinetic data for tracer kinetic models (Chapter 22) and ventricular outlines in cardiac wall-motion studies.

Computer-based acquisition and processing also permits the raw data and processed image data to be stored digitally (on disks or tape) for later analysis and display. Integrated computer systems now are available that incorporate essentially all aspects of a nuclear medicine clinical operation from acquisition, processing, and display of image data to administrative support such as scheduling, report generation, and monitoring of quality control protocols.

In this chapter, we describe general concepts of digital image processing for nuclear medicine imaging. The discussion will focus on applications involving the Anger camera. Additional discussion of specific applications involving tomographic imaging can be found in Chapters 19 and 20.

A. The Digital Image

The Anger camera detector generates analog X and Y position signals that are used to display each event as it occurs at an appropriate location on a CRT monitor (Chapter 15). For digital image processing, these events must be localized within an image consisting of a grid of discrete (usually square) picture elements, or *pixels* (Figure 21-1). Depending on the mode of acquisition (discussed in Section A.3 below), the x–y address of the pixel in which each event occurs, or the total number of counts recorded in each pixel, p(x,y), is stored in computer memory.

Digital numbers, such as event location or number of counts per pixel, usually are represented as *binary numbers* in computer systems. Binary number representation uses powers of two, whereas the commonly used decimal number system uses powers of ten. For example, the decimal number "13," which means $[(1 \times 10^1) + (3 \times 10^0)]$, is represented as the binary number "1101," meaning $[(1 \times 2^3) + (1 \times 2^2) + (0 \times 2^1) + (1 \times 2^0)]$. Each of the digits in the binary number representation is called a bit. Thus, the decimal number "13" is represented by a 4-bit binary number "1101." In general, an n-bit binary number can represent decimal numbers with values between zero and $(2^n - 1)$.

Binary numbers are conveniently represented in computer hardware by electronic components that can exist only in an "on" or "off" state. Thus, an n-bit binary number can be represented by the "on" or "off" state of a sequence of n such components. More complicated mathematical operations involving noninteger numbers (e.g., decimals and frac-

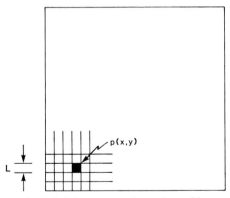

Fig. 21-1. A digital image consists of a grid or matrix of pixels, each of size L × L units. Each pixel has an (x,y) address location, with pixel value, p(x,y), corresponding to the number of counts or other quantity associated with that pixel.

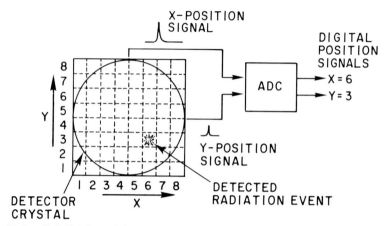

Fig. 21-2.   Subdivision of the Anger camera detector area for generating a digital image. Amplitudes of x- and y-position signals are analyzed using analog-to-digital converters (ADCs) to assign the digital matrix location for each detected event.

tions) require the use of *floating point* numbers. The method by which binary numbers are converted to floating point format is beyond the scope of this presentation and can be found in more advanced texts on computer systems listed at the end of the chapter.

Figure 21-2 illustrates the process by which analog position signals from a gamma camera are transformed into a digital image format. The electronic subdivision of the camera image into a matrix of pixels is accomplished by using an analog-to-digital converter (ADC) on the x–y position signals for each event recorded. The ADCs are identical to the ones used to digitize pulse amplitudes for energy analysis in multichannel analyzers (Chapter 5, Section C.4). For example, in the example illustrated in Figure 21-2, the x- and y-position signals for the event shown have digital amplitudes of 6 and 3, respectively. Thus, the event would be assigned to pixel local ($x = 6$, $y = 3$) in the 8×8 digitized image.

Digital images are characterized by *matrix size* and *pixel depth*. Matrix size determines the number and size of discrete picture elements and hence the degree of spatial detail that can be presented. Matrix sizes used for nuclear medicine images typically range from 32×32 to 512×512 pixels. Pixel depth determines the maximum number of events that can be recorded per pixel. Most systems offer a choice of maximum pixel depths of 8 bits ($2^8 = 256$; counts range from 0 to 255) or 16 bits ($2^{16} = 65536$; counts range from 0 to 65535). In most computer systems in use in nuclear medicine, 8 bits equals a *byte* of memory and 16 bits equals a *word* of memory, although 32-bit words used with newer systems are likely to become the standard. The pixel depth, therefore, frequently is described as "byte" mode or "word" mode.

1. Spatial Resolution and Matrix Size

The spatial resolution of a digital image is governed by two factors: the resolution of the imaging device itself (detector intrinsic resolution, collimator resolution, etc.), and the size of the pixels used to represent the digitized image., i.e., the matrix size. Clearly, a smaller pixel size can display more image detail, but beyond a certain point there is no further improvement, because of resolution limitations of the imaging device itself. A question of practical importance is, At what point does this occur, i.e., how many pixels are needed to ensure that significant detail is not lost in the digitization process?

The situation is entirely analogous to that presented in Chapter 19 for sampling requirements in tomography. In particular, Equation 19-8 applies, i.e., the linear sampling distance, d, or pixel size, must be less than or equal to the inverse of twice the maximum spatial frequency, ν_{max}, to be represented in the image;

$$d \leq 1/(2\nu_{max}) \tag{21-1}$$

Once this sampling requirement is met, increasing the number of pixels with a finer grid size does not improve spatial resolution, although it may produce a cosmetically more appealing image with less evident grid structure. If the sampling requirements are not met (too coarse a grid), spatial resolution is lost. If the resolution of an image is measured in terms of the full width at half-maximum (FWHM) of the line spread function (LSF) (Chapter 18, Section A.2), then the sampling distance (pixel size) should be approximately equal to one third of this value to avoid significant loss of spatial resolution, i.e.,

$$\text{Pixel Size} \simeq \text{FWHM}/3 \tag{21-2}$$

This applies for noise-free image data. With added noise it may be preferable to relax the sampling requirement somewhat (i.e., use larger pixels) to diminish the visibility of noise in the final digitized image.

Example 21-1.
What is the approximate resolution that can be displayed for a 30 cm wide image using a 64 × 64 matrix? A 128 × 128 matrix? Assume the original data are noise free.

Answer:
64 × 64 matrix
64 × 64 image produces a pixel size of 300/64 = 4.69 mm
From Equation 21-2, FWHM = 3 × pixel size = 14.06 mm
128 × 128 matrix
FWHM = 3 × 300/128 = 7.03 mm

The values calculated in Example 21-1 represent the approximate levels of imaging system resolution that could be displayed without loss of imaging resolution for the image and matrix sizes given.

2. Image Display

Digital images in nuclear medicine are displayed on cathode-ray tubes (CRT) or on film exposed from a CRT. CRT monitors must be continuously refreshed from digital memory because the display spot continuously scans the image (Chapter 5, section G). Ordinary television monitors can display digital images if supplied with appropriate input video signals.

Individual pixels in a digital image are displayed with different brightness levels, depending on the pixel value, e.g., number of counts in the pixel. These in turn are transformed into different shades of gray on film images recorded from the display. A linear gray scale is one that transforms count density or pixel value into a linear range of display intensities or film densities. (Note that the CRT display intensity must be calibrated to compensate for the sensitometric properties of the recording film to achieve a linear relationship between pixel value and film image density (see Figure 15-9).

Digital images also can be displayed in color by assigning color hues to represent different pixel values. One such scale, the *pseudocolor* scale, assigns different colors from the visible spectrum, ranging from blue through green, yellow, and red, to progressively increasing pixel values. This is an intrinsically nonlinear scale, since the viewer does not perceive equal significance for successive color steps. A somewhat more natural scale, the so-called "*heat*" scale, assigns different shades of similar colors, e.g., red, yellow, and white, to progressively increasing pixel values, corresponding to the colors of an object heated to progressively increasing temperature. The colors are blended to produce a gradual change over the full range of the scale.

Color scales produce a broader dynamic range than can be achieved by conventional gray scales; however, they are somewhat unnatural and also can produce contours, i.e., apparently sharp changes in pixel values where none actually exist. Color displays sometimes are useful for color-coding different areas of images, e.g., regions of early vs. delayed uptake determined from a sequence of images.

The human eye is capable of distinguishing approximately 40 levels of gray when the levels are presented in isolation and an even larger number of gray levels if they are presented as a sequential series of steps separated by sharp borders. Image displays are characterized by the potential number of gray (or color) levels that they can display. For example, an 8-bit display can potentially display $2^8 = 256$ different gray or color levels. Such a range of gray levels is more than adequate in comparison with the capabilities of human vision. In practice, the effective gray scale often is considerably less than the physical limits of the display device because of image noise. For example, if an image has a root mean square (RMS) noise level of 1%, then there are not more than 100 significant gray levels in the image, regardless of the capabilities of the display device.

Although each pixel in a digital image is assigned a specific level of intensity determined by the pixel value, real displays often do not produce square pixels of uniform brightness. Instead, as illustrated by Figure 21-3, individual pixels usually are displayed with nonuniform intensity profiles, having a maximum intensity at the center and falling off toward the edges of the pixel. As shown by this illustration, the display of a series of pixels representing the same pixel value, p(x,y), will not be of uniform brightness but will consist of a summation of intensity distribution profiles. The perceived uniformity of such a distribution will depend on the grid size and on the shape and width of the display spots themselves. In general, a Gaussian-shaped display spot is preferred to a perfectly square one. Also, the display spot should be at least as wide as the width of the pixels

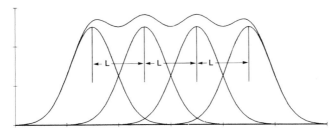

Fig. 21-3. Intensity distribution across four Gaussian-shaped spots of equal intensity. The pixel width is L units. The resulting display is a summation of intensities as shown by the line above the individual intensity distributions.

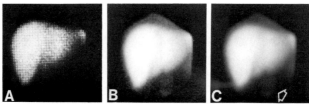

Fig. 21-4. Digitized Anger camera images of the liver. In (A) the discrete matrix elements are visible, while in (B) the display has been altered to produce a more uniform appearance by enlarging the relative widths of the display spots per pixel. In (C) the image has been smoothed. Arrow indicates vertebral body uptake. (Courtesy Brent S. Baxter.)

themselves. Otherwise, a pronounced grid structure may result because of sharp edges of square spots or gaps between pixels. Figure 21-4 illustrates the effects of display spot size on the appearance of a digital image of a ^{99m}Tc-sulfur colloid liver scan.

3. Acquisition Modes

Digital images are acquired either in *frame mode* or in *list mode*. In frame-mode acquisition, individual events are sorted into the appropriate x–y locations within the digital image matrix immediately after their position signals are digitized. After a preset amount of time has elapsed or after a preset number of counts have been recorded, the acquisition of data for the image is stopped and the pixel values (p(x,y) = number of counts per pixel) are stored in computer memory. When a series of such images is obtained sequentially, individual images in the sequence are referred to as "frames." Clearly, the image matrix size (e.g., 64 × 64, 128 × 128, etc.) must be specified before the acquisition begins. Additionally, the time duration of the frame sets a limit on the temporal accuracy of the data. For example, if the frame is acquired over a 1-minute period, the number of counts recorded in each pixel represents the integrated number of counts over the 1-minute acquisition period and cannot be subdivided retrospectively into smaller time intervals. When faster framing rates are used, such as for cardiac blood-pool imaging, temporal sampling accuracy is improved, but the total counts per frame and per pixel are reduced compared with slower frame rates.

In list-mode acquisition, the incoming x and y position pulses from the camera are digitized but they are not sorted immediately into an image grid. Instead, the x and y position coordinate for each individual event are stored, along with periodic and clock markers (e.g., at millisecond intervals). This permits retrospective framing with frame duration chosen after the data are acquired. Most nuclear medicine systems require that matrix size be specified before the acquisition of list-mode data. While list-mode acquisition permits greater flexibility in data analysis, it also requires more computer storage per study, because each event recorded requires a separate storage location in computer memory.

B. PROCESSING TECHNIQUES

A variety of digital processing techniques are used in nuclear medicine, some of which are fully automatic, i.e., performed entirely by computer, such as image smoothing, while others are interactive, i.e., require some observer input such as manually drawing a region of interest on a CRT display. Most computer systems permit the observer to alter the gray-scale of the displayed image in several ways, including changing from a linear to other, e.g., logarithmic or color, relationships between intensity and counts, and limiting the range of pixel values displayed. The latter is referred to as "windowing." For example, if greater contrast is desired in one region of an image, the full brightness range of the display device may be used to display only the range of pixel values found within that region. This increases the displayed contrast for the selected area, but other portions of the image may have diminished contrast as a result (i.e., the counts per pixel may be beyond the upper or lower range of the selected gray-scale window).

While digital images are convenient from an archival point of view, i.e., they can be stored in computer memory or on disks and tapes in digital form, often it is the quantitative aspects of the image that are of greatest use in nuclear medicine. Determination of count densities on a pixel-by-pixel, region-by-region or image-by-image basis is useful in a variety of situations ranging from simple corrections for background activity to tracer kinetic modeling of physiologic data (Chapter 22). Numerical operations performed on individual frames in a sequence of images are known as *frame arithmetic* operations. These operations typically are applied on a pixel-by-pixel basis, e.g., adding, subtracting, multiplying or dividing pixel values in an image by corresponding pixel values in other images or by other constants or functions. Figure 21-5 is an example of a simple frame arithmetic operation: subtraction. The study illustrated is a visual stimulation study using ^{15}0-labeled water as a flow tracer. Visual stimulation resulted in increased blood flow to the occipital (visual) cortex, while flow to the remainder of the brain remained largely unaffected. Subtraction of an image taken from a resting control study from the image obtained in the stimulation study provides a display of the blood flow changes occurring as a result of the stimulation.

Edge detection is useful for generating quantitative estimates of

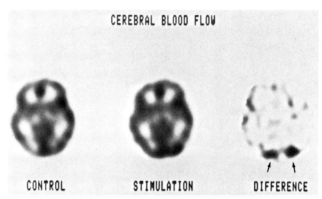

Fig. 21-5. Control, stimulation, and difference images from a visual stimulation study using ^{15}O-labeled water and PET imaging. The control image was subtracted from the stimulation image on a pixel-by-pixel basis. The highest count densities in the difference image are in the posterior occipital (visual cortex) region of the brain (arrows). (Courtesy of J. C. Mazziotta and M. E. Phelps)

isotope concentrations in "regions of interest" (ROI) either interactively with a joystick or similar device (Figure 21-6) or automatically with an edge-detection algorithm. Edge detection algorithms work best with edges that are very clearly defined (Figure 21-7). However, such algorithms can be employed as a time-saving procedure even when manual region identification can produce similar or better results, e.g., establishing ventricular outlines in gated cardiac studies as shown in Figure 21-6. Several algorithms exist for automatic edge detection. One of the most common is the Laplacian technique. The Laplacian is defined by:

$$\text{Laplacian} = \frac{\partial^2}{\partial x^2} + \frac{\partial^2}{\partial y^2} \tag{21-3}$$

where $\partial^2/\partial x^2$ represents the second partial derivative of the function (i.e., the image pixel values, $p(x,y)$), with respect to spatial coordinate x, and similarly for the spatial coordinate y. The local minimum value of the Laplacian represents areas with a high rate of change between neighboring pixel values, i.e., edges. Areas of high count density, such as the left ventricle on a gated blood-pool study, usually have peak count densities in their center, which decrease progressively toward the edge, where the rate of change becomes a minimum. The observer must specify a starting point for the algorithm, which then will search all possible directions and construct a line (edge) where the above relationship is minimized. Eliminating small changes (i.e., setting limits) in the Laplacian reduces

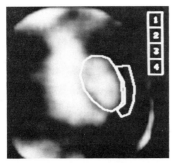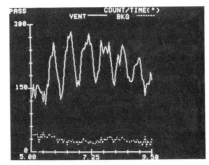

Fig. 21-6. Displays from a cardiac flow study performed with an Anger camera interfaced to a computer (left). The cardiac image has regions of interest superimposed for the left ventricle and for background activity. The ROIs were drawn manually. The plot on the right of the figure is a computer-generated pair of curves representing counting rate versus time for cardiac (top) and background (bottom) regions. (Courtesy of ADAC,Inc.)

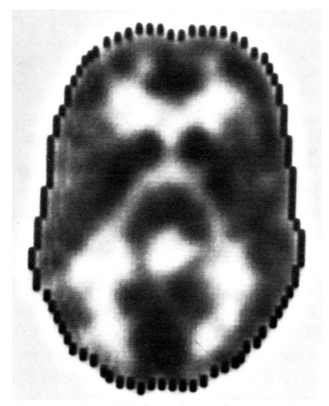

Fig. 21-7. Single PET image from a fluorodeoxyglucose (FDG) study (see Chapters 19, 20, and 22) of a normal brain at the level of the basal ganglia. The dotted line around the periphery of the brain was constructed automatically with a Laplacian algorithm technique.

461

the effect of noise. Figures 21-6 illustrates an image with manually defined edges and Figure 21-7 an image with edges defined by the Laplacian algorithm.

All nuclear medicine computer systems also provide *image-smoothing* algorithms. Figure 21-4 illustrates the effect of smoothing on an image with a prominent grid in the unprocessed state. Smoothing operations are, in essence, techniques that average the local pixel values to reduce the effect of pixel-to-pixel variation. Two common algorithms are the 5-point and 9-point smoothing, in which a pixel value is averaged with its nearest 5 or 9 neighbors. Therefore:

$$\text{smoothed image} = \text{original image} * \text{smoothing filter} \qquad (21\text{-}4)$$

where $*$ represents the operation of convolution (Appendix G). While smoothing frequently produces a more appealing image by reducing noise more than signal (and improving the S/N value), it also results in blurring and potential loss of image detail. Sometimes it is convenient to perform analytical studies (e.g., integrating pixel count values over an area) on an unsmoothed image after identifying regions of interest on a smoothed image. In such applications, a practical compromise between resolution and visual appeal must be reached.

Most digital images in nuclear medicine are, in essence, pictures of the count density in the underlying organ of interest. While many factors, including the sensitivity of the imaging device and method of attenuation correction, influence the accuracy of this representation, the observer is actually looking at the distribution of the tracer in tissue as controlled by underlying physiological or biochemical processes. Instead of presenting the data in this format, one may desire to first process the image data on a pixel-by-pixel basis using a model that represents the functional process and then display the result. The result is a *parametric image*, in which individual pixel values represent the parameter defined by the data-processing method. For example, a digital ventilation image may be divided by a perfusion image to produce a parametric image showing the ventilation/perfusion ratio. Phase processing of gated cardiac blood-pool studies produces parametric images of phase and amplitude of the contraction process. Examples of parametric images obtained by PET imaging and representing glucose metabolism are shown in Figure 20-19.

C. PROCESSING ENVIRONMENT

A digital processing environment in nuclear medicine may be limited to a single gamma camera or encompass a large department with a variety of cameras and tomographic imaging devices. In all cases, digital image processing involves several steps: (1) acquisition, (2) processing, (3) display, (4) archiving (storing the raw or processed data or images), and (5) retrieval. A single analog gamma camera interfaced to a film formatter performs all of these steps (except image retrieval), although processing is limited to varying only the film exposure factors. The archiving capacity of this basic system is limited to a piece of x-ray film. Digital techniques provide a greater and more flexible range of processing and storage options. More elaborate nuclear medicine systems include capabilities of Picture Archival Communications Systems (PACS). PACS systems store and move images from acquisition sites to more convenient viewing stations and are potentially useful for all forms of medical imaging including nuclear medicine. Because they are computer-based, incorporating digital image processing into these systems is a natural extension of the basic task of archiving and transmitting images. A true archival system not only should store the image or processed image data, but also should be organized around a logical retrieval system that permits correlation of images with other types of data (reports, etc.) for a given patient study. That is, it should have the capacity of a computer database system.

Although PACS systems are under investigation in a variety of research centers, commercial development of this concept is still only beginning. Figure 21-8 is a diagram of a general nuclear medicine

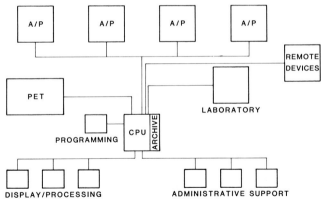

Fig. 21-8. Model of a digitally based nuclear medicine department. A central computer system and archival storage are interfaced to other computers, including those attached to gamma cameras for local acquisition and processing (A/P), a PET system, and remote digital devices such as x-ray CT scanners, digital radiography, and MRI. Administrative, programming, laboratory, and display/processing terminals are also included.

department containing a centralized computer system interfaced to smaller peripheral computers attached to gamma cameras. Also included are other devices such as a PET system, access to remote digital systems such as x-ray CT, digital radiography, and MRI, and terminals dedicated to procesing and display, programming, and administrative tasks. With such a system, most of the administrative and technical aspects of clinical nuclear medicine procedures can be incorporated into a unified computer environment that permits a variety of other tasks such as scheduling, patient tracking, and billing. This approach is well-suited to a database management system that permits storage and retrieval of a variety of types of data for each patient study, including raw and processed image data as well as administrative data.

REFERENCES

Additional information on nuclear medicine computer systems and applications can be found in

Barrett HN, Swindell W: Radiological Imaging—The Theory of Image Formation, Detection and Processing. New York, Academic Press, 1981

Castleman KR: Digital Image Processing Englewood Cliffs, NJ, Prentice-Hall, 1979

Goris ML, Briandet PA: A Clinical and Mathematical Introduction to Computer Processing of Scintigraphic Images New York, Raven Press, 1983

22
Tracer Kinetic Modeling

When interpreting nuclear medicine images, an observer mentally applies a model incorporating his or her knowledge of anatomy and of functional or physiologic processes. For dynamic studies such as first-pass cardiac examinations or serial renal imaging, changes in the images over time are compared with expected temporal patterns. Mathematical descriptions of the underlying processes in such studies are called *tracer kinetic models*. The purpose of these models is to expand the observer's ability to describe the underlying processes. This expanded capability may be in the form of numerical precision, expression of results in physiologic units, e.g., blood flow in units of ml/min, or diagnostic interpretations that are not apparent from simple visual inspection of the images.

Tracer kinetic models may be very simple. For example, one method for evaluating renal function is to measure the uptake of ^{99m}Tc-labeled DMSA using a single region of interest (ROI) positioned over each kidney at one point in time. "Function" in this case is determined in "relative" rather than physiologic units. A more rigorous approach for evaluating kidney function is to measure glomerular filtration rates (GFR), in ml/min, using a tracer that is filtered by the kidneys, such as ^{99m}Tc-labeled DTPA. In this case, it is necessary to obtain serial images of the kidneys and also to collect blood samples to measure tracer concentration in the blood as a function of time. Using these data and applying an appropriate mathematical model, one can then calculate the GFR. In yet another approach, no images are obtained, but both blood and urine samples are collected and tracer concentrations in each are measured as a function of time. In this case, the calculated value of GFR reflects global renal function and cannot be fractionated into separate values for each kidney.

Each of the above examples permits an assessment of "renal function" that is based on a different model for the behavior of the kidneys. The approach of choice depends on the medical or biologic information desired, as well as on the equipment available and the acceptable level of technical complexity. Developing a model requires the investigator to synthesize a large amount of biologic information into a comprehensive description of the process of interest. There is no standardized approach for this stage of model development, although there are a variety of general principles of tracer kinetic analysis applicable in many modeling situations. This chapter summarizes some of these principles and techniques, and presents some examples of tracer kinetic models currently used in nuclear medicine.

The following example illustrates the principle of tracer kinetic techniques. Figure 22-1 represents a hollow tube with a substance flowing through it. If a small amount of tracer is injected at point A and the measured activity at point B is plotted as a function of time, the resultant

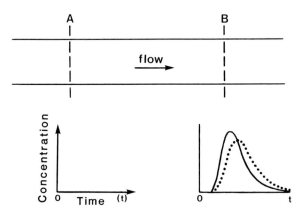

Fig. 22-1.   Illustration of use of tracer kinetics for measurement of flow. System consists of a hollow tube characterized by flow in direction indicated. Bolus of tracer introduced at point A produces a time-activity curve at B with a relatively higher flow rate (smooth line) and lower flow rate (dotted line). [From ref. 1: Phelps ME, Mazziotta JC, Schelbert HR: Positron Emission Tomography and Autoradiography: Principles and Applications for the Brain and Heart. Raven Press, New York, 1986. With permission.]

curve represents the values and relative abundances of particle transit times from point A to point B. It can be shown that the rate of flow through the tube can be calculated if the average time taken by the tracer particle to move from point A to point B is measured (the mean transit time) and the volume of the tube is known. The mean transit time can be determined directly from the time-activity curve at point B. If flow is decreased, the mean transit time is prolonged and the time-activity curve is spread over a wider range of values (dotted curve in Figure 22-1). This simple example illustrates conceptually how the kinetic (i.e., temporal) pattern of tracer and changes in this pattern, allow the identification and measurement of the kinetics (i.e., rates) of processes through which the tracer passes.

A. TRACERS AND COMPARTMENTS

Most applications of tracer kinetic principles in nuclear medicine are based on *compartmental models*. In this section, we review the basic principles of compartmental modeling, and the use of tracers to study them.

1. Definition of a Tracer

A *tracer* is a substance that follows ("traces") a physiologic or biochemical process. In this chapter, tracers are assumed to be radionuclides or compounds labeled with radionuclides, although in a general case this is not required, (e.g., dye dilution techniques). Tracers can be naturally occurring substances, analogs of natural substances (i.e., substances that mimic the natural substance), or compounds that interact with specific physiologic or biochemical processes in the body. Examples include diffusible tracers for blood flow, labeled particulate matter for studying capillary blood flow distribution or trapping of particles by the reticuloendothelial cells of the liver, gases for evaluating ventilation, etc. Some specific requirements for an ideal tracer include: (1) the behavior of the tracer should be identical or related in a known and predictable manner to that of the natural substance, (2) the mass of tracer used should not alter the underlying physiologic process being studied or should be small compared to the mass of endogenous compound being traced (a typical "rule of thumb" is that the mass of tracer should be less than 1 percent of the endogenous compound), (3) the specific activity of the tracer should be sufficiently high to permit imaging and blood or plasma activity assays without violating requirements 1 and 2, and (4) any isotope effect (Chapter 2, Section B) should be negligible or at least quantitatively predictable.

To meet requirement (4), a tracer labeled with an element not originally present in the compound (e.g., ^{99m}Tc, ^{123}I, ^{18}F) must behave similarly to the natural substance or in a way that differs in a known manner. The strictness of this requirement depends on the process under investigation. In most cases, the tracers that are used in nuclear medicine are employed to examine gross function and distribution, such as blood flow, filtration, and ventilation. This is primarily because the commonly available radionuclides (e.g., ^{99m}Tc, ^{67}Ga, ^{111}In, and ^{123}I), represent elements that are not normally present in human biochemistry (iodine is an exception when used to study thyroid metabolism). It is much more difficult to mimic a chemical reaction sequence. The chemical systems of the body are more specific than the processes that move or filter fluids or gases. Chemical systems can selectively require that compounds be of one optical polarity versus the other, that compounds fit within angstroms in the cleft of an enzyme, that chemical bond angles, lengths, and strengths are appropriate, etc. When a compound is labeled with a foreign species, e.g., ^{99m}Tc, one cannot be sure that it will retain its natural properties and a careful examination and characterization of the compound must be undertaken. One of the advantages of radionuclides that represent elements normally involved in biochemical processes, such as ^{11}C, ^{13}N, and ^{15}O, is that they generally do not alter the behavior of the labeled compound. Another example of this situation is the use of radioisotopes of iodine for thyroid studies.

Analog tracers are compounds that possess many of the properties of natural compounds but with differences that change the way the analog interacts with biologic systems. For example, analogs that participate only through a limited number of steps in a sequence of biologic reactions have been developed in biochemistry and pharmacology. Analogs are used to decrease the number of variables that must be measured, to increase the specificity and accuracy of the measurement, or to selectively investigate a particular step in biochemical sequence. Correction factors based upon the principles of competitive substrate or enzyme kinetics are employed in studies using analog tracers to account for differences between the analog and the natural compound. A well-known example, discussed in Section F, is the use of FDG (^{18}F-2-fluoro-2-deoxy-D-glucose) to study glucose metabolism.

Table 22-1 lists some examples of tracers that are used in nuclear medicine and their applications.

2. Definition of a Compartment

A *compartment* is a volume or space within which the tracer rapidly becomes uniformly distributed, i.e., it contains no significant concentration gradients. In some cases, a compartment has an obvious physical interpretation, e.g., the intravascular blood pool, reactants and products in a chemical reaction, substances that are separated by membranes, etc. For other compartments, the physical interpretation may be less obvious, e.g., a tracer may be metabolized or trapped by one of two different cell populations in an organ, thus defining the two populations of cells as separate compartments. Additionally, while the definition of a particular compartment may be appropriate for one tracer, (e.g., the distribution of labeled red blood cells in the intravascular blood pool), it might not apply for a different tracer, (e.g., the distribution of potassium, which has both an intravascular and an extravascular distribution). Thus, the number, interrelationship, organization, and definition of compartments in a compartmental model must be developed from knowledge of physiological and biochemical principles.

3. Distribution Volume and Partition Coefficient

A compartment may be *closed* or *open* to a tracer. A closed compartment is one from which the tracer cannot escape, whereas an open compartment is one from which it can escape to other compartments. Whether a compartment is closed or open depends on both the compartment and the tracer. Indeed, a compartment may be open to one tracer and closed to another.

If a tracer is injected into a closed compartment, such as a nondiffusible tracer in the vascular system, conservation of mass requires that after the distribution of the tracer reaches equilibrium or steady-state conditions, the amount of tracer injected, A (in millicuries or other units of activity), must equal the concentration of the tracer in the compartment, C (in millicuries/ml), multiplied by the *distribution volume*, V_d, of the compartment. Thus,

$$V_d(ml) = [A/C] \text{ at equilibrium} \qquad (22\text{-}1)$$

This is the basis for the *dilution principle*, which provides a convenient

Table 22-1
Examples of Tracers Used in Nuclear Medicine

Process	Tracer
Blood Flow	
Diffusible	^{133}Xe, H_2^{15}O, ^{85m}Kr, ^{77}Kr, [^{11}C]alcohols, CH_3^{18}F
Diffusible (trapped)	^{13}NH$_3$ (heart), ^{82}Rb (heart), [^{123}I]IMP (brain), ^{201}Tl (heart)
Non Diffusible (trapped)	[^{99m}Tc]macroaggregated albumin, labeled microspheres
Effective Renal plasma flow	[^{123}I]hippuran
Blood Volume	
Red Blood Cells (RBC)	[^{99m}Tc]-, [^{51}Cr]-, [C^{15}O]-RBC
Plasma	[^{125}I]-, [^{11}C]-albumin
Tissue pH	[^{11}C]DMO, ^{11}CO$_2$
Transport and Metabolism	
Oxygen	[^{15}O]O$_2$
Glucose, Glucose Analogs, Metabolites	2-deoxy-2-[^{18}F]fluoro-D-glucose, 2-[^{11}C]deoxy-D-glucose, [^{11}C]D-glucose, 3-0-[^{11}C]methyl-D-glucose, [^{11}C]lactate, -pyruvate, -acetate, -succinate, -oxalo-acetate
Amino Acids: ^{13}N	L-[^{13}N]glutamate, -α and ω -glutamine, -alanine, -aspartate, -leucine, -valine, -isoleucine, -methionine
Amino Acids: ^{11}C	L-[^{11}C]aspartate, -glutamate, -valine, -leucine, -phenylalinine, -methionine; D.L-[^{11}C]alanine, -tryptophan, -1-aminocyclopentane carboxylic acid, -1-aminocyclo-butane carboxylic acid

Free Fatty Acids	[^{11}C]palmitic acid, -oleic acid, -heptadecanoic acid, -β-methylheptadecanoic acid, [^{123}I]-hexadecanoic acid
Bile	[^{99m}Tc]HIDA
Osteoblastic Activity	[^{99m}Tc]MDP
Glomeralar Filtration Rate	[^{99m}Tc]DPTA
Molecular Diffision	[^{99m}TcO$_4$], [^{68}Ga]-EDTA, ^{82}Rb(brain)
Protein Synthesis	L-[1-^{11}C]leucine, -methionine, -phenylalanine, L[^{11}C-methyl]methionine
Receptor Systems	
Dopaminergic	[^{18}F]spiperone, [^{11}C]spiperone, [^{11}C]raclopride, [^{75}Br] and [^{76}Br]-p-bromospiperone, [^{18}F]haloperidol, [^{11}C]pimozide, [^{11}C]methylspiperone, L-[^{11}C]dopa, [6-^{18}F]-fluoro-L-dopa
Cholinergic	[^{11}C]imipramine, [^{11}C]-, [^{123}I]-QNB
Benzodiazepine	[^{11}C]flunitrazepam, [^{11}C]diazepam, [^{11}C]R015-1788, [^{18}F]fluorovalium
Opiate	[^{11}C]etorphine, N-methyl-[^{11}C]morphine, [^{11}C]-heroin, [^{11}C]-carfentanil
Adrenergic	[^{11}C]norepinephrine, [^{11}C]propanolol
Anticonvulsants	[^{11}C]valproate, [^{11}C]diphenylhydantoin

Abbreviations used:		
DTPA	—	diethylenetriaminopentaacetate
IMP	—	iodoamphetamine
EDTA	—	ethylenediaminetetraacetate
HIDA	—	hepatobilary iminodiacetate
MDP	—	methylenediphosphonate
HIPDM	—	hydroxyliodobenzylpropanediamine
DMO	—	dimethyloxazolidinedione
QNB	—	quinuclidinyl bezilate

method for determining the distribution volume of a closed compartment, as shown by the following example.

Example 22-1.

What is the distribution volume of the red blood cells (RBCs) if 30 μCi ^{51}Cr-labeled RBCs are injected into the blood stream and an aliquot of blood taken after an equilibration period (10 minutes) contains 6×10^{-3} μCi/ml? Assume the hematocrit, H (fraction of blood volume occupied by RBCs), is 0.4.

Answer.

From Equation 22-1:

$$V_d = (30 \ \mu Ci)/(6 \times 10^{-3} \ \mu Ci/ml)$$

$$= 5000 \ ml$$

This result gives the total distribution volume, i.e., total blood volume. The RBC volume is given by

$$V_{RBC} = H \times V_d$$

$$= 0.4 \times 5000 \ ml$$

$$= 2000 \ ml$$

More commonly, a compartment will be open, i.e., the tracer will be able to escape from it. This applies, for example, to tracers that are distributed and exchanged between blood and tissue. In this case, after the tracer reaches its equilibrium distribution,* the concentration in blood will typically be different from that in the tissue (Figure 22-2A). The ratio of tissue-to-blood concentration, at equilibrium, is called the *partition coefficient*, λ, defined by

$$\lambda \ (ml/gm) = C_t(\mu Ci/gm)/C_b(\mu Ci/ml) \tag{22-2}$$

In actual measurements, it is usually the blood concentration, C_b, that is measured. If one assumes that the concentration of tracer in tissue is the same as the concentration in blood (Figure 22-2B), and applies Equation

---

* Note that "equilibrium" in this case means that the concentration of the tracer in the compartments has reached a constant value with time. It does not imply equilibrium in the thermodynamic sense, i.e., that there is no further transport of tracer between tissue and blood. Thus, tracer equilibrium is synonymous with the term "steady state" (see Section A.6).

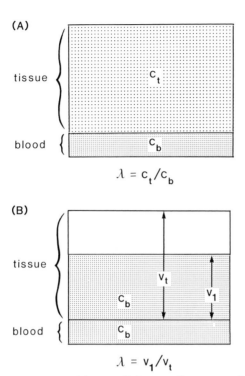

Fig. 22-2. (A): Partition coefficient, λ, for tracers that can diffuse or be transported into tissue from blood. Value of λ is given by the ratio of tissue-to-blood concentrations of the tracer when it has reached a equilibrium or steady-state condition. (B): Partition coefficient also equals the ratio of the apparent distribution volume in tissue, V_1, assuming same tracer concentration as blood, to tissue volume (or mass) V_t. [From ref. 1: Phelps ME, Mazziotta JC, Schelbert HR: Positron Emission Tomography and Autoradiography: Principles and Applications for the Brain and Heart. Raven Press, New York, 1986. With permission.]

22-1, this leads to an apparent distribution volume in tissue given by $V_1 = A_t/C_b$, where A_t is the activity in the tissue. One also knows that $A_t = C_t \times V_t$, where V_t is the volume (or mass) of tissue; therefore, combining these relationships and Equation 22-2 yields

$$\lambda = V_1/V_t \qquad (22\text{-}3)$$

Thus, another interpretation of the partition coefficient is that it is the

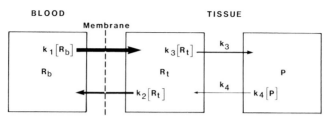

Fig. 22-3. A three-compartment system consisting of reactants in blood (R_b) and tissue (R_t) and product in tissue (P) is shown. The fluxes between the compartments, indicated by arrows, are products of the first-order rate constants and the respective compartmental concentrations. Width of arrows represent comparative magnitude of fluxes between compartments. [From ref. 1: Phelps ME, Mazziotta JC, Schelbert HR: Positron Emission Tomography and Autoradiography: Principles and Applications for the Brain and Heart. Raven Press, New York, 1986. With permission.]

distribution volume per unit mass of tissue for a diffusible substance or tracer. This interpretation is employed in some models for estimating blood flow and perfusion, as discussed in Section D.

4. Flux

Flux refers to the amount of substance that crosses a boundary or surface per unit time, e.g., mg/min or moles/min (Figure 22-3). It also can refer to the transport of a substance between different compartments in terms of flux/unit volume or mass of tissue, e.g., moles/min/ml or mg/min/gm.

Flux is a general term that can refer to a variety of processes. For example, the total mass of red blood cells moving through a blood vessel per unit time is a flux. The "boundary" or "surface" in this case could be any transverse plane through the vessel. The amount of glucose moving across a cell membrane per unit time also is a flux. Fluxes therefore may either be closely related or unrelated to blood flow.

5. Rate Constants

Rate constants describe the relationships between the concentrations and fluxes of a substance between two compartments. For simple *first-order processes*, the rate constant, k, multiplied by the amount (or concentration) of a substance in a compartment determines the flux:

$$\text{flux} = k \times \text{amount of substance} \qquad (22\text{-}4)$$

For first-order processes, the units of k are $(time)^{-1}$. If "amount" refers to the mass of tracer in the compartment, the units of flux are mass/time, e.g., mg/min. If "amount" refers to concentration of tracer in the compartment, the units of flux are mass/time per unit of compartment volume, e.g., mg/min/ml, or mass/time per unit of compartment mass, e.g., mg/min/gm. Note that, as illustrated by Figure 22-3, different directions of transport between two compartments can be characterized by different rate constants.

Another interpretation of a first-order rate constant is that it represents the fractional rate of transport of a substance from a compartment per unit time. For example, a rate constant of 0.1 min^{-1} corresponds to a transport of 10 percent of the substance from the compartment per minute. The inverse of the rate constant, 1/k, is sometimes referred to as the *turnover time*, or *mean transit time*, τ, of the tracer in the compartment (in this example 10 minutes). Similarly, the *half-time of turnover*, $t_{1/2}$, i.e., the time required for the original amount of tracer in the compartment to decrease by 50 percent (assuming no back transfer into the compartment) is given by:

$$t_{1/2} = 0.693/k \qquad (22\text{-}5)$$

Thus, the rate constant k is analogous to the decay constant λ for radioactive decay, while the mean transit time is analogous to the average lifetime of a radionuclide (Chapter 3, Section B). In first-order models, transport out of a compartment through a single pathway (without back transport) is described by an exponential function, e^{-kt}, analogous to the radioactive decay factor $e^{-\lambda t}$.

If there is more than one potential pathway for a tracer to leave a compartment, each characterized by a separate rate constant, k_i, then the turnover time of the tracer in the compartment is the inverse of the sum of all these rate constants and the halftime of turnover is:

$$t_{1/2} = 0.693/(k_1 + k_2 + \cdots + k_i) \qquad (22\text{-}6)$$

Most compartment models used in nuclear medicine are based on the assumption that first-order kinetics describe the dynamics of the system of interest. The tracer kinetics of such systems are linear. That is, doubling the input (amount or concentration) doubles the output (flux) of the system. As shown in Section F, linear first-order tracer kinetic models adequately describe many systems even when the dynamics of the natural substances are nonlinear.

A more general expression for the relationship between rate constants, fluxes and concentrations (or masses) is:

$$\text{flux} = k \times [\text{mass or concentration of substance}]^n \qquad (22\text{-}7)$$

where n refers to the *order* of the reaction. The units of rate constants for nth order reactions (in terms of concentration) are [concentrations]$^{(1-n)}$[time]$^{-1}$. Thus, only first-order rate constants represent a constant fractional turnover and Equations 22-5 and 22-6 apply only to first-order processes.

Figure 22-3 illustrates a three-compartment system consisting of a blood compartment separated by a membrane barrier (e.g., capillary wall) from two sequential tissue compartments. R and P refer to chemical reactant and product while the subscripts b and t refer to reactant in blood and tissue compartments, respectively. $[R_b]$, $[R_t]$, and $[P]$ are the blood and tissue concentrations of reactant and product, while the fluxes between the compartments are the first-order rate constants, k_1, k_2, k_3, and k_4, multiplied by corresponding concentrations. The widths of the arrows are proportional to the magnitude of the corresponding flux. In this example, the fluxes into and out of tissue are larger than corresponding fluxes between the reactant and product compartments in tissue. Thus, the majority of the substrate initially transported into the tissue space is back transported into blood without undergoing any biochemical reactions. This is a common occurrence in real biochemical systems and introduces a reserve capacity into the system that can accommodate changes in metabolic supply and demand.

Figure 22-4 illustrates the relationship between first-order rate con-

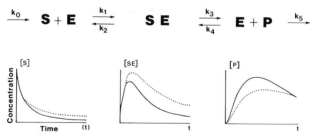

Fig. 22-4. Illustration of tracer kinetics of a chemical reaction sequence. First order rate constants (k_0, k_1, k_2, k_3, k_4, and k_5) characterize the various reaction steps, while S refers to substrate, E refers to enzyme, P is product and SE is the substrate-enzyme complex. The time (t) activity relationships for concentrations of labeled S, SE and P are shown below for a given value of k_3 (smooth lines) and with k_3 decreased by 50%. [From ref. 1: Phelps ME, Mazziotta JC, Schelbert HR: Positron Emission Tomography and Autoradiography: Principles and Applications for the Brain and Heart. Raven Press, New York, 1986. With permission.]

stants and the relative concentrations of the substrates in a biochemical sequence. If a substrate (S) and enzyme (E) combined to form a substrate-enzyme complex (SE) which then dissociates into a product (P) with release of the enzyme, the fluxes of the first-order reaction steps are concentrations multiplied by the corresponding rate. If a small amount of labeled substrate is introduced into the system at time zero, the tracer will go through the reaction steps, producing concentrations of labeled S, SE, and P as shown in the graphs in Figure 22-4. If k_3 (the forward rate constant for the reaction converting SE to E and P) is reduced by 50 percent with all the other rate constants remaining unchanged, the concentrations of labeled S, SE, and P are then represented by the dotted lines in Figure 22-4. Decreasing k_3 causes a slower accumulation of P and causes a compensatory increase in labeled S and SE.

6. Steady State

The term *steady state* refers to a condition in which a process, parameter, or variable is not changing with time. For example, a flux through a biochemical pathway is said to be in steady state when the concentration of reactants and products are not changing with time. In all tracer kinetic models, it is assumed that the underlying process that is being measured by the tracer is in a steady state. Because of biorhythms, steady states almost never exist in the body; however, if the magnitude or temporal period of change is small compared to the process being measured, then the steady state assumption is reasonable. In many cases, the experimental temporal sampling rate is slow compared to the biorhythm (e.g., blood sampling rate vs. pulsatile nature of blood flow) and it is not perceived in the measured data. In these cases, the measured parameters represent average values of the function measured. If the period of the biorhythm is large compared to the temporal sampling rate or the average rate of the process observed, this can produce significant errors in the model calculations. In this case, the calculated parameters typically do not represent a simple average of the non-steady-state values.

Steady state of a process should not be confused with steady state of the tracer. Measurements of the tracer commonly are made when the tracer itself is not in steady state, but rather while it is distributing through the process under study. Some tracer kinetic models are used in which measurements are made when both the tracer and process studied are in a steady state. These methods usually are referred to as "equilibrium" models (Section G).

An important and useful property of a steady-state condition is that the rates (fluxes) of all steps in a nonbranching transport or reaction sequence are equal. Thus, if a tracer technique is used to measure one

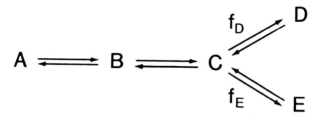

Fig. 22-5. Example of a multistep reaction sequence that branches into two pathways. The terms f_D and f_E are the branching fractions for the corresponding pathways.

step in a sequence, the rate for each step in the entire sequence can be determined. If the reaction branches into two or more separate pathways then the sum of each pathway must equal the rate of the preceding step. In this case, if one determines the rate of any of the preceding steps and also knows the branching fractions, then the rate of each branch can be determined by multiplying the rate of the preceding step by the branching fraction. For example, if the reaction sequence in Figure 22-5 is in a steady state and the rate of disappearance of A is R_A, the rates of formation of B,C,D, and E are R_B, R_C, R_D, and R_E, respectively, and f_d and f_E are the branching fraction down the corresponding pathways, then:

$$R_A = R_B = R_C = (R_D + R_E) \qquad (22\text{-}8)$$

and

$$R_D = f_D \times R_C \qquad (22\text{-}9)$$

$$R_E = f_E \times R_C \qquad (22\text{-}10)$$

where

$$f_D + f_E = 1 \qquad (22\text{-}11)$$

B. TRACER DELIVERY AND TRANSPORT

A tracer that is injected into the body must follow several steps in sequence before it can enter a biochemical pathway: delivery to the capillary via blood flow, extraction across the capillary wall into the tissue space, and finally, incorporation into a biochemical reaction sequence. Although only one of the steps in a process may be of interest in a particular application, it may be influenced by other steps in the process of tracer delivery. In this section we examine tracer techniques for describing these processes.

1. Blood Flow, Extraction, and Clearance

Blood flow through vessels is described in units of volume per unit time, ml/min. With regional tissue measurements it is blood flow per mass of tissue that is determined (ml/min/gm). Blood flow per mass of tissue is more properly referred to as *perfusion*; however, in the literature the term blood flow is used to indicate both blood flow and blood flow per mass of tissue. In both cases the basic phenomenom is still blood flow. Thus, relationships involving blood flow apply equally to blood flow and perfusion, provided that care is taken to ensure that the units are consistent. For example, in the relationship between blood flow and blood volume (Section D), if blood flow is in unit of ml/min then blood volume must be in units of ml. If blood flow is in units of ml/min/gm, then blood volume must be in units of volume per mass of tissue, ml/gm. In this text, the term blood flow, symbolized by F, will be used to denote either blood flow or blood flow per mass of tissue. The units will indicate which quantity is being discussed.

In addition to its dependence on blood flow, the uptake of a tracer by tissue depends on tissue extraction and clearance. Extraction is defined in two different contexts: net and unidirectional. *Net extraction* refers to the difference in steady state tracer concentrations between the input and output blood flow of an organ. If the input (arterial) concentration is C_A, and the output (venous) concentration is C_V, the net extraction fraction, E_n, is defined as

$$E_n = (C_A - C_V)/C_A \qquad (22\text{-}12)$$

If there is no metabolism of the tracer, i.e., if all the tracer delivered to the tissue eventually is returned to the blood, the net extraction is zero. This situation applies, for example, to inert diffusible blood flow tracers when steady state conditions for the tracer are reached.

Unidirectional extraction refers to the amount of tracer extracted only from blood to tissue. It does not include the amount transferred back from tissue to blood. Thus, the unidirectional extraction fraction, E_u, generally is larger than the net extraction fraction. An exception to this general rule occurs with O_2. Virtually all oxygen extracted by tissue is metabolized; thus, the net and unidirectional extraction fractions are the same. For essentially all other substances, a major portion of what is extracted by the tissue is transported back to blood. This is the situation represented by the bidirectional transport in the model shown in Figure 22-3.

Extraction fractions are expressed as fractions or as percentages and can be measured using tracer kinetic techniques. To determine net extraction, it is necessary to measure the input and output concentrations of the tracer in the blood under steady-state conditions, i.e., after the concentrations have reached constant values. The route of administration of the tracer is unimportant in this case. For example, the tracer can be administered by constant infusion or as a bolus into a peripheral vein.

Unidirectional extraction can be measured by observing the rate of uptake by the tissue or organ immediately after injection of the tracer, i.e., when the blood concentration is maximum and the tissue concentration is zero. Measurements of unidirectional extraction are useful for studying the transport properties of substrates and drugs.

An important concept relating the processes of blood flow, flux, and extraction is the *Fick principle*. This principle is based on the conservation of mass and states that, under steady-state conditions, the net uptake of a tracer (or other substance) is simply the difference between the input to and output from the organ or tissue. If the input (arterial) concentration of the tracer is C_A(mg/ml) and the output (venous) concentration is C_V(mg/ml), and the blood flow to the organ is F(ml/min), then the net uptake rate, U(mg/min), is given by

$$U = F \times (C_A - C_V) \tag{22-13}$$

As an example, if the arterial and venous concentrations of oxygen, and the blood flow to an organ are measured, Equation 22-13 can be used to determine the oxygen utilization rate for that organ. If blood flow F in Equation 22-13 is replaced by blood flow per mass of tissue (perfusion), then the uptake or utilization is given in units of utilization per mass of tissue (mg/min/gm).

The Fick principle can be employed only under steady-state conditions. An alternative approach that is applicable to non-steady-state conditions is the Kety-Schmidt method, which is discussed in Section D.

The extraction of tracers generally occurs across membranes or through the fenestrations of capillaries. The extraction fraction of a tracer depends on the capillary surface area, S, the capillary permeability for the tracer, P, and blood flow through the capillaries, F. A simple model relating these quantities was developed by Renkin and Crone.[2,3] Figure 22-6 illustrates an idealized capillary (i.e., rigid tube) through which is passing a tracer with flow F. It is assumed that the concentration of tracer across the cross-section of the capillary at any point along its length is constant, and that the extraction of tracer from the capillary to the tissue at any point is proportion to the concentration of the tracer in the blood. It is further assumed that extraction is unidirectional, i.e., no back transfer of the tracer from tissue to blood. For this simple model, it can be shown[1] that the unidirectional extraction fraction E_u for the capillary is given by

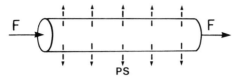

Fig. 22-6. Renkin-Crone capillary model. The capillary is assumed to be a rigid tube, and extraction from blood to tissue is characterized by the product of permeability, P, and surface area, S. Blood flow through the capillary is F.

$$E_u = [1 - e^{-(PS/F)}] \tag{22-14}$$

Thus, the extraction fraction depends only on the permeability-surface area product, PS (ml/min), and on flow. This equation also can be stated in terms of perfusion, by replacing blood flow with perfusion (ml/min/gm) and the permeability-surface area product with PS for a capillary network per mass of tissue (ml/min/gm).

Example 22-2.
What is the unidirectional extraction fraction for a diffusible tracer such as $^{13}NH_3$ in the brain if PS = 0.25 ml/min/gm and blood flow to the brain (perfusion) is 0.50 ml/min/gm?

Answer.
From Equation 22-14:

$$E_u = 1 - e^{-(0.25/0.50)} = 0.39$$

The Renkin-Crone model is not completely realistic, because it assumes no back transfer of tracer from tissue to blood, that the permeability-surface area product, PS, does not depend on blood flow, and that the capillary is a rigid tube. Nevertheless, it is instructive for illustrating the relationships between extraction fraction, blood flow, and the permeability-surface area product.

The ratio (PS/F) sometimes is referred to as the *extraction coefficient*. One interpretation of the product, PS, is that it represents the flow of the tracer from blood to tissue through the capillary wall, whereas F represents flow through the capillary itself. These two "flows" represent competing processes for removal of the tracer from the capillary. Thus, the fraction of a substance that is extracted by tissue can be increased either by increasing the "flow" through the capillary wall, PS, or

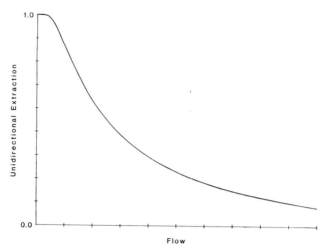

Fig. 22-7. Unidirectional extraction fraction versus flow for the Renkin-Crone model. The extraction fraction is 1.0 when flow is near zero, and decreases toward zero as flow increases.

decreasing the blood flow through the capillary. For a given value of PS, the greater the flow, F, the shorter the residence time of the tracer in the capillary, and, thus, the less the chance that the tracer will escape through the capillary wall. This is illustrated graphically in Figure 22-7.

On the other hand, the *amount* of material entering the tissue depends on the product of blood flow times extraction fraction, $F \times E$. This product is sometimes referred to as *clearance*, and has the same units as flow, i.e., ml/min (or ml/min/gm). In essence, it represents a "virtual flow" from the capillary into the tissue. Typically the increased amount of tracer that is delivered to the capillary with increasing blood flow more than offsets the decrease in the extraction fraction, with the net result that clearance increases with flow. This is illustrated graphically in Figure 22-8. Note that for small values of PS, i.e., low "flow" across the capillary membrane, clearance is low and reaches a plateau value for relatively low values of capillary blood flow, F, whereas for large values of PS, clearance continues to increase with increasing flow through the capillaries. This indicates that the clearance or deposition of a tracer into tissue will have a high or low dependence on blood flow, depending on whether it has a high or low value of PS.

Clearance of tracers from tissue to blood also is used in tracer kinetic modeling. The most common use of tissue to blood clearance is in the measurement of bidirectional transport and blood flow.

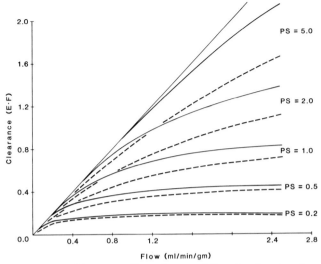

Fig. 22-8. Clearance (flow times unidirectional extraction fraction) vs. flow for various values of permeability-surface area product, PS, for the Renkin-Crone model (smooth lines, Equation 22-14) and for a compartmental model description (dotted lines, Equation 22-19). PS is in units of ml/min/gm. [From ref. 1: Phelps ME, Mazziotta JC, Schelbert HR: Positron Emission Tomography and Autoradiography: Principles and Applications for the Brain and Heart. Raven Press, New York, 1986. With permission.]

2. Transport

Three different mechanisms exist for the transport of substances across a membrane or capillary wall. *Active* transport mechanisms require energy and can move substances against concentration gradients. Usually the energy source is ATP. Examples of active transport are the sodium-potassium "pump" that maintains the difference in between intra- and extracellular concentrations of these ions, and renal tubular reabsorption of glucose.

Passive transport mechanisms do not require energy and move substances in the same direction as the concentration gradient. The passive mechanisms include *carrier-mediated* diffusion, e.g., glucose and amino acid transport from blood to brain, and *passive diffusion*, which depends only the existence of a concentration gradient, e.g., the diffusion of ^{99m}Tc-pertechnetate from blood to brain through a disrupted blood-brain barrier. Bulk flow across fenestrations in capillaries also accounts for a fraction of passive transport but varies from tissue to tissue, e.g., it is insignificant in the brain when the blood brain barrier is intact, but it is a major source of capillary/tissue transport in heart.

Simple molecular diffusion for a given membrane and molecule is characterized by a *diffusion constant*, D. Membrane permeability is related to the diffusion constant by:

$$P(cm/min) = D(cm^2/min)/X(cm) \qquad (22\text{-}15)$$

where X is the thickness of the membrane or the diffusion path length. One usually deals with the PS product rather than P itself because in most applications the regional capillary surface area S is not known accurately. The larger the value of D (or PS), the more rapid the passive diffusion process and the greater the clearance of the substance from blood to tissue or from tissue to blood (Figure 22-8). Many substances and in vivo processes depend on passive diffusion mechanisms, e.g., water, oxygen, ammonia, and carbon dioxide.

Carrier-mediated diffusion is somewhat more complicated. It also transports substances in the same direction of a concentration gradient, and is characterized by the following reaction process:

$$S + C \underset{k_2}{\overset{k_1}{\rightleftarrows}} SC \underset{k_4}{\overset{k_3}{\rightleftarrows}} C + S \qquad (22\text{-}16)$$

where S is the substrate and C is the carrier molecule. SC is a carrier/substrate complex that physically moves across the membrane and then dissociates into C and S, and k_1, k_2, k_3, and k_4 are first-order rate constants that characterize the respective steps of the process. Because only a finite number of carrier molecules are available, this type of transport process can be saturated. The rate of the process increases as the substrate concentration S increases, but only to the point of saturating the number of available carrier sites. Generally, the carrier C is a protein enzyme that is neither created nor destroyed in the reaction but only enhances its rate. The kinetics of carrier-mediated diffusion are described further in Section F.

C. FORMULATION OF A COMPARTMENTAL MODEL

Most models commonly in use in nuclear medicine are compartmental models with first-order rate constants describing the flux of material between compartments. Consider the simple two compartment models

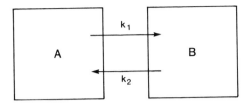

Fig. 22-9. Transport between two compartments, A and B, is described by rate constants k_1 and k_2.

illustrated in Figure 22-9. If a tracer is present in compartment A with concentration defined by A(t) (e.g., a tracer administered as a bolus so that the concentration in A is time dependent), then the rate of change in concentration of compartment B [dB(t)/dt] is described by:

$$dB(t)/dt = \text{flux into B} - \text{flux out of B} \qquad (22\text{-}17)$$

Because first order kinetics apply, the flux into B is simply $k_1A(t)$ and the flux out of B is $k_2B(t)$; therefore:

$$dB(t)/dt = k_1A(t) - k_2B(t) \qquad (22\text{-}18)$$

This first-order ordinary differential equation with constant coefficients is a typical, although simple, example of the equations necessary to mathematically define a tracer kinetic model. The time course of the tracer in the delivery compartment (usually the blood) [A(t)] is the "input function," while the rate constants k_1 and k_2 are model "parameters."

The parameters k_1 and k_2 can be estimated numerically with a technique known as "regression analysis." The input function A(t) is measured and the time course of activity in tissue B(t) is determined from images or other counting measurements. A discussion of regression analysis and other numerical methods related to tracer kinetic models is beyond the scope of this chapter but the interested reader is referred to reference 1.

A simple compartmental model illustrated in Figure 22-10 also can be used to describe the relationship between extraction and blood flow discussed in Section B.1 in reference to the Renkin-Crone model (Equation 22-14). In the compartmental model, the vascular space in the capillary is assumed to be a compartment of uniform concentration. The extraction and venous blood flow compete through the common vascular pool for removal of tracers. According to this compartmental model the extraction E is related to flow F and the PS product as[1]:

$$E = PS/(PS + F) \qquad (22\text{-}19)$$

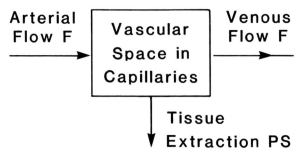

Fig. 22-10. Compartmental model of capillary in which tissue extraction is competing with the venous flow for the tracer that is delivered by the arterial blood flow. [From ref. 1: Phelps ME, Mazziotta JC, Schelbert HR: Positron Emission Tomography and Autoradiography: Principles and Applications for the Brain and Heart. Raven Press, New York, 1986. With permission.]

Tissue extraction as a function of blood flow for this compartmental model is illustrated by the dashed lines in Figure 22-8. The amount of extraction predicted with the compartmental model is lower than that predicted with the Renkin-Crone model for a given PS value. In addition, the change in extraction with blood flow is somewhat different. In most modeling applications of interest in nuclear medicine, the Renkin-Crone model (Equation 22-14) and the compartmental model (Equation 22-19) of capillary extraction yield substantially equivalent results.

In most of the modeling approaches of interest in nuclear medicine and in most of the examples presented in this chapter, two sources of data occur: the time course of the injected radiotracer in whole blood or plasma (the input function), and the measured amount of activity in tissue (the tissue response), usually obtained from region of interest (ROI) analysis from images. The ROI count values are equivalent to local tissue concentrations of the tracer of interest if appropriate corrections are made for attenuation and for other causes of counting inaccuracy. Additionally, the systems used to measure radioactivity in blood and tissue (e.g., a well counter and a camera) must be calibrated so corrections can be made to account for their differences in counting efficiencies.

Figure 22-11 illustrates several relationships between the input function and tissue response curves for two different model configurations. The curves for the first model (a three-compartment model with three rate constants) illustrate how the shape of the tissue reponse curve changes as the shape of the input function changes. In both cases, the kinetics of the tracer in tissue are identical but the temporal response in tissue is

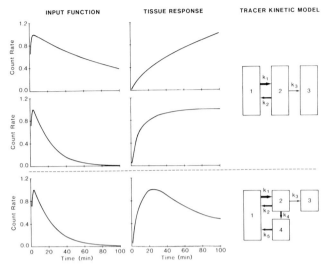

Fig. 22-11.   Input function and tissue response (time course of activity in tissue) with two different models and different shapes of input functions. Different input functions produce different tissue responses for a given model configuration (first two rows), while the same input function with different model configurations (bottom two rows) also produces different tissue responses. [From ref. 1: Phelps ME, Mazziotta JC, Schelbert HR: Positron Emission Tomography and Autoradiography: Principles and Applications for the Brain and Heart. Raven Press, New York, 1986. With permission.]

influenced by the input function (e.g., changing the rate of injection could produce this pattern). The parameters of the model (the rate constants) are unchanged in these two situations. If one did not measure the input function in this example and only measured the tissue response function, the different tissue response functions might be interpreted incorrectly as a change in the rate of the physiologic or biochemical process in the tissue. In the second example (bottom row in the figure) a four-compartment model representing a more complicated biologic process produces a different tissue response than the first model even when presented with the same input function. Thus, the observed shape of the tissue response is a function of both the input function and a characteristic of the tissue "system" called the impulse response. The impulse response of a linear system is the system's response when presented with an impulse as an input function. An impulse is in essence a function of infinitely short duration with an undefined magnitude at the origin and that has an integrated value of one if summed over all time. It can be thought of as an "idealized bolus" input given instantaneously (i.e., beyond zero time it has a zero value). In reality, a practical "impulse" delivery of tracer to a system has a duration shorter than the shortest vascular transit time through the organ. For example, when a tracer begins to clear from the organ the input of the tracer into the organ has dropped to zero.

D. BLOOD FLOW MODELS

Many tracer kinetic methods and models to measure blood flow exist.[1] Virtually all such methods are included in one of three categories: *trapping*, *clearance*, and *equilibrium* techniques. These techniques can be implemented by administering compounds labeled with either gamma emitting or positron emitting isotopes and imaging their distribution with gamma cameras, SPECT, or PET tomographs (Table 22-1). All techniques require measuring the concentration of tracer in arterial blood if quantitative estimates of blood flow in units of ml/min or ml/min/gm (perfusion) are desired.

In trapping methods, tracers are attached to particles that are distributed to organs in proportion to blood flow but that are then trapped, either physically in the circulation (e.g., trapping of macroaggregated albumin labeled with ^{99m}Tc in the pulmonary capillaries in lung perfusion studies), or metabolically in tissue (e.g., $^{13}NH_3$ and ^{123}I-iodoamphetamine).

Clearance methods require injecting metabolically inert labeled tracers that also are distributed in proportion to flow but that do not remain trapped in the vascular or tissue spaces. The rate of washout, or clearance, of these tracers is dependent upon blood flow. Either nondiffusible tracers that remain within the vascular compartment or diffusible tracers that distribute in both the tissue and vascular compartments can be used. As discussed below, with both classes of tracers, the mathematical approach to measuring blood flow is similar.

Equilibrium techniques require administering a continuous supply of a diffusible blood flow tracer, waiting until a tracer steady state has been reached, and then imaging the distribution. This approach uses very short half-life radioisotopes in which equilibrium is established between removal of the tracer from tissue by the rate of blood flow vs. the rate of radioactive decay.

1. Microsphere and Tracer Trapping Models

A simple trapping method for measuring blood flow employing nondiffusible tracers is the *labeled microsphere* technique. Microspheres are spherical or irregularly shaped small particles that are larger than capillaries and embolize the first capillary bed they encounter. They remain within the capillary system for a time that is sufficiently long so that particle breakdown and excretion is insignifient during the measurement period.

If labeled microspheres are injected into the left atrium, they are distributed to individual organs in proportion to the blood flow to the organ. If the total activity of microspheres injected is A_t, blood flow to an organ can be calculated from:

$$F(ml/min) = C.O. (ml/min) \times (A_o/A_t) \qquad (22\text{-}20)$$

where A_o is the activity of microspheres accumulated in the organ, (assuming 100 percent trapped), and C.O. is the cardiac output. A_o is determined by tissue sampling or from quantitative imaging measurements. Cardiac output must be measured independently. Organ perfusion, i.e., blood flow per gram of tissue, is given by

$$F(ml/min/gm) = C.O. \times [(A_o/m_o)A_t] \qquad (22\text{-}21)$$

where A_o/m_o is the concentration of activity in the organ or the measured tissue sample.

If the labeled microspheres are not 100 percent trapped, A_o will be reduced and Equations 22-20 and 22-21 will lead to underestimations of flow or organ perfusion. This effect is illustrated graphically in Figure 22-8 for tracers with a PS product below the value required for 100 percent clearance over the blood flow range studied.

Frequently, cardiac output is difficult to measure. In such cases, flow to a single organ can be determined by a modification of the above method known as the *reference sample technique*. In this technique, arterial blood is withdrawn at a rate $S(ml/min)$ during the time when the microspheres are flowing to the organ, and the total activity of the blood sample withdrawn, A_s, is determined. Blood flow to the organ then is calculated from

$$F = S(ml/min) \times (A_o/A_s) \qquad (22\text{-}22)$$

where A_o is the activity of microspheres trapped in the organ. *Perfusion* of the organ is calculated from

$$F = S \times [(A_o/m_o)/A_s] \qquad (22\text{-}23)$$

Although the microsphere technique is conceptually simple, it requires injection of the tracer into the left atrium to avoid extraction of particles by the lungs and causes microembolization of capillaries exposed to the particles. To minimize perturbation of the system being studied, only a small number of microspheres are injected. An example of the labeled microsphere technique is the use of labeled albumin (which dissolves with time) to determine lung perfusion or to detect right-to-left cardiac shunts. The microsphere technique is infrequently used in humans and is more commonly used in research studies involving animals.

Other non-diffusible tracers that do not embolize the capillary beds, e.g., labeled red blood cells, labeled non-aggregated albumin, and diffusible tracers that do not remain exclusively within the vascular space also are used to trace and quantitate blood flow. Indeed, all tracers injected into the vascular system initially behave as "blood flow tracers" to some degree, but not all tracers permit convenient quantitation of blood flow independent of other processes such as extraction, metabolism, etc.

Example 22-3.

Suppose that microspheres are labeled with a radionuclide that permits quantitative measurement of concentrations in tissues, e.g., ^{11}C measured by PET. For simplicity, assume that these measurements can be related to the actual number of microspheres present. Calculate blood flow per gm of tissue (i.e., perfusion) to the brain if 500,000 microspheres are injected into the left atrium, and the average concentration of microspheres measured in the brain is 50 microspheres/gm. Assume the cardiac output is 5 liters/min.

Answer.

From Equation 22-21, blood flow per gram of tissue is given by

$$F = \frac{(5000 \text{ ml/min}) \times (50 \text{ microspheres/gm})}{500,000 \text{ microspheres}}$$

$$= 0.50 \text{ ml/min/gm}$$

Example 22-4.

Assume in the situation of example 22-2 the cardiac output is unknown. After injecting 500,000 microspheres into the left atrium, radial arterial blood is sampled at a rate of 10 ml/min. The average microsphere concentration in the whole brain is again 50 microspheres/gm. Assume the microspheres are 100 percent trapped in capillaries in one pass through the circulation (i.e., in one minute). A total of 1000 microspheres are counted in the radial arterial sample obtained in a one minute period. What is the average brain blood flow per gm of tissue?

Answer.

From equation 22-23:

$$F = \frac{(10 \text{ ml/min}) (50 \text{ microspheres/gm})}{(1000 \text{ microspheres})}$$

$$= 0.50 \text{ ml/min/gm}$$

---

2. Clearance Techniques

Most clearance techniques for measuring blood flow are based on the *Central Volume Principle*, which is defined as follows:

$$F = V/\tau \qquad (22\text{-}24)$$

where V is the volume in which the tracer is distributed and τ is the mean transit time of the tracer through this volume. In the case of blood flow in units of ml/min, V is in units of ml. For blood flow in units of ml/min/gm, V is in units of ml/gm (volume per mass of tissue).

For a nondiffusible tracer, i.e., one that stays within the vascular space, V is the blood volume in ml or ml/gm, depending upon the units of blood flow. The determination of F with a nondiffusible tracer requires the measurement of both τ and V. Normally, with nondiffusible tracers only τ is measured, which thus provides a measure of F/V. Since F changes with both τ (τ decreases as F increases) and V (V increases as F increases) there is a nonlinear relationship between F/V and τ, with the magnitude of changes in τ being less than the magnitude of changes in F.

It is more common and easier to measure blood flow with diffusible tracers. Diffusible tracers are those that have 100 percent extraction from blood to tissue during a single transit through the vascular bed of the tissue, almost exclusively occurring at the level of capillaries because of their large vascular surface area. If the tracer is chemically inert, it will be cleared from tissue in proportion to blood flow and F can be determined by Equation 22-24. For diffusible tracers, V is the volume into which the tracer is distributed. The fraction of the total tissue that a diffusible tracer will occupy depends upon the specific diffusion and solubility properties of the tracer. This volume is denoted by V_1, as described in Section A.3. Thus, by substituting V_1, for V in Equation 22-24 and rearranging,

$$F/V_1 = 1/\tau \qquad (22\text{-}25)$$

Multiplying each side of Equation 22-25 by V_1/V_t, where V_t is the total tissue volume, gives

$$F/V_1 \, (V_1/V_t) = (1/\tau) \, (V_1/V_t)$$

$$F/V_t = \lambda/\tau \tag{22-26}$$

where V_1/V_t is the partition coefficient (λ) for the tracer as given by Equation 22-3. As discussed earlier λ typically is measured using Equation 22-2. F/V_t is blood flow per volume or mass of tissue (perfusion). As discussed in B.1, by convention in the literature F/V_t is also referred to as blood flow, F. Thus, Equation 22-26 also may be written as $F = \lambda/\tau$.

The problem of V varying with flow, discussed above for nondiffusible tracer, does not exist to any significant degree with diffusible tracers. The term V with diffusible tracers is the tissue volume that does not change to any appreciable degree with changes in blood flow. Thus, changes in $1/\tau$ are directly proportional to flow. In addition, τ is longer for diffusible (i.e., 30–100 seconds for brain) than nondiffusible (3–6 seconds for brain) tracers that are commonly used. Thus, because of the longer values of τ and the linear relationship between τ and blood flow with diffusible tracers, they usually provide more accurate and convenient measurements of blood flow than obtained with nondiffusible tracers. However, λ usually is measured in normal tissue and it may vary from this value in pathologic tissues. For example, ^{15}O-labeled water has little variability,[1] while ^{133}Xe has considerable variability[4] between normal and diseased tissue.

An example of the Central Volume Principle for measuring flow is the Kety-Schmidt method for measuring cerebral blood flow (CBF) with inhaled, diffusible, inert gasses (e.g., nitrous oxide, krypton, etc.). This approach is based upon the assumption of a constant partition coefficient of 1.0 ml/gm in the case of nitrous oxide and krypton[1] in the brain. Thus CBF is given by (Equation 22-26):

$$CBF = \lambda/\tau = 1.0 \text{ ml/gm}/\tau(min) = \tau^{-1} \text{ (ml/min/gm)} \tag{22-27}$$

The technique thus requires measuring the mean transit time of the gas through the brain. The original technique involved giving a subject a continuous inhalation of the gas and sampling the gas concentrations in the arterial supply to the brain (i.e., any convenient arterial source) and the venous drainage (internal jugular bulb). Gas was breathed until an equilibrium (or near equilibrium) concentration was reached in the brain and blood. The law of conservation of mass states that the total amount of tracer remaining within the brain at equilibrium must be the difference between the cumulative input and output. Therefore:

$$VC_E = F \int_0^\infty C_A(t)dt - F \int_0^\infty C_V(t)dt \tag{22-28}$$

But $\lambda/F = \tau$ (Equation 22-26); therefore, rearranging Equation 22-28 yields:

$$\lambda/F = \int_0^\infty [C_A(t) - C_V(t)]dt/C_E = \tau \qquad (22\text{-}29)$$

where $C_A(t)$ and $C_V(t)$ are the arterial and venous concentrations as a function of time and C_E is the equilibrium concentration in the blood, usually approximated by a venous value at a selected time (e.g., 10 minutes) after the initiation of the inhalation. Typical values for this approach are $\tau = 2$ minutes, which, from Equation 22-27 yields a flow of about 0.5 ml/min/gm or 50 ml/min/100gm of brain tissue. A completely analogous approach with nuclear medicine imaging devices (e.g., PET and SPECT) permits one to perform the above calculations regionally in the brain or other tissues and also produces estimates of blood flow using compartmental modeling approaches with a measured arterial input function and serial images of the tissue (i.e., venous efflux concentration measurements are not necessary).

For example, consider a diffusible tracer such as ^{133}Xe. With a bolus injection followed by imaging the wash out of the tracer from an organ, it can be shown that the mean transit time through a compartment described by distribution volume V is[1]:

$$\lambda/F = \tau = \int_0^\infty A(t)\, dt/A(0) \qquad (22\text{-}30)$$

where $A(t)$ is the amount of the tracer in tissue as a function of time after the injection and $A(0)$ is the amount originally injected at time zero. Figure 22-12 illustrates Equation 22-30 graphically. This approach is often referred to as an "area/height" method for determining CBF.

Labeled water is a convenient tracer for measuring blood flow. If $C^{15}O_2$ gas is inhaled, it is converted to $H_2^{15}O$ by carbonic anhydrase in the lungs and then delivered to the body by the systemic circulation. Alternatively, a bolus of $H_2^{15}O$ can be injected intravenously. Imaging its distribution with PET together with measurements of the input function (blood activity concentration over time) permits calculation of regional blood flow using the Central Volume Principle.

Most non-PET nuclear medicine determinations of blood flow by clearance techniques involve relative, rather than absolute, estimations of flow. For example, a dynamic study of ^{99m}Tc DTPA flow through the abdominal aorta and its branches yields a qualitative representation of blood flow to each kidney. A significant reduction or delay in flow to one

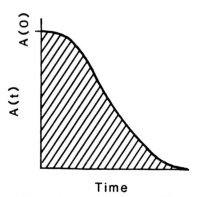

Time

Fig. 22-12. Tissue time-activity curve following bolus injection of a blood flow tracer. The total amount of activity detected in a given tissue region is plotted as a function of time. The maximum activity at time zero represents $A(0)$. From Equation 22-30, the mean transit time, τ is given by the area under the curve divided by the height of the curve, $A(0)$. This method is often referred to as the "area/height" method.

kidney will produce a less intense pattern of uptake over that kidney. As discussed in the introduction of this chapter, DTPA is extracted from the blood by glomerular filtration and the dynamics of renal uptake of this tracer therefore represent a combination of flow and extraction processes. ^{99m}Tc agents (including ^{99}TcO$_4$) also are useful for qualitative studies of cerebral blood flow. Because such agents normally are excluded from the brain parenchyma by an intact blood brain barrier, they act as nondiffusible flow tracers.

3. Equilibrium Techniques

^{15}O-labeled water is another convenient tracer for quantitatively measuring blood flow with PET using an equilibrium method. The constant infusion method originally developed by Jones and coworkers[5] is a good example of an approach that simplifies the data acquisition because it produces a flat input function and a constant tissue concentration of the tracer once the tracer steady state has been reached. The novel aspect of this approach is that the steady state is one between the blood flow delivery of H$_2$^{15}O to tissue and removal by venous outflow and by radioactive decay of the short half-life of ^{15}O ($t_{1/2}$ = 2 min). This method works for any diffusible tracer with a very short half-life. The principle has been used in single photon imaging with ^{81m}Kr ($t_{1/2}$ = 13 sec) but required intraarterial infusion because of the low solubility of Kr in blood.

The principle of conservation of mass states that the flux into the tissue must equal the flux out in a tracer steady state. Adding a factor to account for removal by radioactive decay of the isotope yields the following equation:

$$Q = FC_i/[(0.693/t_{1/2}) + F/\lambda] \qquad (22\text{-}31)$$

$$F = (0.693/t_{1/2})Q \, \lambda/(C_i\lambda - Q) \qquad (22\text{-}32)$$

where Q is the tissue radioactivity concentration, blood flow is F, $t_{1/2}$ is the radioactive half-life (2 min) for ^{15}O, C_i is the arterial blood concentration of ^{15}O and λ is the partition coefficient of $H_2^{15}O$. This approach includes the assumption that the partition coefficient is a constant (typically assumed to be 1.0 ml/gm) and requires a continuous delivery of ^{15}O-labeled water from a cyclotron. This usually is accomplished by having the subject breath $C^{15}O_2$ continuously. The $C^{15}O_2$ immediately is converted to ^{15}O-water by carbonic anhydrase in the lung. Tomographic images are obtained after the tracer steady state has been reached and blood flow is calculated from Equation 22-32. If the blood level reaches a constant level instantaneously, steady state will be approached with a half time, h, given by

$$h = 0.693/[(0.693/t_{1/2}) + (F/\lambda)] \qquad (22\text{-}33)$$

It should be noted that the time to reach equilibrium is dependent upon both the value of the radioactive half-life and value of blood flow. In practice, time is required for the blood level to reach a constant level so longer times than indicated by Equation 22-33 are required. A period of about 10 minutes usually is employed. It also is possible to measure oxygen metabolism with a similar method based on the same principle by having the patient continuously breath $^{15}O_2$ rather than $C^{15}O_2$.[1]

Example 22-5.
Given that the half-life of ^{15}O is 2 minutes and assuming an instantaneous constant blood level of $H_2^{15}O$, how long does it take to reach 93.75 percent of the equilibrium tissue concentration of ^{15}O if the blood flow is 0.25 ml/min/gm or 1 ml/min/gm? Assume partition coefficient $\lambda = 1$ ml/gm

Answer.
Equilibrium is approached with a half time h given by Equation 22-33. The number of half times to reach 93.75% of equilibrium is:

$$1 - 0.0625 = 0.9375 = [1 - (1/16)] = [1 - (1/2)^4]$$

Therefore, four half times are required to reach 93.75 percent of the equilibrium concentration.

For ^{15}O, $t_{1/2}$ = 2 minutes

$$\frac{0.693}{t_{1/2}} = \frac{0.693}{2} \text{ min}^{-1} = 0.347 \text{ min}^{-1}$$

For blood flow of 0.25 ml/min/gm, the time required is:

$$\text{time} = \frac{4 \times 0.693}{0.347 \text{ min}^{-1} + (0.25\text{ml/min/gm})/(1\text{ml/gm})}$$

$$\text{time} = \frac{4 \times 0.693}{0.347 + 0.25}$$

$$\text{time} = 4.6 \text{ minutes}$$

For a blood flow of 1 ml/min/gm,

$$\text{time} = \frac{4 \times 0.693}{0.347 + 1} \text{ minutes} = 2.1 \text{ minutes}$$

The relationship between tissue radioactivity and blood flow in Equation 22-32 is not linear. The degree of nonlinearity is related to the decay constant of the isotope used (see Figure 22-13). This results in more accurate flow measurements at low, rather than high flow rates.

E. BLOOD VOLUME AND EJECTION FRACTION

When tracers that remain within the vascular compartment are used, the initial, first pass distribution reflects blood flow while the steady state (equilibrium) distribution represents blood volume. This is an example of a static tracer equilibrium study as compared to a dynamic tracer equilibrium study described in Section D.3. Two commonly performed techniques in nuclear medicine based upon static tracer equilibrium states include determination of cerebral blood volume and the measurement of left ventricular ejection fraction.

1. Cerebral Blood Volume

If a tracer is administered that binds to red cells and remains within the vascular compartment, the volume of distribution and blood volume can be calculated as shown by Equation 22-1 and Example 22-1. A

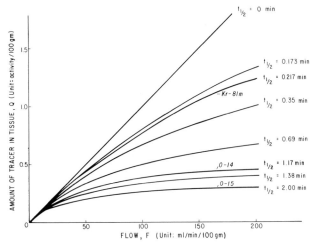

Fig. 22-13. Amount of radioactivity in tissue during an equilibrium study as a function of blood flow for various radioactive decay half-lives of the radionuclide. The shorter the half life, the more linear the relationship. [From ref. 1: Phelps ME, Mazziotta JC, Schelbert HR: Positron Emission Tomography and Autoradiography: Principles and Applications for the Brain and Heart. Raven Press, New York, 1986. With permission.]

related, but different, quantity of interest is the amount of blood in a given volume or mass of tissue. For example, in the brain, the cerebral blood volume per unit mass of tissue consists of arterial, capillary, and venous blood. Because of the large volume of the dural venous sinuses, most of the cerebral blood volume (averaged over the entire brain) is venous, although the relative distribution between arterial, capillary, and venous changes in different locations within the brain. If carbon monoxide labeled with ^{11}C or ^{15}O is inhaled, it will bind tightly to hemoglobin and the resultant PET images will represent regional blood volume (rCBV). Correspondingly, in SPECT, red blood cells are labeled with ^{99m}Tc for measurement of rCBV. The rCBV (blood volume per mass of tissue) is given by:

$$rCBV(ml/gm) = \frac{C_t}{C_b \times 0.85 \times d} \qquad (22\text{-}34)$$

where C_t is the tissue activity concentration, C_b is the peripheral venous blood activity concentration, 0.85 is a correction factor for the difference between peripheral and central hematocrits, and d is the density of brain tissue (1.04 gm/ml). The value of rCBV usually is expressed in units of ml/gm or ml/100 gm of brain tissue.

Example 22-6.
Thirty mCi of ^{11}CO are inhaled as a bolus and the activity is allowed to equilibrate in the blood pool for about three minutes. PET tomographic images of the brain are obtained and a sample of blood is assayed in a well counter for determination of ^{11}C activity. A region of interest drawn over a representative section of gray matter yields a count density of 700 cpm/ml. A blood sample is determined to have 18,000 cpm/ml, after correction for different efficiencies of the well counter and tomograph. What is the rCBV for this region?

Answer.
From Equation 22-34:

$$rCBV = \frac{700 \text{ cpm/ml}}{18000 \text{ cpm/ml} \times 0.85 \times 1.04 \text{ gm/ml}} = 0.044 \text{ ml/gm}$$

---

2. Ejection Fraction

^{99m}Tc-labeled red blood cells (RBCs) are used for dynamic (first pass) and equilibrium gated studies of the heart. If a bolus of ^{99m}Tc-labeled RBCs is injected intravenously and their distribution through the thorax is imaged with a gamma camera interfaced to a computer, the initial distribution will map the direction of blood flow through the venous system into the right atrium and right ventricle, to the lungs and then to the left atrium, left ventricle and out through the aorta to the systemic circulation. Abnormalities in this flow pattern (such as those produced by structural defects in the heart that result in intracardiac shunts) result in an abnormal distribution of the bolus of activity. For example, a ventricular septal defect with shunting of blood from the right to the left ventricle will result in an early appearance of the bolus of activity in the left ventricle as some of the blood (and labeled RBCs) bypass the lungs and travel directly to the left ventricle. The amount of shunting can be estimated if time activity curves of the activity distribution are generated and an appropriate model is applied.

More commonly, the distribution of activity over the left ventricle is plotted as a function of time. Superimposed on the pattern of the distribution of the bolus is the change in ventricular volume caused by

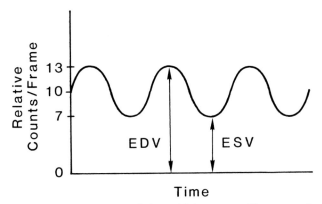

Fig. 22-14.   Example of sinusoidal curve to illustrate relative counts per frame in a gated blood image. Background
counts have been subtracted. EDV and ES are end diastolic
and end systolic volumes, respectively.

cardiac contractions (Figure 21-6). This permits calculation of the ventricular ejection fraction because the relative number of counts within the
ventricle is proportional to the blood volume of the ventricle (see Section
A.3). Precisely the same principle applies in equilibrium gated cardiac
studies, where a changing amount of activity within the ventricle throughout the cardiac cycle (Figure 22-14) permits calculation of the cardiac
ejection fraction. With the equilibrium approach, however, the initial
pattern of the distribution of flow is lost. Only the equilibrium blood
volume information is present.

Example 22-7.
Twenty mCi of ^{99m}Tc-labeled red blood cells are injected intravenously and the number of counts within the left ventricle are
plotted as a function of time (Figure 22-14) after the labeled red
blood cells have equilibrated within the blood pool. Calculate the
left ventricular ejection fraction using the data obtained through
three cardiac cycles.

Answer.
The counts per frame (a typical frame is about 0.04 seconds) over
the left ventricle are plotted in Figure 22-14. Background activity
has been subtracted and the data are represented as a sinusoidal
curve. Real data, of course, consist of a series of discrete values
for frame counts that do not vary in a truly sinusoidal manner. The

ejection fraction (EF) is defined by (end diastolic volume, EDV) − (end systolic volume, ESV) divided by end diastolic volume. Therefore:

$$EF = (EDV - ESV)/EDV = (13 - 7)/13 = 46\%$$

F. ENZYME KINETICS: GLUCOSE METABOLISM

Enzymes catalyze many biochemical reactions that are of interest from the modeling standpoint. An example is the hexokinase catalyzed phosphorylation of glucose that is the step initiating glycolysis and also is the focal reaction for the deoxyglucose and fluorodeoxyglucose (FDG) model for determining rates of glucose metabolism (see below and references 1 and 6).

1. Michaelis-Menten Equation

The Michaelis-Menten hypothesis states that an intermediate complex is formed between a reactant and an enzyme that is then converted to the chemical product with release of the enzyme. This reaction can be written in form similar to that for carrier-mediated transport (Equation 22-16) in Section B.2:

$$S + E \underset{k_2}{\overset{k_1}{\rightleftarrows}} SE \overset{k_3}{\rightleftarrows} P + E \tag{22-35}$$

where S is the substrate, P is the product, E is the enzyme and k_1, k_2, and k_3 are the rate constants for the steps of the reaction process. Note that it is generally assumed that there is no reverse association of P and E, therefore no k_4 rate constant is present. However, in biological systems there usually are separate enzymes for conversion of P back to S for additional regulation of reaction sequences.

The reaction rate (conversion of S to P) is:

$$R = \frac{V_m[S]}{[S] + K_m} \tag{22-36}$$

The term V_m (mg/min) is the maximum rate of the reaction while K_m is the

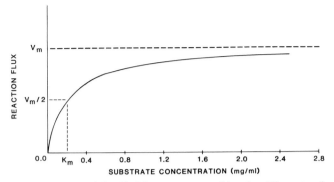

Fig. 22-15. Michaelis-Menten enzyme kinetics. The rate of a reaction, the reaction flux, is plotted against substrate concentration using Equation 22-36. Note that when the substrate concentration equals K_M, the reaction rate is $V_m/2$. As the substrate concentration increases, the reaction rate gradually approaches V_m. [From ref. 1: Phelps ME, Mazziotta JC, Schelbert HR: Positron Emission Tomography and Autoradiography: Principles and Applications for the Brain and Heart. Raven Press, New York, 1986. With permission.]

concentration of S that produces a reaction rate of one half the maximum value, as shown in Figure 22-15. The brackets indicate concentration.

The Michaelis-Menten relationship (e.g., Equation 22-36) predicts that the reaction rate approaches the maximum value V_m as [S] approaches infinity. It is clear from Equation 22-36 and Figure 22-15 that the reaction rate is not a linear function of [S]; however, it still is possible to model such processes with linear tracer compartmental models because of the following relationship. If more than one substrate is competing for the enzyme E (i.e., S and S'), it can be shown[1] that the reaction rates R and R' for the competing processes are:

$$R = \frac{V_m[S]/K_m}{([S]/K_m) + ([S']/K'_m) + 1} \quad (22\text{-}37)$$

$$R' = \frac{V'_m[S']/K'_m}{([S]/K_m) + ([S']/K'_m) + 1} \quad (22\text{-}38)$$

Where V'_m and K'_m are the Michaelis-Menten constants for the reaction with substrate S'. If S' represents a tracer of the original substrate S, then [S'] is of a much lower value than [S]. Therefore:

$$R = \frac{V_m[S]}{[S] + K_m} \tag{22-39}$$

$$R' = \frac{V'_m K_m / K'_m}{[S] + K_m} [S'] \tag{22-40}$$

R is simply the original rate of the process (Equation 22-36) unaffected by the presence of the tracer S', while R' is a linear function of [S'] as long as [S'] remains much less than [S] (i.e., as long as the tracer condition holds). Therefore, the tracer concentration [S'] is linearly related to the reaction rate R' and linear modeling techniques are appropriate for describing this process. Dividing Equation 22-40 by Equation 22-39 yields:

$$R'/R = \frac{V'_m K_m [S']}{V_m K'_m [S]} \tag{22-41}$$

The rate of the measured or "traced" process, R', is therefore directly related to the "natural" or unknown rate R by a ratio of the Michaelis-Menten constants and the relative concentrations of S and S'. In some cases (e.g., isotopic substitution labeling of biological compounds such as ^{11}C for ^{12}C, ^{15}O of ^{16}O, and ^{13}N for ^{14}N and ^{15}N) the Michaelis-Menten constants for the tracer and natural substance are essentially the same and the above equation would reduce to a simple ratio of [S'] to [S]. With analog tracers the Michaelis-Menten constants are different than the natural substance but Equation 22-41 still applies.

2. Deoxyglucose Model

As an example of an analog tracer approach to biochemical modeling, consider the Sokoloff deoxyglucose method or the analogous approach with PET using ^{18}F labeled fluorodeoxyglucose (FDG) for measuring glucose metabolism in the brain.[1] Glucose supplies approximately 95–99 percent of the brain's energy in normal physiologic states and the rate of glucose utilization is an excellent indicator of energy-requiring functions of the brain.

FDG is an analog of glucose (Section A.1) that is similar to glucose in several respects. Like glucose, it is transported from the blood to the brain by a carrier-mediated diffusion mechanism. Hexokinase catalyzes the phosphorylation of glucose to glucose-6-PO_4 and FDG to FDG-6-PO_4. In both the transport and phosphorylation steps, FDG is a competitive substrate with glucose. FDG-6-PO_4; however, is not a significant sub-

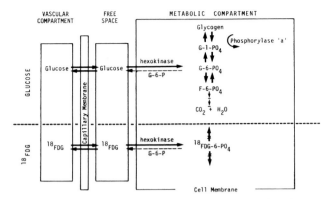

Fig. 22-16. Transport and metabolic pathways for glucose and 2-deoxy-2[^{18}F]fluoro-D-glucose (FDG). Physically, the free space represents a combination of the interstitial space and the cytosol where unphosphorylated glucose and FDG are uniformly distributed. G-6-P is glucose-6-PO$_4$, G-1-P is glucose-1-PO$_4$, F-6-PO$_4$ is fructose-6-PO$_4$. [From ref. 1: Phelps ME, Mazziotta JC, Schelbert HR: Positron Emission Tomography and Autoradiography: Principles and Applications for the Brain and Heart. Raven Press, New York, 1986. With permission.]

strate for further metabolism. It is not converted into glycogen to any significant extent and is not further metabolized in the glycolytic pathway, as shown in (Figure 22-16). The FDG-6-PO$_4$ also does not diffuse across cell membranes and is therefore metabolically trapped in tissues, which is convenient both from an imaging and modeling view point.

If glucose metabolism in the tissue of interest (brain) is assumed to be in a steady state (i.e., it has a constant rate), then the rate of the hexokinase reaction will be the rate of the entire process of glycolysis (Section A.6). A compartmental configuration for the FDG model is shown in Figure 22-17. The three-compartment model consists of FDG in plasma, FDG in tissue, and FDG-6-PO$_4$ in tissue corresponding to comparable distributions of glucose, although glucose continues on through metabolism. The first-order rate constants k_1^* and k_2^* describe the transport of FDG from the blood to brain and brain to blood, respectively, while the first-order rate constants k_3^* and k_4^* describe the phosphorylation of FDG and dephosphorylation of FDG-6-PO$_4$. The asterisk refers to FDG indices while the corresponding terms for glucose do not have an asterisk.

Let CMRGlc* refer to the cerebral metabolic rate of FDG and CMRGlc be the metabolic rate for glucose. If C_E is the concentration of

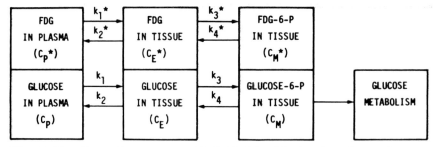

Fig. 22-17. Three Compartment FDG Model with the four first order rate constants describing transport between the compartments. C_p, C_E, and C_M are the concentrations of glucose in plasma, tissue and glucose-6-PO_4 in tissue, respectively, while C_p^*, C_E^*, and C_m^*, are the corresponding concentrations for FDG. [From ref. 1: Phelps ME, Mazziotta JC, Schelbert HR: Positron Emission Tomography and Autoradiography: Principles and Applications for the Brain and Heart. Raven Press, New York, 1986. With permission.]

free (unphosphorylated) glucose in the tissue space and C_E^* is the corresponding concentration for FDG (2nd compartment of Figure 22-17), then, from Equation 22-41 and the fact that the rate of phosphorylation (i.e., flux as described in Sections A.4 and A.5) equals $k_3[C_E]$ for glucose and $k_3^*[C_E^*]$ for FDG, it follows that:

$$\frac{\text{CMRGlc}^*}{\text{CMRGlc}} = \frac{V_m^* K_m [C_E^*]}{V_m K_m^* [C_E]} = \frac{k_3^* [C_E^*]}{k_3 [C_E]} \tag{22-42}$$

Equations 22-42 assumes that k_4^* and k_4 are very small and the forward rate of phosphorylation of glucose and FDG approximate the net metabolic rates. V_m and K_m are the Michaelis-Menten constants for the hexokinase mediated phosphorylation of FDG (*) and glucose (no*).

If the ratio of terms defined by Equation 22-42 is a constant, then:

$$\text{CMRGlc} = \text{CMRGlc}^*/\text{constant} \tag{22-43}$$

If plasma glucose (C_p) and plasma FDG (C_p^*) concentrations are constant and both sides of Equation 22-42 are multiplied by C_p/C_p^*, then:

$$\frac{\text{CMRGlc}^*/[C_p^*]}{\text{CMRGlc}/[C_p]} = \frac{V_m^* K_m [C_E^*]/[C_p^*]}{V_m K_m^* [C_E]/[C_p]} \tag{22-44}$$

But, from Equation 22-2, the ratios C_E^*/C_p^* and C_E/C_p are the partition coefficients (i.e., tissue-to-blood concentration ratios) of FDG (λ^*) and glucose (λ). If the numerator and denominator of the left side of Equation 22-44 are divided by cerebral blood flow (CBF), the numerical value of the equation does not change; thus, with these substitutions:

$$\frac{CMRGlc^*/([C_p^*] \times CBF)}{CMRGlc/([C_p] \times CBF)} = \frac{V_m^* \, K_m \, \lambda^*}{V_m \, K_m^* \, \lambda} \qquad (22\text{-}45)$$

This ratio of terms is defined as the "lumped constant," LC, of the FDG model. The left side of Equation (22-45) is simply the net extraction of FDG (E'_{net}) divided by the net (i.e., steady state) extraction of glucose (E_{net}). Therefore:

$$LC = (E'_{net})/(E_{net}) \qquad (22\text{-}46)$$

That is, the lumped constant of the FDG model is just the steady state ratio of the net extraction of FDG to that of glucose at constant plasma levels of FDG and glucose. The lumped constant (LC) is a direct consequence of Equation 22-41 and illustrates the principle of competitive enzyme kinetics applied to tracer kinetic modeling. Intuitively, the lumped constant is simply a correction term that measures the net difference in the way a tissue utilizes FDG and glucose. The full expression of LC also includes an additional term including the influence of dephosphorylation of glucose on the net metabolic rates of FDG and glucose.[1] This latter term is normally quite close to 1.0 but is intrinsically included in the measured values of LC by Equation 22-46.

While the lumped constant describes the differences between FDG and glucose metabolism, it is actually glucose metabolism itself that is of interest physiologically. It can be shown that CMRGlc is given by[1]:

$$CMRGlc = \frac{C_p}{LC} \left(\frac{k_1^* k_3^*}{(k_2^* + k_3^*)} \right) \qquad (22\text{-}47)$$

The term $k_1^*/(k_2^* + k_3^*)$ is the partition coefficient (λ) for FDG. To understand this, consider the tracer steady state when the flux of FDG into tissue is balanced by the flux out. Thus:

$$\text{flux in} = \text{flux out} \qquad (22\text{-}48)$$

$$k_1^* \, [C_p^*] = k_2^* [C_E^*] + k_3^* \, [C_E^*] \qquad (22\text{-}49)$$

$$\frac{k_1^*}{k_2^* + k_3^*} = \frac{[C_E^*]}{[C_p^*]} \qquad (22\text{-}50)$$

It is apparent from Equation 22-50 that the partition coefficient, $k_1^*/(k_2^* + k_3^*)$, is simply the tissue-to-plasma concentration ratio. Since LC is the correction factor that converts the transport and phosphorylation steps measured with FDG to those for glucose, one can perform the following transformation from values for FDG to those for glucose:

$$\frac{[k_1^*/(k_2^* + k_3^*)]k_3^*}{LC} = [k_1/(k_2 + k_3)]k_3 \qquad (22\text{-}51)$$

Since $k_1/(k_2 + k_3) = C_E/C_P$, the tissue concentration of glucose, C_E, can be obtained from the plasma concentration, C_p by:

$$C_p[k_1/(k_2 + k_3)] = [C_E/C_p]C_p = C_E \qquad (22\text{-}52)$$

Thus from the general equation for calculating fluxes (Equation 22-3)

$$CMRGlc = k_3[C_E] \qquad (22\text{-}53)$$

Equations 22-47 and 22-53 are valid only if the dephosphorylation rate is negligible compared to the rate of phosphorylation. Models including dephosphorylation have been developed by Phelps, Huang, and colleagues and are described in reference 1.

Equation 22-47 produces a local estimate of GMRGlc if C_p (the steady state plasma glucose value) is measured, if LC is known and if the rate constants for FDG (k_1^*, k_2^*, and k_3^*) are determined for each region of the brain. The equations and procedures for measuring these rate constants are given in reference 1. While this technique generates local estimates of CMRGlc, it does require scanning the brain over time and iteratively solving for the rate constants in Equation 22-47. In actual practice, an operational equation for the FDG model usually is employed that utilizes predetermined population values for the FDG rate constants and requires only a single tissue measurement of the total tissue concentration of ^{18}F ($^{18}FDG + ^{18}FDG\text{-}6\text{-}PO_4$) obtained from region of interest analysis from the image data. This operational equation originally was developed by Sokoloff and coworkers[6] for autoradiographically determining CMRGlc with $^{14}C\text{-}DG$. The operational equation used for FDG and PET was developed by Phelps, Huang, and colleagues,[1] and includes the dephosphorylation reaction. This technique still requires knowledge of the time course of FDG input function ($C_p^*(t)$), the plasma glucose concentration C_p, the lumped constant value (LC) and average values of the rate constants.

The Sokoloff operational equation of the deoxyglucose model, which does not include the dephophorylation of DG-6-PO_4, is given by

$$\text{CMRGlc} = \frac{C_i^*(T) - k_1^* \, e^{-(k_2^*+k_3^*)T} \displaystyle\int_0^{\infty} C_p^*(t)e^{(k_2^*+k_3^*)t}dt}{LC\left[\displaystyle\int_0^T \frac{(C_p^*(t))dt}{C_p} - e^{-(k_2^*+k_3^*)T}\int_0^T \frac{C_p^*(t)e^{(k_2^*+k_3)t}dt}{C_p}\right]}$$

$$(22\text{-}54)$$

where $C_i^*(T)$ is the ^{18}F tissue concentration at time, T.

In this approach, only the quantities in bold type in Equation 22-54 are measured in each experiment. Average estimates of the rate constants and LC obtained from separate experiments are used as a part of the routine calculation of CMRGlc with Equation 22-54. It can be shown[1] that the use of average estimates of the rate constants over the normal range of CMRGlc values cause little error at late times (i.e., 40 min) after injection because they appear with terms in Equation 22-54 with negative exponentials which become small when T becomes large.

In words, Equation 22-54 can be expressed as:

$$\left(\begin{array}{c}\text{Regional Glucose}\\\text{Metabolic Rate}\end{array}\right) = \left(\frac{\text{Plasma Glucose}}{\text{LC}}\right)\left[\frac{\left(\begin{array}{c}\text{Total }^{18}\text{F}\\\text{in Region}\end{array}\right)-\left(\begin{array}{c}\text{Free }^{18}\text{FDG}\\\text{in Region}\end{array}\right)}{\left(\begin{array}{c}\text{Total Net }^{18}\text{FDG Concentration}\\\text{Transported to the Region}\end{array}\right)}\right]$$

$$(22\text{-}55)$$

The total ^{18}F minus free ^{18}FDG equals the tissue concentration of the reaction product, FDG-6-PO$_4$.

The operational equation given by Equation 22-54 requires knowledge of the typical kinetics of the transport and phosphorylation processes in order to make intelligent decisions about scan duration and imaging time. Typically, approximately 40 minutes are required for the tracer to reach a near steady state in tissue after a bolus intravenous injection of FDG. A series of images usually is obtained at this time with PET, each one of which is characterized by a different time of acquisition (if they are obtained serially). This information, with the ROI data and other model parameters described above, is then used to calculate local values of CMRGlc. Figure 20-19 illustrates images of the brain obtained with FDG and PET.

The FDG model contains several simplifications based upon the approaches outlined in the previous sections. The strategy of using an analog tracer effectively eliminates many alternatives biochemical pathways for glucose metabolism and makes possible the simple three-compartment mode. Additionally, the transport (between the first two compartments) and phosphorylation steps (between the second two compartments) represent "combined" steps of more complicated multistep processes. The exchange between substructures within each compartment is assumed to be rapid compared to exchange between compartments.

Even though blood flow has a major impact on tracer delivery it is not included in the FDG model explicitly. The extraction of FDG normally is low enough (i.e., low value of the PS product) that the delivery of FDG has a low dependence on blood flow. In addition, the initial flow dependence on the delivery of FDG progressively diminishes with time after injection. Figure 22-18 illustrates the distribution of FDG reflects

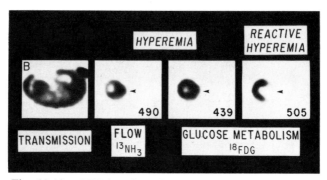

Fig. 22-18. PET imaging of a cross-section of heart in an open-chest dog, illustrating the independence of the FDG/FDG-6-PO$_4$ distribution at late times (50 min postinjection) from blood flow. At left is transmission scan of the cross-section of chest. Other images are distributions of blood flow and FDG + FDG-6-PO$_4$ under the conditions indicated above the images. Numbers on the PET images are blood flow in ml/min/100g in left circumflex distribution (arrows) as determined by microspheres. Flow in rest of left ventricle was about 85 ml/min/100g in each experiment. In images marked hyperemia, uniform glucose metabolism throughout ventrical is correctly indicated by FDG even though blood flow in the left circumflex distribution is locally increased 5.5 times, as also seen in ^{13}NH$_3$ flow image. In study marked "reactive hyeremia," true glucose metabolic rate in left circumflex distribution is 20% of value in the rest of myocardium while blood flow in the left circumflex (505 ml/min/100g) is six times higher than the remainder of the myocardium. Arrowheads identify region of myocardium supplied by left circumflex coronary artery. Note that with various rates of flow, glucose utilization measured by FDG is not closely linked to flow rates. [From ref. 1: Phelps ME, Mazziotta JC, Schelbert HR: Positron Emission Tomography and Autoradiography: Principles and Applications for the Brain and Heart. Raven Press, New York, 1986. With permission.]

glucose metabolism rather than variations in flow at later times after injection.

In the tracer kinetic model, the FDG concentration in the vascular compartment shown in Figure 22-17 is measured by taking blood samples from the systemic circulation. Typically, it is assumed that the measured tissue data does not contain any significant activity from the vascular space. In the operational equation of Equation 22-54 this is a good approximation at the typical imaging time of 40 minutes after injection. Models have been developed that add the vascular compartment to equations describing the tissue time-activity curve since in kinetic studies for measuring the rate constants, the amount of FDG in the tissue vascular pool is significant at early times after injection.[1]

The deoxyglucose and fluorodeoxyglucose methods have been used to measure exogenous glucose utilization in many organs and tissues. Examples include brain, heart, tumor, liver, kidney and peripheral tissues.

G. EQUILIBRIUM DISPLACEMENT TECHNIQUES FOR LIGAND ASSAYS

Equilibrium displacement techniques, also known as competitive binding assays, are based on the principle that a tracer and another substance that compete for the same binding site (usually a protein) will be distributed in bound and unbound fractions in proportion to their relative concentrations in the binding environment. The approach is thus similar in concept to carrier-mediated diffusion and Michaelis-Menten enzyme kinetics. Both of these approaches are based on "saturation kinetics" (Figure 22-15). A tracer competing with another substance for a carrier site, a binding site on an enzyme or a binding site in an assay system is essentially the single phenomenon of a tracer and a competitor binding to a protein.

In these assay techniques, the tracer is present in known quantities and its bound/free ratio (B/F ratio) in the assay system thus is related directly to the unknown concentration of the competing substance. Thus, measuring the B/F ratio of the tracer (once it is calibrated relative to competitor concentrations) yields a measurement of the competitor concentration. There are a number of formalized approaches to analyzing such data but the most common is by Scatchard plots. Both in vitro (e.g., radioimmunoassay) and in vivo applications of this technique exist.

Consider the example of the [^{11}C] carfentanil method for imaging opiate receptors in the brain. Endogenous neurotransmitters and labeled neurotransmitters or neurotransmitter analogs compete for the same binding sites. Figure 22-19 illustrates a PET brain study using [^{11}C] carfentanil with and without pretreatment with the active isomer (+) of

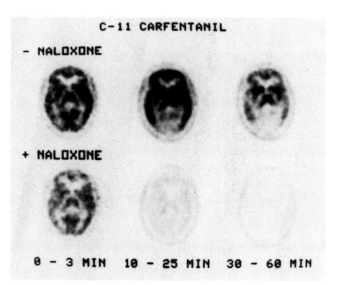

Fig. 22-19. PET images of the brain after intravenous injection of the labeled opiate ligand C-11 carfentanil. Images were obtained with the addition of inactive (−) and active (+) forms of the opiate antagonist naloxone on the first and second row of images, respectively. The initial image (0–3 minutes) primarily reflects tracer delivery (blood flow and diffusion) while the 10–25 minute image and 30–60 minute image primarily reflect tracer binding to opiate receptors in the subject not pretreated with (+) naloxone. Courtesy of Frost JJ, Wagner HN, Dannals RF et al.

naloxone (an opiate antagonist). Opiate receptors are distributed fairly uniformly in the brain with the exception of localized areas such as the visual cortex in the occipital lobe that has a very low concentration of opiate receptors. Figure 22-19 illustrates that in subjects not pretreated with (+) naloxone, the distribution of the tracer maps the known distribution of these receptors quite well after an initial distribution phase (0–3 minute image) that predominantly reflects the distribution of blood flow and diffusion from blood to tissue. In subjects pretreated with (+) naloxone, the initial distribution phase is quite similar as would be expected, but at later times when the images are dependent upon specific binding to opiate receptors, there is now a lack of binding due to the competitive blocking effect of (+) naloxone.

The same fundamental approach, as well as kinetic modeling schemes for quantifying receptor-ligand interactions with PET, with other labeled ligands (Table 22-1) are rapidly being developed at this time.[1]

H. CEREBRAL PROTEIN SYNTHESIS

A model for the measurement of protein synthesis in the brain with PET illustrates many of the modeling principles and strategies developed in this chapter. In addition, it illustrates an approach to simplifying the tracer kinetic model by the choice of the radioactive label and where it is placed in a compound. The purpose of this model is to estimate the rate of protein synthesis in the brain or more specifically, the rate of incorporation of amino acids into proteins.

Desirable properties of a tracer for measuring protein synthesis in the brain include a high blood-brain barrier permeability, a rapid turnover rate of the amino acid in the brain precursor pool (i.e., rapid incorporation into protein) and a relatively simple biochemical fate and a rapid clearance of the labeled amino acid from the blood pool. L-[^{11}C]-leucine satisfies these requirements reasonably well.

A difficulty is encountered because leucine is both incorporated into proteins and metabolized through an alternate pathway as shown in Figures 22-20 and 22-21. This branching pathway can not be differentiated by simply measuring total rate at which the brain uses leucine. To remove this confounding factor, Smith, Sokoloff, and colleagues used leucine with ^{14}C in the carboxyl (i.e., number 1) position.[7] Thus labeled leucine enters the brain by carrier-mediated diffusion with a portion being incorporated into proteins and the remainder entering the metabolic pathway.

In the metabolic pathway, leucine is transaminated to alpha ketoisocaproic acid, which then is decarboxylated in the mitochondria with release of the label in the form of ^{11}CO$_2$. The labeled ^{11}CO$_2$ diffuses through the brain tissue and then is removed by blood flow. As the decarboxylation process and clearance of labeled ^{11}CO$_2$ proceeds, there is an increasing fraction of the label remaining in the protein pool relative to the metabolic pool (Figure 22-22). Thus, labeling with ^{11}C in the carboxyl position produces effectively a "shunt" that removes the label in the metabolic pathway by decarboxylation and clearance from the tissue by diffusion and blood flow.

The tracer kinetic model must include these processes with appropriate definition of the compartments or pools of interest. Figure 22-21 illustrates such a compartment model composed of activity in the cerebral vascular space and extravascular space while Figure 22-22 is an example of the compartmental kinetics in a normal volunteer. In this study from a subject fed a carbohydrate meal with a supplement of oral glucose, the ratio of label in proteins compared to that in the precursor pool and in the metabolic pathway is dominant for times later than about 20 minutes after injection.

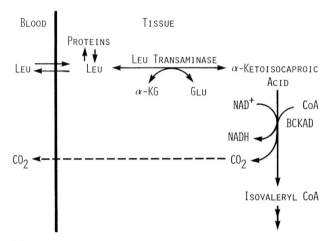

Fig. 22-20. Leucine biochemical pathways in brain. Leucine can be incorporated into proteins or metabolized. If leucine is labeled in the carboxyl position (L−[1−^{11}C]leucine), then the ^{11}C label is eliminated in the metabolic pathway at the decarboxylation step as labeled carbon dioxide ($^{11}CO_2$) that diffuses out of the tissue and is removed by cerebral blood flow. Leu = leucine; α-KG = alpha-ketoglutaric acid; GLU = glutamic acid; NAD = nicotinamide adenine dinucleotide; NADH = reduced form of NAD; CoA = coenzyme A; BCKAD = branched-chain ketoacid dehydrogenase. [From ref. 1: Phelps ME, Mazziotta JC, Schelbert HR: Positron Emission Tomography and Autoradiography: Principles and Applications for the Brain and Heart. Raven Press, New York, 1986. With permission.]

With this compartmental model, one can estimate the various rate constants with nonlinear regression if the tissue time-activity curve and input functions (plasma time-activity curve for ^{11}C-leucine and plasma concentration of leucine) are measured. Because both protein synthesis and metabolism originate from the same tissue precursor pool, the relative ratio of the fluxes of these processes is:

$$\frac{\text{rate of protein synthesis}}{\text{rate of leucine metab.}} = \frac{k_5 \text{ [leucine in tissue]}}{k_3 \text{ [leucine in tissue]}} = \frac{k_5}{k_3} \quad (22\text{-}56)$$

The protein synthesis rate (PSR) or flux of leucine incorporated into proteins is:

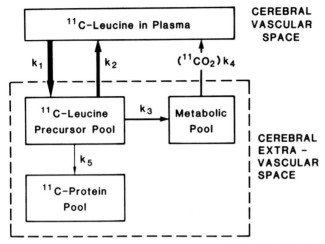

Fig. 22-21. Leucine compartmental model. The kinetics described include bidirectional transport (k_1, k_2), incorporation into proteins (k_5), metabolism (k_3), and clearance of labeled carbon dioxide (CO_2) from tissue to blood (k_4) after intravenous injection of L-leucine labeled with ^{11}C in the carboxyl position (^{11}C leucine). The widths of the arrows indicate the normal relative mass flux (i.e., k × [reactant concentration]), through each of the functional pathways. [From ref. 1: Phelps ME, Mazziotta JC, Schelbert HR: Positron Emission Tomography and Autoradiography: Principles and Applications for the Brain and Heart. Raven Press, New York, 1986. With permission.]

$$PSR = [^{11}C\text{-leucine in tissue}] \times k_5 \qquad (22\text{-}57)$$

The metabolic rate for leucine (MRL) also can be determined and is given by

$$MRL = [^{11}C\text{-leucine in tissue}] \times k_3 \qquad (22\text{-}58)$$

Analogous to the approach developed above for the FDG model, the concentration of leucine in the tissue precursor pool is:

$$[\text{Leucine in tissue}] = \text{Partition Coefficient} \times \text{plasma concentration}$$

$$= [k_1/(k_2 + k_3 + k_5)] \times [\text{plasma leucine}] \quad (22\text{-}59)$$

Note that because ^{11}C leucine is just an isotopic label of leucine, no

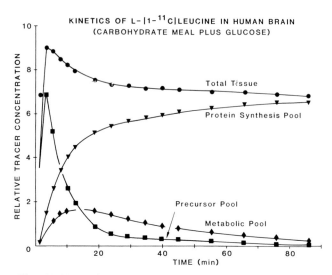

Fig. 22-22. Kinetic PET study in a normal human volunteer after the intravenous injection of L-leucine labeled with ^{11}C in the carboxyl position. Circles indicate the actual measured tissue concentration with the tomograph. Squares, triangles, and diamonds indicate the concentrations of the tracer in the indicated compartments, as calculated from fitting the tissue kinetic data (solid line) with the model in Figure 22-21. [From ref. 1: Phelps ME, Mazziotta JC, Schelbert HR: Positron Emission Tomography and Autoradiography: Principles and Applications for the Brain and Heart. Raven Press, New York, 1986. With permission.]

"lumped constant" as used with the analog tracer FDG (Equation 22-47) is necessary and the kinetics of ^{11}C leucine are identical with the natural substrate. The protein synthetic rate thus results directly from Equation 22-57 and the precursor concentration calculated with Equation 22-59.

Leucine also can be labeled with [13]N. In this case the ^{13}N-labeled leucine will be transported into tissue and incorporated into proteins in an identical manner and rate as ^{11}C-leucine. However, as ^{13}N-leucine proceeds down the metabolic pathway, the ^{13}N label is transferred to glutamate at the transamination step shown in Figure 22-20. Since ^{13}N-glutamate has a very slow clearance rate from tissue (Figure 22-23) there is no way by tracer kinetic methods to separate the protein synthesis and metabolic pathways and only the sum of these two processes could be measured if leucine were labeled with [13]N.

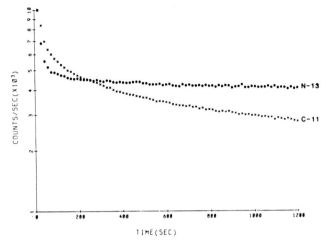

Fig. 22-23.   Time activity curves subsequent to intracarotid bolus injections of ¹³N-leucine (N-13) and L−[1−¹¹C]-leucine (C-11) in a monkey. The temporal sequence illustrates how a portion of ¹³N and ¹¹C labeled leucine remains in blood and passes through the brain (initial peak) and a portion is transported into tissue. Both labeled compounds are transported into the brain at the same rate. However, ¹³N activity is retained in tissue while a portion of ¹¹C activity is cleared. [From ref. 1: Phelps ME, Mazziotta JC, Schelbert HR: Positron Emission Tomography and Autoradiography: Principles and Applications for the Brain and Heart. Raven Press, New York, 1986. With permission.]

I. SUMMARY

This chapter on tracer kinetic modeling techniques in nuclear medicine has stressed some of the principles of these techniques and their relationship to measurements and descriptions of underlying physiologic processes. Many modeling approaches exist. The first, and most important step in developing a model or choosing among the available modeling techniques is to clearly define the endpoint or goal of such a model. The examples included in this chapter illustrate that "models" are not finished products but rather organized frameworks from which data can be critically evaluated.

Many of the more quantitative models currently of interest in nuclear medicine apply to PET, because of its ability to accurately quantify regional tissue activity concentrations (see Chapters 19 and 20) and because of its abundance of biologically active labeled compounds. The same tracer kinetic principles, however, apply in non-PET tracer studies. Careful integration of all factors related to the model (i.e., goal, data acquisition characteristics, tracer selection, and modeling technique) will result in models that not only describe the underlying processes but that predict the response of the system in normal and diseased states.

It is difficult, if not impossible to define and structure a tracer kinetic model by kinetic measurements alone. Biochemical measurements and knowledge are required to achieve this. However, once a model is properly formulated tracer kinetics can provide extremely accurate measurements of the local processes for which the model was developed. Tracer kinetic approaches provide unique and accurate methods for measuring rates of physiologic, biochemical, and pharmakokinetic processes. Measurements can be performed with processes having concentrations of reactants and products down to picomolar values or lower without disturbing the process. This is a powerful feature of all radioassay techniques. Probably no other single technique has contributed more knowledge about biochemical and physiologic systems than the tracer kinetic method as it is used across the spectrum of biologic sciences.

Once rigorous investigative studies are carried out, more simplified and even qualitative approaches can be used in a clinical setting. However, even the qualitative use of the tracer technique is no more justifiable than the degree of knowledge that exists to establish the principles upon which qualitative observations are made.

REFERENCES

1. Phelps ME, Mazziotta JC, Schelbert HR: Positron Emission Tomography and Autoradiography: Principles and Applications for the Brain and Heart. Raven Press, New York, 1986.
2. Renkin EM: Transport of potassium-42 from blood to tissue in isolated mammalian skeletal muscles. Am J Physiol 197:1205–1210, 1959.
3. Crone C: Permeability of capillaries in various organs as determined by use of the indicator diffusion method. Acta Physiol Scan 58:292–305, 1963
4. Lassen NA, Perl W: Tracer Kinetic Methods in Medical Physiology. Raven Press, New York, 1979.
5. Jones T, Chesler DA and Ter-Pogossian MM: The continuous inhalation of oxygen-15 for assessing regional oxygen extraction in the brain of man. Br J Radiol 49:339–343, 1976.
6. Sokoloff L, Reivich M, Kennedy C, DesRosiers MH, Patlak CS, Pettigrew KD, Sakurada O, Shinohara M: The [C-14] Deoxyglucose method for the measurement of local cerebral glucose utilization: theory, procedure, and normal values in the conscious and anesthetized albino rat. J Neurochem 28:897–916, 1977.

7. Smith CB, Davidsen L, Deibler G, Patlak C, Pettigrew K and Sokoloff L: A method for the determination of local rates of protein synthesis in brain. Trans Am Soc Neurochem 11:94, 1980.

Additional discussion of the theory, mathematical formulation and application of compartmental modeling and mathematical techniques in estimation theory for modeling can be found in the following:

Jacquez JA: Compartmental Analysis in Biology and Medicine, 2nd edition, The University of Michigan Press, 1985.

Carson ER, Cobelli C, Finkelstein L: The Mathematical Modeling of Metabolic and Endocrine Systems, John Wiley & Sons, New York, 1985.

23
Radiation Safety and Health Physics

All nuclear medicine laboratory personnel are exposed to radiation in their normal working environment. Stored radioactive materials, radioactive preparations for patients, and patients to whom these preparations have been administered all are potential sources of radiation exposure. An additional problem is the potential for radiation exposure to nonlaboratory personnel, such as patient relatives, attending nursing staff, and even passers-by in the hallways adjacent to the laboratory.

The quantities of radioactive material used and radiation levels encountered in a nuclear medicine laboratory are generally well below what is necessary to cause any type of "radiation sickness." Of more concern are the potential long-term effects that can result from chronic exposures to even low levels of radiation. The most important of these effects are genetic damage to reproductive cells and carcinogenesis. At the present time, there is no demonstrable "threshold dose" for these long-term effects. Thus although the risks may be small, common sense dictates that radiation exposures in and around the nuclear medicine laboratory be kept as small as is reasonably practicable.

The analysis of problems in the handling of radiation sources and the development of safe handling practices are the general concerns of the broad field of *health physics*. The practices that are prescribed by this analysis are sometimes expressed formally, as regulations, and sometimes as "common sense" recommendations. In this chapter we will discuss aspects of health physics and radiation safety practices as they apply to the nuclear medicine laboratory.

A. QUANTITIES AND UNITS

1. Dose-Modifying Factors

For health physics purposes, specification of the radiation absorbed dose in rads (Chapter 10) is inadequate for a complete and accurate assessment of potential radiation hazards. Although the relative risk of potential injury increases with increasing absorbed dose values, several other *dose-modifying factors* must also be taken into account:

1. *The part of the body exposed.* Total-body exposure carries a greater risk than partial-body exposure. Exposure of major organs in the trunk of the body is more serious than exposure to the extremities. The active blood-forming organs, the gonads, and the lens of the eye are especially sensitive to radiation damage. A superficial dose to the skin—e.g., from an external source of β particles—is less hazardous than the same dose delivered to greater depths—e.g., from an external source of γ rays or from internally deposited radioactivity.
2. *The time span over which the radiation dose is delivered.* A given number of rads delivered over a short time period (e.g., minutes or hours) has a greater potential for damage than the same dose delivered over a long time period (e.g., months or years).
3. *The age of the exposed individual.* Children are more susceptible to injurious radiation effects than adults. The developing embryo and fetus are especially sensitive.
4. *The type of radiation involved.* In general, densely ionizing radiation (i.e., high-LET radiation; Chapter 8, Section A.4), such as α particles, fission fragments, and other nuclear particles, are more damaging per rad of absorbed dose than less densely ionizing radiation, such as β particles and γ rays.

The dose-modifying factors listed above are taken into account in preparing regulations and making recommendations for handling of radioactive materials. For example, regulations specify different dose limits for different parts of the body (item 1), for different time periods (item 2), and for different age groups (item 3). To account for the differing hazards of different types of radiation (item 4), an additional quantity for specifying radiation dose, called *dose equivalent*, is introduced.

2. Dose Equivalent: The Rem

The basic unit of dose equivalent is the *rem*. Dose equivalent H in rems is related to absorbed dose D in rads by

$$H = DQ \tag{23-1}$$

Table 23-1
Quality Factors for Different Types of Radiation

Type of Radiation	Q
X rays, γ rays, electrons, and β particles	1.0
Neutrons and protons, $E \leq 10$ MeV	10
	(30 for irradiation of the eyes)
α particles	20

where Q is the *quality factor* for the particular type of radiation involved. The SI unit for dose equivalent is the *sievert* (Sv). One sievert is the dose equivalent for an absorbed dose of one gray (100 rads), with $Q = 1$. Thus 1 Sv = 100 rem and 1 rem = 10^{-2}Sv.

Values of Q assigned to different types of radiation are based on recommendations provided by various advisory bodies, such as the ICRU, NCRP and ICRP (Section B.7). They are meant to provide, in a general way, a means for evaluating the relative hazards of different types of radiation. Currently used values are summarized in Table 23-1. Note that for γ rays, x rays, and β particles, $Q = 1$. Thus for most of the radiation encountered in nuclear medicine, the dose equivalent in rems is numerically equal to the absorbed dose in rads. For α particles, however, the dose equivalent in rems is 20 times the absorbed dose in rads. This is one reason why α-particle emitters are not used in diagnostic nuclear medicine.

3. Exposure: The Roentgen

For the purpose of describing radiation *levels* in a radiation environment, an additional quantity—*exposure*—is used. Exposure refers to the amount of ionization of air caused by γ-ray or x-ray beam. The basic unit of exposure is the *roentgen* (R), with subunits of milliroentgens (1 mR = 10^{-3} R), microroentgens (1 μR = 10^{-6} R), etc. An exposure of 1 R implies ionization liberating an amount of charge equal to 2.58 $\times$ 10^{-4} coulombs/kg of air, or about 2 $\times$ 10^9 ionizations per cc of dry air at STP. An *exposure rate* of 1 R/min implies that this amount of ionization is produced during a 1 min period. The SI unit for exposure is the coulomb/kg, with no special name. Thus 1 coulomb/kg $\approx$ 3876R and 1 R = 2.58 $\times$ 10^{-4} coulombs/kg.

Exposure is a useful quantity because it can be *measured* using ionization chambers, which are basically ionization-measurement devices

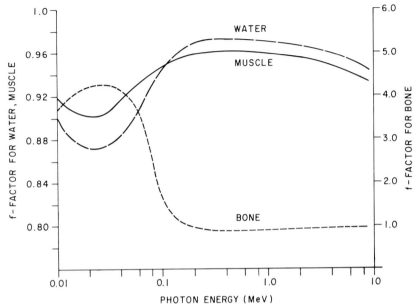

Fig. 23-1.   The *f* factor (rads/roentgen) versus photon energy water, muscle, and bone.

(Chapter 4, Section A.2). Instruments used for health physics measurements are described in Section E of this chapter.

If the exposure level in roentgens is known at a certain location, the absorbed dose in rads that would be delivered to a person at that location can be estimated by means of the *f* factor. Figure 23-1 shows the *f* factor as a function of energy for bone and for soft tissues. For soft tissues (muscle and water), $f \approx 1$. For low-energy photons ($E \lesssim 100$ keV), the *f* factor for bone is greater than unity. Because of photoelectric absorption by the heavier elements in bone (Ca and P), energy absorption in bone is greater than energy absorption by air at these energies; however, for most of the γ-ray energies commonly employed in nuclear medicine, the *f* factor for bone is also about unity.

Thus for practical purposes the exposure level measured in roentgens is approximately equal numerically to the absorbed dose in rads that would be received by an individual at that location, and in turn, as described in Section A.2, the absorbed dose in rads is numerically equal to the dose equivalent in rems. Because of their approximate numerical equivalence, roentgens, rads, and rems are sometimes (mis)used as approximately interchangeable quantities; however, one should be aware that they represent distinctly different quantities.

B. REGULATIONS PERTAINING TO THE USE OF RADIONUCLIDES

1. NRC Licensing and Regulations

The use and distribution of radioactive materials in the United States is under the primary control of the Nuclear Regulatory Commission (NRC). The NRC issues licenses to individuals and to institutions to possess and use radioactive materials. In addition to medical uses, industrial, research, educational, and other uses of radioactive materials also require NRC licensing. In some states, the NRC has entered into an agreement to transfer its regulatory and licensing functions to a radiation control agency within the state. Such states are called *agreement states*. About half of the states fall into this category at the present time.

Medical licenses generally fall into one of two categories: specific licenses of limited scope or specific licenses of broad scope. Limited scope licenses are for limited kinds and quantities of radionuclides, which are listed specifically in the license. They may be issued to individual physicians (e.g., in private offices) or to institutions (e.g., hospitals). Licenses issued to institutions will list the names of individuals authorized to practice under the license.

Broad scope licenses are issued to larger institutions that require greater licensing flexibility (e.g., basic research as well as medical uses in a university setting). Broad scope licenses generally cover more radionuclides and greater quantities than do limited scope licenses. The NRC permits the institutional radiation safety committee to authorize individuals to use radionuclides under the license, rather than requiring them to be listed specifically on the license.

The NRC also issues regulations that must be observed by licensees in the use of radioactive materials. These regulations are published in Title 10 of the Code of Federal Regulations. Two of the more relevant sections of these regulations for nuclear medicine are Part 20 (10CFR20), covering radiation protection, and Part 35 (10CFR35), covering medical uses. The NRC regulations are based primarily on the recommendations of two advisory bodies, the ICRP and the NCRP, as discussed in Section B.7. The NRC also periodically issues regulatory guides to assist licensees in the interpretation of and implementation of its regulations.

In addition to the NRC, several other Government agencies are involved in the regulation of radioactive materials, e.g., the Department of Transportation (shipping regulations) and the Food and Drug Administration (FDA) (pharmaceutical aspects). A complete discussion of the many regulations involved is beyond the scope of this chapter. Also, the regulations are under constant review and subject to periodic changes.

Therefore, only a brief discussion of the more important regulations will be presented here. Further information may be obtained in the references at the end of the chapter or from institutional health physicists.

2. Restricted and Unrestricted Areas

The NRC regulations prescribe different maximum radiation limits for restricted and unrestricted areas. A restricted area is one ". . . access to which is controlled by the licensee for the purposes of protection of individuals from exposure to radiation and radioactive materials. . . ." Normally, restricted areas are not accessible to the general public, and generally they are occupied only by individuals whose employment responsibilities require them to work with radioactive materials and other radiation sources. Such individuals are said to be *occupationally exposed*—e.g., nuclear medicine physicians, technicians, and pharmacists. Secretaries and receptionists generally are not included in this category. Restricted areas must be clearly marked with radiation warning signs.

3. Maximum Permissible Doses (MPD)

Maximum permissible dose (MPD) values specified in 10CFR20 are based on the general recommendations by the ICRP and NCRP (Section B.7) that an individual's average occupational dose to the whole body or to radiation-sensitive organs should not exceed 5 rems per year. Specifically, the NRC recommends that an individual's lifetime cumulative occupational dose should not exceed $(N - 18) \times 5$ rems, where N is the individual's age in years. Higher MPD values are accepted for exposures to limited areas of the body.

MPD values specified in 10CFR20 are based on quarterly equivalents of these average annual values; they are summarized in Table 23-2. NRC regulations state specifically that ". . . no licensee shall possess, use, or transfer licensed materials in such a manner as to cause any individual in a restricted area to receive in any one calendar quarter from radioactive material and other sources of radiation in the licensee's possession a dose in excess of . . ." these limits. These dose limits, which apply to

Table 23-2
Maximum Permissible Doses (According to 10CFR20)
(rems per Calendar Quarter)

Whole body; head and trunk; active blood-forming organs; lens of eyes; or gonads	1.25
Hands and forearms; feet and ankles	18.75
Skin of whole body	7.5

occupationally exposed personnel, are called *occupational dose* limits. Occupational dose limits do not include radiation doses received by the occupationally exposed individual while that individual is undergoing a medical examination, nor do they include any radiation dose from natural radiation sources, e.g., cosmic rays and naturally occurring radioactivity in the environment.

Note that the regulations require the licensee to control radiation doses not only from the license materials but from "other sources in the licensee's possession" as well (e.g., nonlicensed sources or an x-ray generator). Thus a licensee would be in violation of the regulations if the MPD value for occupational dose were exceeded even if most of the radiation dose were caused by nonlicensed sources.

The MPD for the whole body, gonads, active blood-forming organs, and lens of the eye is the most restrictive limit. The 1.25 rem/quarter is equivalent to 5 rem/year, or about 0.1 rem/week. The quarterly limit may be exceeded occasionally (up to 3 rem/quarter), provided that the individual's cumulative lifetime occupational dose does not exceed ($N -$ 18) $\times$ 5 rems, where N is the individual's age in years. Well-documented records of previous radiation doses received (e.g., personnel dosimeter records, Section E.2) must be available to apply this rule. If not, it must be assumed, for purposes of the regulations, that an occupational dose of 1.25 rems was received during those calendar quarters for which the records are not available.

Note that for persons age 18 years and under, the cumulative occupational dose limit is zero. The interpretation of this rule is simply that persons under age 18 cannot receive occupational exposures.

Maximum permissible doses for *persons under age 18*, and for persons in *unrestricted areas*, are reduced by a factor of 10 from those for restricted areas. Thus radiation levels in unrestricted areas must deliver a radiation dose of less than 125 mrem/quarter, or an average of only about 0.25 mrem/hour, assuming 40 hours per week occupation of the area. Transient radiation levels of up to 2 mrem/hour or 100 mrem/week are permitted, provided that the 125 mrem/quarter limit is not exceeded.

4. Maximum Permissible Concentrations for Airborne Radioactivity (MPC$_{air}$)

A particular problem in nuclear medicine laboratories is the potential for leakage or escape of radioactive gases (e.g., ^{133}Xe used in pulmonary function studies) or volatile radioactive material (e.g., concentrated ^{131}I solutions). The NRC regulations specify *maximum permissible concentrations* for airborne radioactive materials (MPC$_{air}$).

Table 23-3
Maximum Permissible Concentrations in Air (MPC$_{air}$)
for Some Radionuclides of Interest to Nuclear Medicine

Radionuclide	MPC$_{air}$ (μCi/cm^3)	
	Restricted Area	*Unrestricted Area*
^{125}I	5×10^{-9}	8×10^{-11}
^{131}I	9×10^{-9}	1×10^{-10}
^{99m}Tc	4×10^{-5}	1×10^{-6}
^{133}Xe	1×10^{-5}	3×10^{-7}

MPC$_{air}$ values for restricted areas taken from 10CFR20 for some radionuclides used in nuclear medicine are summarized in Table 23-3. They assume 40 hours per week occupancy. Levels in unrestricted areas (e.g., in a hallway adjacent to the laboratory) are smaller by factors of about 10–60. Longer occupation is assumed for unrestricted areas, and they may involve exposure of minors and other nonoccupationally exposed persons. The regulations state that concentrations may be averaged over a 1 year period. Thus transient concentrations in excess of the MPC values are allowed. Some useful examples of calculations based on MPC values are found in ref. 1.

5. Maximum Permissible Concentrations for Sewage Disposal (MPC$_{water}$)

The NRC regulations also specify maximum permissible concentrations for radionuclides disposed of into sewage water (MPC$_{water}$). Radioactive concentrations in sewage are of concern because they may eventually reach public water supplies. MPC$_{water}$ values and methods for calculating concentrations are described in 10CFR20. In addition, the regulations specify an annual limit of one curie for the *total* amount of radioactivity disposed of into the sewer system by any licensee. In many situations, this is the most restrictive limit.

6. Record-Keeping Requirements

The NRC regulations require that rather extensive records be kept by the licensee. These include, among others, personnel dosimetry and radiation survey records (Section E), wipe testing records for sealed sources, summaries of quality control checks on radiation monitoring equipment, inventory and disposal records, minutes of radiation safety committee meetings, and records of training in radiation safety of laboratory personnel. Maintenance of proper records is one of the major activities of an NRC licensee.

7. Recommendations of Advisory Bodies

The NRC regulatory MPD limits are based on recommended radiation dose limits published by various advisory bodies. These bodies include the *National Council on Radiation Protection* (NCRP), a U.S. organization, and two international groups, the *International Commission on Radiation Protection* (ICRP) and the *International Commission on Radiological Units* (ICRU). The last group is concerned mostly with definitions of radiologic units, such as rems, rads, and roentgens.

Recommendations from these groups do not carry the force of law; however, there is a tendency of regulatory agencies such as the NRC to convert them into law. Therefore it is worthwhile keeping abreast of their recommendations.

Some titles of NCRP reports that are applicable to nuclear medicine are listed in the references at the end of the chapter. Table 23-4 lists some MPD values currently recommended by the NCRP. Note that their coverage is somewhat broader than those appearing in the NRC regulations. Note also the restrictive limits placed on pregnant women with respect to the fetus. A pregnant, occupationally exposed woman may

Table 23-4
Maximum Permissible Dose Limits Recommended by the NCRP

Maximum permissible dose equivalent for occupational exposure	
Whole Body	5 rem in any one year after age 18
Skin	15 rem in any one year
Hands	75 rem in any one year (not more than 25 rem per quarter)
Forearms	30 rem in any one year (not more than 10 per quarter)
Other organs	15 rem in any one year
Pregnant women (with respect to the fetus)	0.5 rem during gestation period
Dose Limits for the general public or occasionally exposed persons†	
Whole body	0.5 rem in any one year

†Nonoccupational exposures.
From NCRP Report No. 39, Basic Radiation Protection Criteria, p. 106.

require special work restrictions to ensure that this dose limit for the fetus is not exceeded during her pregnancy.

C. SAFE HANDLING OF RADIOACTIVE MATERIALS

1. The ALARA Concept

Radiation dose limits, MPC values, and other restrictions specified in NRC regulations are legal limits that must not be exceeded at any time by an NRC licensee; however, they should not be considered as thresholds below which the hazards may be assumed to be "zero." At the present time, although the radiation hazards associated with MPD and MPC limits in the regulations are very small, they are not assumed to be totally risk free, and any reasonable technique for reducing radiation dose may have potential benefits in the long run.

Recognizing this, the NCRP as early as 1954, and more recently the NRC Regulations, have recommended as an operating philosophy that the objective of radiation safety practices should be not simply to keep radiation doses within legal limits but to keep them *"as low as reasonably achievable"* (ALARA). In its regulations, the NRC has defined ALARA to mean ". . . as low as reasonably achievable taking into account the state of technology and economics of improvement in relation to benefits to the public health and safety, and other societal and socioeconomic considerations, and in relation to the use of atomic energy in the public interest . . ." Several changes may be anticipated in future NRC regulations in light of the move toward ALARA philosophy. For example, the term "maximum permissible dose" may be replaced by "dose-limiting recommendation" or similar terminology to reflect the fact that under ALARA, the specified dose limit is in many cases not "permissible." NRC Regulatory Guides 8.10 ("Operating Philosophy For Maintaining Occupational Exposures As Low As Reasonably Achievable") and 8.18 ("Information Relevant To Ensuring That Occupational Radiation Exposures At Medical Institutions Will Be As Low As Reasonably Achievable") provide practical advice on implementation of ALARA principles.

The concept of ALARA has long been the operational objective of radiation safety practices in well-run nuclear medicine laboratories, and they have now taken on regulatory force. ALARA principles can be applied to the handling of radiation sources, to storage and shielding techniques, and to the design and layout of the laboratory. Some of the basic techniques for keeping radiation doses "ALARA" are discussed below.

2. Reduction of Radiation Doses From External Sources

Types of sources. External sources are those that deliver a radiation dose from outside the body. The principle sources are γ-ray- and x-ray-emitting radionuclides in patients, syringes, vials, waste disposal areas, etc. Unshielded β emitters emitting particles of sufficient energy to travel some distance in air (e.g., ^{32}P, but not ^{14}C) also constitute an external hazard, although β particles generally deliver only a superficial radiation dose to the skin.

Exposure rate constant Γ. Radiation exposure levels caused by γ-ray and x-ray emitters can be estimated from the *exposure rate constant*, Γ. The exposure rate constant has a specific value for each radionuclide, the exposure due to γ- and x-ray emissions, in R/hour, at a distance of 1 cm from an unshielded 1 mCi source of that radionuclide. The units for Γ are R·cm²/mCi·hr. Calculation of the exposure rate constant is based on the number of γ- and x-ray emissions from the radionuclide (number per disintegration) and their energies and on the absorption coefficient of air at these energies. For practical health physics purposes, this calculation should include only γ and x rays above a certain minimum energy value—say, 20 keV—because photons of lower energy have such low penetrating power (e.g., through the walls of a syringe or a vial) as to constitute a negligible external hazard. The value calculated for a 20 keV lower energy limit is symbolized by Γ_{20}. Values of Γ_{20} for some radionuclides used in nuclear medicine are summarized in Table 23-5.

To estimate the exposure rate E(R/hr) at a distance d(cm) from an activity n(mCi) of a radionuclide having an exposure rate constant Γ(R·cm²/mCi·hr), the following equation is used:

$$E = n\Gamma/d^2 \qquad (23\text{-}2)$$

The appearance of d^2 in the denominator of Equation 23-2 is an expression of the *inverse-square law* (Chapter 12, Section A.1). Because γ rays and x rays are emitted isotropically (e.g., with no preferred direction) radiation intensity and exposure levels decrease as the square of the distance from the source.

Example 23-1.
  Calculate the exposure rates at 10 cm and 300 cm distances from a syringe containing 30 mCi of ^{99m}Tc.

Answer.

The exposure rate constant Γ_{20} is 0.6 R·cm^2/mCi·hr (Table 23-5). Therefore from Equation 23-2, at 10 cm.

$$E(R/hr) = 30 \text{ mCi} \times 0.6(R \cdot cm^2/mCi \cdot hr)/(10 \text{ cm})^2$$

$$= 0.18 \text{ R/hr}$$

$$= 180 \text{ mR/hr}$$

and at 300 cm,

$$E(R/hr) = 30 \text{ mCi} \times 0.6(R \cdot cm^2/mCi \cdot hr)/(300 \text{ cm})^2$$

$$= 0.0002 \text{ R/hr}$$

$$= 0.2 \text{ mR/hr}$$

The strong effect of distance on radiation exposure is illustrated by Example 23-1.

Equation 23-2 is accurate for distances that are large in comparison to the physical size of the source; however, it is not valid at very small distances. For example, it predicts that the exposure rate becomes infinite as d approaches zero. A practical situation in which this problem arises is

Table 23-5
Γ_{20} Values for Some Radionuclides of Interest to Nuclear Medicine

Radionuclide	Γ_{20} (R · cm^2/mCi · hr)
^{51}Cr	0.18
^{57}Co	0.58
^{60}Co	12.96
^{67}Ga	0.80
^{75}Se	1.91
^{99}Mo	1.45
^{99m}Tc	0.60
^{123}I	1.53
^{125}I	1.41
^{131}I	2.16
^{127}Xe	2.15
^{133}Xe	0.15

Adapted from ref. 1: Anger RT: Radiation protection in nuclear medicine, in: The Physics of Clinical Nuclear Medicine. Chicago, American Association of Physics in Medicine, 1977. With permission.

in the estimation of exposure levels on contact with the source, e.g., exposure and dose rates to the hand while handling syringes and vials. These exposure rates have been determined experimentally for ^{99m}Tc. They range from about 600 mR/mCi·hr on the surface of larger syringes (10–20 cc) up to about 3000 mR/mCi·hr for smaller syringes (1–2 cc).[1] Exposure rates on contact with syringes containing 20–30 mCi of ^{99m}Tc can be in the range of *several R/min*, an obvious matter of concern in operations requiring handling of these sources.

Time, distance, shielding (TDS rules). The basic principles for reducing radiation doses from external sources are described by the "TDS" rules, for *t*ime, *d*istance, and *s*hielding:

1. Decrease the *time* of exposure.
2. Increase the *distance* from the source.
3. Use *shielding* where necessary.

Time of exposure is decreased by working with or in the vicinity of radiation sources as rapidly as possible, consistent with good technique. Personnel should spend as little time as possible in "hot labs" and other high-level radiation areas. In particular, these areas should not be used for visiting, discussing problems unrelated to activities in the area, etc. Laboratory monitors should be used in these areas to warn personnel when high-level radiation sources are present.

As shown by Example 23-1, *distance* can have a marked effect on radiation levels. Increasing distance always has a dose reduction effect. Direct contact with radiation sources should be avoided by any available means, e.g., by using tongs to handle vials. Patient study areas (e.g., imaging rooms) should be arranged to permit the technician to operate instrumentation at reasonable distances (e.g., 2 meters) from the patient. Separate waiting areas should be provided for patients who have been injected with radioactivity and for relatives, orderlies, and patients not requiring radioactive injections. Reception areas should not be used as waiting areas for radioactive patients. Storage areas for generators, radioactive trash, and other high-level sources should be located remote from regularly occupied areas of the laboratory. Special attention should be given to their location in relation to unrestricted areas. (They should also be located remote from imaging rooms and counting rooms to minimize instrument background levels.)

Examples of effective use of *shielding* are lead pigs for storage of vials and generators, lead-lined syringe holders, lead aprons, lead bricks for lining storage areas, and lead-lined drawing stations (Figure 23-2). Leaded glass provides comfortable viewing and radiation protection simultaneously, especially for low-energy γ- and x-ray emitters (≤200

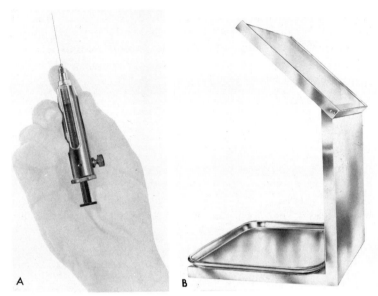

A   B

Fig. 23-2. Examples of protective shielding devices used in nuclear medicine. (A) Shielded syringe holder. (B) Lead-lined drawing station for preparing and handling radioactive materials. Lead-lined glass provides a good view of the work area. [Courtesy of Atomic Products Corp.]

keV). Dose calibrators should be enclosed in a shielded area, using lead sheet or bricks, to avoid unnecessary exposure during measurement of radiopharmaceutical activity.

Table 9-4 lists tenth-value thicknesses of lead for several γ- and x-ray emitters. Small thicknesses of lead (≤ 1 mm) provide effective shielding for low-energy emitters, e.g., ^{133}Xe and ^{99m}Tc. Lead-lined aprons, which usually contain 0.25 or 0.5 mm equivalent lead thicknesses, provide a modest amount of radiation protection, but probably not enough to warrant their routine use in the nuclear medicine laboratory; however, they may be useful for specific applications, such as during handling of large quantities of ^{133}Xe or during elution of a ^{99m}Tc generator. Greater thickness (> 1 cm) are required for higher-energy γ-ray emitters, such as ^{131}I; however, lead is still an effective shielding material at these energies. Concrete and similar materials find limited use for general purpose shielding in nuclear medicine.

Shielding is very effective for β emitters. A few millimeters of almost any solid material will stop even the most energetic β particles (see Figure 8-10). In this case, however, low-Z materials (e.g., plastic, ordinary glass) are preferred over high-Z materials (e.g., leaded glass) to minimize bremsstrahlung production (Equation 8-1). A good shielding arrangement for a high-energy β emitter, such as ^{32}P, is to use a plastic or glass container for the radioactive material to stop the β particles and then to place this in a lead container to absorb the bremsstrahlung (Figure 8-3).

3. Reduction of Radiation Doses From Internal Sources

Types of sources. Nearly all nuclear medicine personnel are required at one time or another to work with radioactive sources in open or poorly sealed containers. There is always the possibility that in these operations some of the radioactive material will find its way into the body, where it delivers a radiation dose as an internal radiation source. Patient sweat or excreta, linens used on imaging tables, spillage occurring during transfer of activity between containers and syringes, radioactive trash, and radioactive gases released during pulmonary function tests are examples of potential sources.

A radioactive material that has been accidentally or carelessly ingested is an "uncontrolled source"; once it is inside the body, there is very little that can be done to reduce the radiation dose that it will delivery. (Techniques developed by the weapons and reactor industries for speeding the elimination of radioactive materials from the body are generally slow to act and thus are useful only for very long-lived radionuclides and are not practical for nuclear medicine.) The cardinal rule for keeping radiation doses from internal sources "ALARA" is to prevent the entry of the radioactive material into the body in the first place. To a certain extent, this is a matter of careful design of laboratory facilities, but equally as important it is a matter of developing good laboratory work habits.

Some basic rules for avoiding internal radiation doses are

1. No eating, drinking, smoking, or applying cosmetics in areas where open sources may be present (e.g., "hot labs" and patient study areas).
2. Lab coats and gloves should be worn when handling radioactive sources. Gloves should be handled so as to avoid contamination of their inside surfaces. Lab coats, aprons, and other protective clothing should stay in the lab overnight—i.e., they should not be taken home.
3. No foodstuffs or drinks should be stored where radioactive sources are kept—e.g., in laboratory refrigerators.
4. Absolutely no pipetting by mouth.
5. Personnel should wash their hands after working with radioactive sources (a sink should be available in the laboratory), and they should be checked for contamination on a laboratory radiation

monitor (Section E.1). Hands should also be monitored before going to lunch or on breaks and before leaving at the end of the day.

6. Work should be performed on absorbent pads to catch spills and prevent spattering of liquids.
7. Work with radioactive gases or other volatile materials (e.g., concentrated iodine solutions) should be performed in a ventilated fume hood. These materials also should be stored in a hood.
8. Work areas should be kept tidy. Radioactive trash, contaminated pads, etc. should be disposed of promptly.
9. Radioactive storage areas (e.g., hot labs) should not be used to store other materials, such as office supplies or linens.
10. Needless contamination of light switches, doorknobs, and other items that could result in unsuspected contamination to personnel should be avoided.
11. Containers with sharp or broken edges should not be used for radioactive materials.
12. Radioactive materials should be stored when they are not in use.

Studies with radioactive gases, such as ^{133}Xe, require special attention because of the potential for escape of radioactivity into the laboratory and beyond. Optimally, the laboratory ventilation system should be designed to maintain the laboratory under negative pressure relative to its surroundings and should be separate from other ventilation systems to prevent spread of airborne activity into other areas of the hospital. A gas-trapping system should be used to collect gases exhaled by the patient (Figure 23-3).

Most of the rules listed above are of the "common sense" variety and perhaps seem obvious; however, it is surprising how often they are violated through forgetfulness or indifference. This may explain the surprisingly high incidence of internal radionuclides found in some studies of nuclear medicine laboratory personnel (e.g., over 70 percent incidence of radioactive iodine in thyroid glands[1]). Clearly, adherence to proper laboratory work rules is fundamental to the ALARA concept.

4. Laboratory Design

The principles of ALARA are enhanced by careful attention to laboratory design. Several design aspects have been mentioned already in relation to other problems—e.g., negative relative air pressure in laboratories employing volatile or gaseous radioactive materials, and availability of a fume hood with its own exhaust system for storage of these materials. Some additional principles to be considered in laboratory design are the following:

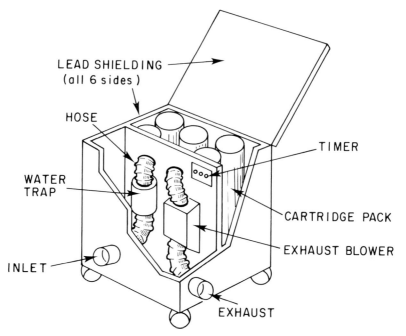

Fig. 23-3.   Gas-trapping system used to collect and trap radioactive gases from patients during studies with ^{133}Xe, etc. Cartridge packs contain activated charcoal to absorb ^{133}Xe. [Courtesy of Nuclear Associates.]

1. Hot labs and radioactive storage areas should be located away from other busy work areas, public corridors, secretarial offices, etc. and away from imaging and low-level counting rooms.
2. Work surfaces and floors should be constructed using smooth, nonabsorbent materials free from cracks and crevices.
3. Workbenches should be sufficiently sturdy to support lead shielding.
4. Wash basins and sinks should be conveniently available where unsealed radioactive materials are handled. It is desirable that sinks in hot labs have foot- or elbow-operated controls.
5. The laboratory design should permit separate storage of glassware and work tools (e.g., tongs, stirring devices, etc.) not used with radioactive materials to prevent needless contamination or mixture with similar items used with radioactive preparations.

5. Procedures for Handling Spills

Accidental spills of radioactive materials are infrequent occurrences in well-run nuclear medicine laboratories. Also, the quantities of radioactivity used in nuclear medicine do not create ''life-threatening'' hazards. Nevertheless, radioactive spills should not be treated as events completely without hazard, the laboratory personnel should be aware of the appropriate procedures to follow when spills do occur.

The steps to follow in dealing with a radioactive spill are (1) to *inform*, (2) to *contain*, and (3) to *decontaminate*.

1. Individuals in the immediate work area should be informed that a spill has occurred so they can avoid contamination if possible. Individuals outside the immediate area should be warned so they do not enter it. The radiation officer should be informed so that he/she may begin supervising further action as soon as possible.

2. By whatever means are reasonably possible, without risking further hazards to themselves, laboratory personnel should attempt to control the spill to prevent further spread of contamination. A flask that has been tipped over should be uprighted. Absorbent pads should be thrown over a liquid spill. Doors should be closed to prevent the escape of airborne radioactivity (gases, powders, etc.). The spill area should be closed off to prevent entry, especially by persons who might not be aware of the spill. Personnel monitoring for contamination should be started as soon as possible, so that contaminated and uncontaminated persons can be segregated. To prevent the further spread of radioactivity, contaminated individuals should be not allowed to leave the area until they are decontaminated, and uncontaminated individuals should not be allowed to enter the spill area. Contamination monitoring should be done using a sensitive radiation monitoring intstrument appropriate for the type of radioactivity involved. It is advisable that each laboratory have on hand a thin-window GM counter survey meter (Section E.1) for handling such situations.

3. Personnel decontamination procedures should receive first priority, followed by decontamination of work areas, etc. Personnel involved in decontamination procedures should wear protective clothing to avoid becoming contaminated themselves in the process.

    Contaminated skin should be flushed thoroughly with water. Special attention should be given to open wounds and contamination around the eyes, nose, and mouth. Contaminated clothing should be removed and placed in plastic bags for storage. After major localized areas of personnel contamination have been attended to, a shower bath may be required to remove more widely distributed contamination.

    Decontamination of laboratory and work areas should not be attempted except under the supervision of the radioactive safety officer or radiation health physicist. If the work surfaces and floors are constructed from a nonabsorbent material, soap and water is generally all that is needed for decontamination. Contaminated areas should be cleaned "from outside in" to minimize the spread of contamination. Porous or cracked surfaces may create difficult problems. If complete decontamination is not possible, it may be necessary to cover and shield the affected surfaces, or perhaps even to remove and replace them.

D. DISPOSAL OF RADIOACTIVE WASTE

There are three general techniques for disposing of radioactive wastes:

1. *Dilute and disperse.*   Small quantities of radioactive materials may be released into the environment—e.g., radioactive gases into the ventilation system or liquid wastes into the sink—provided that the concentrations do not exceed MPC values specified in 10CFR20. In keeping with the ALARA concept, however, this technique should not be used if reasonable alternatives are available (e.g., 2 and 3 below).

2. *Store and decay.*   For materials having reasonably short half-lives (e.g., a few weeks or less), and if suitable storage space is available, this may be an economical and effective disposal technique. After a decay period of ten half-lives has elapsed, only 0.1 percent of the initial activity remains. It is advisable to separate waste materials into two categories: those having half-lives shorter than 3 days and those having half-lives longer than 3 days, so that long-term accumulation of large volumes of waste material can be avoided. Disposal by decay of materials with half-lives longer than about a month is frequently impractical because of the long storage period required.

3. *Concentrate and bury.*   This is frequently the only effective means of disposal of long-lived radioactivity, particularly if storage space is limited. A number of commercial companies provide this type of disposal service.

E. RADIATION MONITORING

1. Survey Meters and Laboratory Monitors

Survey meters are used in monitor radiation levels in and near laboratories in which radioactive materials or other radiation sources are present. Generally, they are battery operated and portable. The radiation detector is usually an ionization chamber or a GM tube (Figures 4-3 and 4-12).

Ionization chamber types are calibrated to read exposure levels. The full-scale reading and range on the meter display is switch selectable, typically from 0–3 mR/hr up to 0–300 mR/hr. Some types have very thin mica or aluminum entrance windows for the ionization chamber and can be used to detect β particles as well as x or γ rays. Ionization chamber survey meters give reasonably accurate estimates of exposure rates (± 10 percent) over most of the nuclear medicine energy range. Most ionization chamber survey meters do not have sealed chambers. Thus for greatest accuracy their readings should be corrected for ambient temperature and pressure variations (Chapter 4, Section A.2, Equation 4-1). These corrections are small at sea-level pressures and room temperatures; however, the pressure correction factor may be significant at higher elevations (≈ 20 percent at 1600 meters or 1 mile).

The accuracy of an ionization chamber survey meter should be checked periodically (e.g., annually, or following major repairs) using a radiation source producing a known radiation exposure level. Sealed sources used in radiation therapy departments (e.g., ^{137}Cs, $\Gamma = 3.23$ R·cm^2/mCi·hr, or ^{226}Ra, $\Gamma = 8.25$ R·cm^2/mCi·hr, with 0.5 mm Pt filtration) are useful for this purpsoe.

GM tube types of survey meters are more sensitive than ionization chamber types because they respond to individual ionizing radiation events. Most of these instruments have meters that display event counting rates (cpm). Some types with thin mica or aluminum entrance windows are suitable for detecting α and β particles as well as γ and x rays. Because of their relatively high sensitivity, GM-type survey meters are most useful for detecting small quantities of radioactivity from minor spills, in waste receptacles, etc.

Laboratory monitors are very similar to survey meters, but they are designed to be used at a fixed location rather than as portable units. They are operated continuously; thus they are generally plugged into the wall rather than battery operated. Most have GM tube detectors and produce an audible clicking noise when radiation is detected in addition to having a meter display of counting rate. A laboratory monitor should be used in any area where large quantities of radioactivity are handled (e.g., in a radiopharmacy lab) to warn of the presence of high radiation levels. They also are useful for monitoring hands after operations requiring the handling of radioactivity.

2. Personnel Dosimeters

Personnel dosimeters are devices worn by laboratory personnel to monitor radiation doses from external sources. There are two general types: *dosimeter badges*, which are used to measure cumulative doses

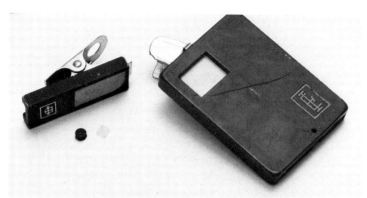

Fig. 23-4.   Examples of personnel dosimeter badges. At left is a TLD badge, with a TLD chip and a black plastic insert lying in front of it. At right is a film badge containing a small packet of x-ray film.

over periods of weeks or months, and *pocket dosimeters*, which are generally used for monitoring over a shorter term.

Dosimeter badges monitor radiation doses using either a small piece of x-ray film or thermoluminescent dosimeter (TLD) chips (Figure 23-4). With the film badge types, the amount of x-ray film blackening is used to estimate the radiation dose received by the person wearing the badge. Thermoluminescent dosimeters generally use small "chips" of lithium fluoride, a material that gives off light when heated after it has been exposed to ionizing radiation. The amount of light given off is measured using a PM tube while the chip is heated in an oven inside a light-tight enclosure. The amount of light given off is used to estimate the radiation dose received.

Dosimeter badge services are provided by a number of commercial suppliers. New badges are supplied at regular (e.g., monthly) intervals, and readings for the preceding period are reported back to the user, typically within about a month. The reports provided by most companies are satisfactory for NRC record-keeping purposes.

Pocket dosimeters were described in Chapter 4, Section A.2 (see Figures 4-4 and 4-5). They are essentially ionization chamber devices that provide an immediate readout of radiation doses and thus are especially useful for measuring over short periods of time or when a rapid indication of results is needed, e.g., during complicated radiopharmaceutical preparation procedures.

3. Wipe Testing

Wipe testing is used to detect small amounts of radioactive contamination on bench-top surfaces, on the outside of shipping packages, etc., or to detect small amounts of radioactive leakage from sealed radioactive sources. The surface is wiped with an alcohol-soaked patch of gauze or cotton-tipped swab, which is then counted in a well counter (for γ-emitting nuclides) or a liquid scintillation counter (for β emitters). Contamination well below the microcurie level can be detected by wipe testing. NRC regulations require periodic wipe testing of work areas.

REFERENCES

1.   Anger RT: Radiation protection in nuclear medicine, in: The Physics of Clinical Nuclear Medicine. Chicago, American Association of Physicists in Medicine, 1977 [a general reference, with discussion of problems in ^{133}Xe disposal]

A general discussion of radiation protection techniques and regulations is found in the following:

Shapiro J: Radiation Protection. A Guide for Scientists and Physicians (2nd Ed.). Cambridge, Mass. Harvard University Press, 1981.

Some NCRP publications relevant to nuclear medicine are the following:

Safe Handling of Radionuclides. NCRP Report No. 30, 1964

Precautions in the management of patients who have received therapeutic amounts of radionuclides. NCRP Report No. 37, 1970

Basic Radiation Protection Criteria. NCRP Report No. 39, 1971

Review of Current State of Radiation Protection Philosophy. NCRP Report No. 43, 1975

Radiation Protection for Medical and Allied Health Personnel. NCRP Report No. 48, 1976

Review of NCRP Radiation Dose Limit for Embryo and Fetus in Occupationally Exposed Women. NCRP Report No. 53, 1977

Medical Radiation Exposure of Pregnant and Potentially Pregnant Women. NCRP Report No. 54, 1977

Management of Persons Accidentally Contaminated with Radionuclides. NCRP Report No. 65, 1980.

Operational Radiation Safety Training. NCRP Report No. 71, 1983.

Protection In Nuclear Medicine and Ultrasound Diagnostic Procedures in Children. NCRP Report No. 73, 1983.

Appendix A

Properties of the Elements

Name	Symbol	At. No.	At. Wt.† (^{12}C scale)	Density† (g/cm^3)	K_B‡ (keV)
Actinium	Ac	89	~227	—	106.759
Aluminum	Al	13	26.982	2.702	1.559
Americium	Am	95	~243	—	124.876
Antimony	Sb	51	121.75	6.684	30.486
Argon	Ar	18	39.948	1.784*	3.203
Arsenic	As	33	74.922	5.727	11.863
Astatine	At	85	~210	—	95.740
Barium	Ba	56	137.33	3.51	37.410
Berkelium	Bk	97	~247	—	131.357
Beryllium	Be	4	9.012	1.85	0.116
Bismuth	Bi	83	208.981	9.80	90.521
Boron	B	5	10.81	(2.34–2.37)	0.192
Bromine	Br	35	79.904	3.119	13.475
Cadmium	Cd	48	112.41	8.642	26.712
Calcium	Ca	20	40.08	1.54	4.038
Californium	Cf	98	~251	—	134.683
Carbon	C	6	12.011	(1.8–3.5)	0.283
Cerium	Ce	58	140.12	(6.657–6.757)	40.449
Cesium	Cs	55	132.905	1.879	35.959
Chlorine	Cl	17	35.453	3.214*	2.819
Chromium	Cr	24	51.996	7.20	5.988
Cobalt	Co	27	58.933	8.9	7.709
Copper	Cu	29	63.546	8.92	8.980
Curium	Cm	96	~247	—	128.088
Dysprosium	Dy	66	162.50	8.550	53.789
Einsteinium	Es	99	~254	—	138.067
Erbium	Er	68	167.26	9.006	57.483
Europium	Eu	63	151.96	5.243	48.515
Fermium	Fm	100	~257	—	141.510
Fluorine	F	9	18.998	1.69*	0.687
Francium	Fr	87	~223	—	101.147
Gadolinium	Gd	64	157.25	7.900	50.229
Gallium	Ga	31	69.72	(5.9–6.1)	10.368
Germanium	Ge	32	72.59	5.35	11.103
Gold	Au	79	196.967	19.3	80.713
Hafnium	Hf	72	178.49	13.31	65.313
Helium	He	2	4.003	0.179*	0.0246
Holmium	Ho	67	164.930	8.795	55.615
Hydrogen	H	1	1.008	0.090*	0.0136
Indium	In	49	114.82	7.30	27.928
Iodine	I	53	126.905	4.93	33.164
Iridium	Ir	77	192.20	22.421	76.097

Appendix A
Properties of the Elements
(Continued)

Name	Symbol	At. No.	At. Wt.† (^{12}C scale)	Density† (g/cm^3)	K_B‡ (keV)
Iron	Fe	26	55.847	7.86	7.111
Krypton	Kr	36	83.80	3.736*	14.323
Lanthanum	La	57	138.905	(6.145–6.17)	38.931
Lawrencium	Lr	103	~257	—	—
Lead	Pb	82	207.2	11.344	88.001
Lithium	Li	3	6.939	0.534	0.055
Lutetium	Lu	71	174.97	9.840	63.304
Magnesium	Mg	12	24.312	1.74	1.303
Manganese	Mn	25	54.938	7.20	6.537
Mendelevium	Md	101	~256	—	—
Mercury	Hg	80	200.59	13.594	83.106
Molybdenum	Mo	42	95.94	10.2	20.002
Neodymium	Nd	60	144.24	(6.80–7.004)	43.571
Neon	Ne	10	20.179	0.900*	0.874
Neptunium	Np	93	237.00	(18.0–20.5)	118.619
Nickel	Ni	28	58.71	8.90	8.331
Niobium	Nb	41	92.906	8.57	18.987
Nitrogen	N	7	14.007	1.251*	0.399
Nobelium	No	102	~259	—	—
Osmium	Os	76	190.2	22.48	73.860
Oxygen	O	8	15.999	1.429*	0.531
Palladium	Pd	46	106.4	(11.4–12.0)	24.347
Phosphorus	P	15	30.974	(2.34–2.70)	2.142
Platinum	Pt	78	195.09	21.45	78.379
Plutonium	Pu	94	239.05	(15.9–19.8)	121.720
Polonium	Po	84	210.05	9.4	93.112
Potassium	K	19	39.098	0.86	3.607
Praseodymium	Pr	59	140.908	6.773	41.998
Promethium	Pm	61	~145	7.22	45.207
Protactinium	Pa	91	231.10	15.37	112.581
Radium	Ra	88	226.025	5	103.927
Radon	Rn	86	~222	9.73*	98.418
Rhenium	Re	75	186.2	20.53	71.662
Rhodium	Rh	45	102.906	12.4	23.224
Rubidium	Rb	37	85.468	1.532	15.201
Ruthenium	Ru	44	101.07	12.30	22.118
Samarium	Sm	62	150.35	7.520	46.846
Scandium	Sc	21	44.956	2.989	4.496
Selenium	Se	34	78.96	4.81	12.652
Silicon	Si	14	28.086	(2.32–2.34)	1.838

Appendix A
Properties of the Elements
(Continued)

Name	Symbol	At. No.	At. Wt.† (^{12}C scale)	Density† (g/cm³)	K_B‡ (keV)
Silver	Ag	47	107.868	10.5	25.517
Sodium	Na	11	22.990	0.97	1.08
Strontium	Sr	38	87.62	2.6	16.106
Sulfur	S	16	32.06	2.07	2.470
Tantalum	Ta	73	180.948	(14.4–16.6)	67.400
Technetium	Tc	43	98.906	—	21.054
Tellurium	Te	52	127.60	6.25	31.809
Terbium	Tb	65	158.925	8.229	51.998
Thallium	Tl	81	204.37	11.85	85.517
Thorium	Th	90	232.038	11.7	109.630
Thulium	Tm	69	168.934	9.321	59.335
Tin	Sn	50	118.69	(5.75–7.28)	29.190
Titanium	Ti	22	47.90	4.5	4.964
Tungsten	W	74	183.85	19.35	69.508
Uranium	U	92	238.029	19.05	115.591
Vanadium	V	23	50.941	5.96	5.463
Xenon	Xe	54	131.30	5.887*∗	34.579
Ytterbium	Yb	70	173.04	6.965	61.303
Yttrium	Y	39	88.906	4.469	17.037
Zinc	Zn	30	65.38	7.14	9.660
Zirconium	Zr	40	91.22	6.49	17.998

†Reprinted with permission from The Handbook of Chemistry and Physics (ed 60). Cleveland, The Chemical Rubber Co., CRC Press, Inc., 1979–1980. Density values in parentheses are given for elements that may exist in different crystalline forms.

‡Values for K-shell binding energies taken from The Radiological Health Handbook. Rockville, Md., U.S. Dept. H.E.W., 1970, pp. 161–162.

∗Densities for gases in g/liter.

Appendix B
Characteristics of Some Medically Important Radionuclides

Except as noted, each of the following figures represent decay scheme and dosimetry data reproduced with permission from Dillman LT, Von der Lage FC: Radionuclide Decay Schemes and Nuclear Parameters for Use in Radiation-Dose Estimation. New York, The Society of Nuclear Medicine, 1975. Note that $\overline{E}_i$ is the mean energy per disintegration per particle *or* photon.

HYDROGEN-3
BETA-MINUS DECAY

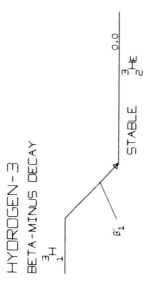

$^3_1$H

β^-_1

STABLE $^3_2$He

0.0

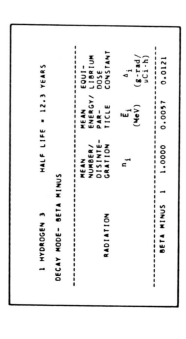

1 HYDROGEN 3   HALF LIFE = 12.3 YEARS

DECAY MODE- BETA MINUS

RADIATION	MEAN NUMBER/ DISINTE- GRATION n_i	MEAN ENERGY/ PAR- TICLE $\bar{E}_i$ (MeV)	EQUI- LIBRIUM DOSE CONSTANT Δ_i (g-rad/ μCi·h)
BETA MINUS 1	1.0000	0.0057	0.0121

CARBON-11
BETA-PLUS DECAY

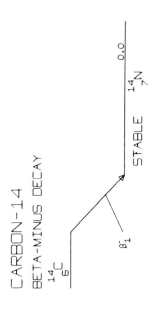

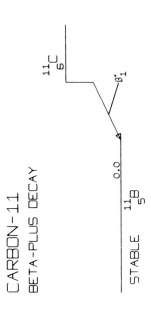

6 CARBON 11	HALF LIFE = 20.3 MINUTES		
DECAY MODE- BETA PLUS			
RADIATION	MEAN NUMBER/ DISINTE- GRATION n_i	MEAN ENERGY/ PAR- TICLE $\bar{E}_i$ (MeV)	EQUI- LIBRIUM DOSE CONSTANT Δ_i (g-rad/ µCi-h)
BETA PLUS 1	0.9980	0.3942	0.8380
ANNIH. RADIATION	1.9960	0.5110	2.1725

CARBON-14
BETA-MINUS DECAY

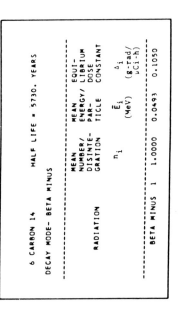

6 CARBON 14	HALF LIFE = 5730. YEARS		
DECAY MODE- BETA MINUS			
RADIATION	MEAN NUMBER/ DISINTE- GRATION n_i	MEAN ENERGY/ PAR- TICLE $\bar{E}_i$ (MeV)	EQUI- LIBRIUM DOSE CONSTANT Δ_i (g-rad/ µCi-h)
BETA MINUS 1	1.0000	0.0493	0.1050

NITROGEN-13
BETA-PLUS DECAY

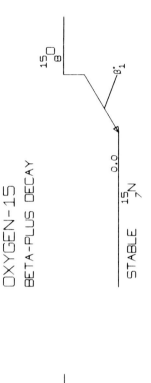

STABLE $^{13}_{6}$C

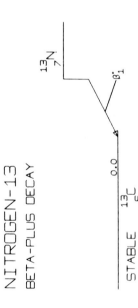

7 NITROGEN 13	HALF LIFE = 10.0 MINUTES		
DECAY MODE- BETA PLUS			
RADIATION	MEAN NUMBER/ DISINTE- GRATION n_i	MEAN ENERGY/ PAR- TICLE $\bar{E}_i$ (MeV)	EQUI- LIBRIUM DOSE CONSTANT Δ_i (g-rad/ µCi-h)
BETA PLUS 1	1.0000	0.4880	1.0395
ANNIH. RADIATION	2.0000	0.5110	2.1768

OXYGEN-15
BETA-PLUS DECAY

STABLE $^{15}_{7}$N

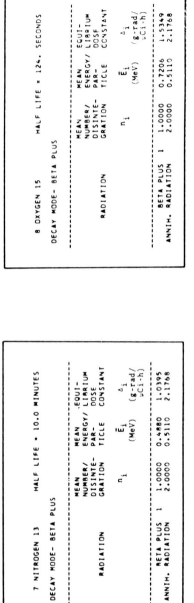

8 OXYGEN 15	HALF LIFE = 124. SECONDS		
DECAY MODE- BETA PLUS			
RADIATION	MEAN NUMBER/ DISINTE- GRATION n_i	MEAN ENERGY/ PAR- TICLE $\bar{E}_i$ (MeV)	EQUI- LIBRIUM DOSE CONSTANT Δ_i (g-rad/ µCi-h)
BETA PLUS 1	1.0000	0.7206	1.5349
ANNIH. RADIATION	2.0000	0.5110	2.1768

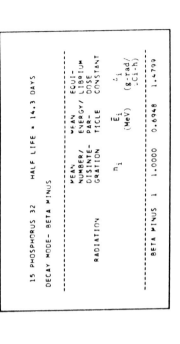

PHOSPHORUS-32
BETA-MINUS DECAY

$^{32}_{15}P$

β^-_1

STABLE $^{32}_{16}S$

0.0

---

15 PHOSPHORUS 32   HALF LIFE = 14.3 DAYS

DECAY MODE- BETA MINUS

RADIATION	n_i MEAN NUMBER/ DISINTE- GRATION	$\bar{E}_i$ (MeV) MEAN ENERGY/ PAR- TICLE	Δ_i (g-rad/ μCi-h) EQUI- LIBRIUM DOSE CONSTANT
BETA MINUS 1	1.0000	0.6948	1.4799

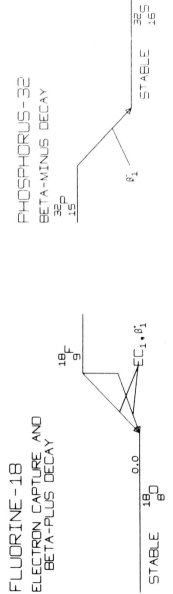

FLUORINE-18
ELECTRON CAPTURE AND BETA-PLUS DECAY

$^{18}_{9}F$

EC_1, β^+_1

0.0

STABLE $^{18}_{8}O$

---

9 FLUORINE 18   HALF LIFE = 109. MINUTES

DECAY MODES- ELECTRON CAPTURE AND BETA PLUS

RADIATION	n_i MEAN NUMBER/ DISINTE- GRATION	$\bar{E}_i$ (MeV) MEAN ENERGY/ PAR- TICLE	Δ_i (g-rad/ μCi-h) EQUI- LIBRIUM DOSE CONSTANT
BETA PLUS 1	0.9700	0.2496	0.5157
ANNIH. RADIATION	1.9400	0.5110	2.1115

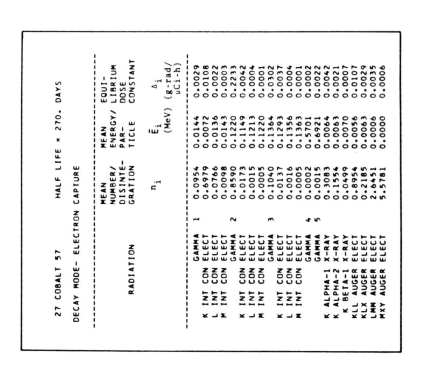

RADIATION	MEAN NUMBER/ DISINTE- GRATION n_i	MEAN ENERGY/ PAR- TICLE $\bar{E}_i$ (MeV)	EQUI- LIBRIUM DOSE CONSTANT Δ_i (g-rad/ μCi-h)
GAMMA 1	0.0954	0.0144	0.0029
K INT CON ELECT	0.6979	0.0072	0.0108
L INT CON ELECT	0.0766	0.0136	0.0022
M INT CON ELECT	0.0098	0.0143	0.0003
GAMMA 2	0.8590	0.1220	0.2233
K INT CON ELECT	0.0173	0.1149	0.0042
L INT CON ELECT	0.0015	0.1213	0.0004
M INT CON ELECT	0.0005	0.1220	0.0001
GAMMA 3	0.1040	0.1364	0.0302
K INT CON ELECT	0.0137	0.1293	0.0037
L INT CON ELECT	0.0016	0.1356	0.0004
M INT CON ELECT	0.0005	0.1363	0.0001
GAMMA 4	0.0002	0.5701	0.0002
GAMMA 5	0.0015	0.6921	0.0022
K ALPHA-1 X-RAY	0.3083	0.0064	0.0042
K ALPHA-2 X-RAY	0.1554	0.0063	0.0021
K BETA-1 X-RAY	0.0499	0.0070	0.0007
KLL AUGER ELECT	0.8954	0.0056	0.0107
KLX AUGER ELECT	0.2185	0.0063	0.0029
LMM AUGER ELECT	2.6451	0.0006	0.0035
MXY AUGER ELECT	5.5781	0.0000	0.0006

27 COBALT 57   HALF LIFE = 270. DAYS

DECAY MODE- ELECTRON CAPTURE

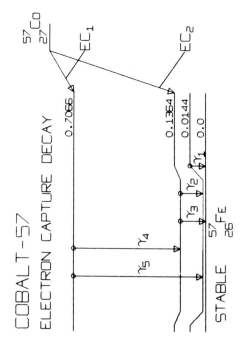

COBALT-57
ELECTRON CAPTURE DECAY

GALLIUM-67
ELECTRON CAPTURE DECAY

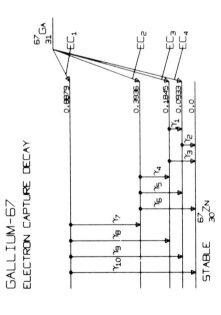

31 GALLIUM 67   HALF LIFE = 78.1 HOURS

DECAY MODE- ELECTRON CAPTURE

RADIATION	MEAN NUMBER/ DISINTE- GRATION n_i	MEAN ENERGY/ PAR- TICLE $\bar{E}_i$ (MeV)	EQUI- LIBRIUM DOSE CONSTANT Δ_i (g-rad/ µCi-h)
GAMMA 1	0.0326	0.0913	0.0063
K INT CON ELECT	0.0021	0.0816	0.0003
GAMMA 2	0.3797	0.0933	0.0754
K INT CON ELECT	0.2830	0.0836	0.0504
- INT CON ELECT	0.0379	0.0922	0.0074
M INT CON ELECT	0.0126	0.0932	0.0025
GAMMA 3	0.2388	0.1846	0.0939
K INT CON ELECT	0.0026	0.1749	0.0009
L INT CON ELECT	0.0004	0.1835	0.0001
GAMMA 4	0.0247	0.2090	0.0110
GAMMA 5	0.1613	0.3002	0.1031
K INT CON ELECT	0.0005	0.2905	0.0003
GAMMA 6	0.0429	0.3936	0.0359
GAMMA 7	0.0009	0.4943	0.0010
GAMMA 8	0.0001	0.7036	0.0002
GAMMA 9	0.0006	0.7947	0.0010
GAMMA 10	0.0015	0.8880	0.0029
K ALPHA-1 X-RAY	0.3075	0.0086	0.0056
K ALPHA-2 X-RAY	0.1534	0.0086	0.0028
K BETA-1 X-RAY	0.0553	0.0095	0.0011
KLL AUGER ELECT	0.5185	0.0075	0.0083
KLX AUGER ELECT	0.1410	0.0085	0.0025
KXY AUGER ELECT	0.0067	0.0094	0.0001
LMM AUGER ELECT	1.7722	0.0008	0.0033
MXY AUGER ELECT	3.7779	0.0000	0.0006

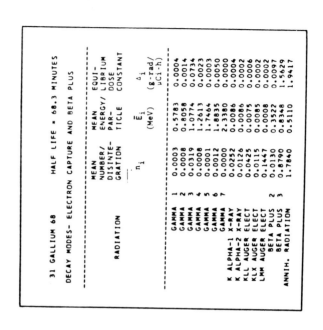

31 GALLIUM 68   HALF LIFE = 68.3 MINUTES

DECAY MODES- ELECTRON CAPTURE AND BETA PLUS

RADIATION	MEAN NUMBER/ DISINTE- GRATION n_i	MEAN ENERGY/ PAR- TICLE $\bar{E}_i$ (MeV)	EQUI- LIBRIUM DOSE CONSTANT Δ_i (g-rad/ µCi·h)
GAMMA 1	0.0003	0.5783	0.0004
GAMMA 2	0.0008	0.8058	0.0014
GAMMA 3	0.0319	1.0774	0.0734
GAMMA 4	0.0008	1.2613	0.0023
GAMMA 5	0.0001	1.7464	0.0003
GAMMA 6	0.0012	1.8835	0.0050
GAMMA 7	0.0000	2.3380	0.0000
K ALPHA-1 X-RAY	0.0252	0.0086	0.0004
K ALPHA-2 X-RAY	0.0126	0.0086	0.0002
KLL AUGER ELECT	0.0425	0.0075	0.0006
KLX AUGER ELECT	0.0115	0.0085	0.0002
LMM AUGER ELECT	0.1447	0.0008	0.0002
BETA PLUS 2	0.0130	0.3522	0.0097
BETA PLUS 3	0.8790	0.8348	1.5629
ANNIH. RADIATION	1.7840	0.5110	1.9417

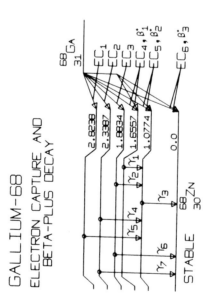

GALLIUM-68
ELECTRON CAPTURE AND
BETA-PLUS DECAY

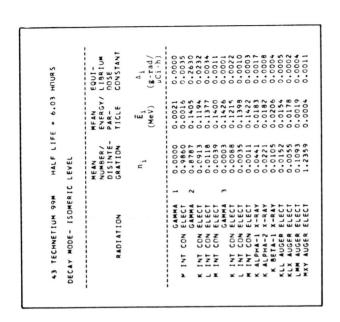

43 TECHNETIUM 99M   HALF LIFE = 6.03 HOURS

DECAY MODE- ISOMERIC LEVEL

RADIATION		n_i MEAN NUMBER/DISINTEGRATION	$\bar{E}_i$ (MeV) MEAN ENERGY/PARTICLE	Δ_i (g-rad/μCi·h) EQUILIBRIUM DOSE CONSTANT
M INT CON GAMMA	1	0.0000	0.0021	0.0000
ELECT		0.9860	0.0016	0.0035
GAMMA	2	0.8787	0.1405	0.2630
K INT CON ELECT		0.0913	0.1194	0.0232
L INT CON ELECT		0.0118	0.1377	0.0034
M INT CON ELECT		0.0039	0.1400	0.0011
GAMMA	3	0.0003	0.1426	0.0001
K INT CON ELECT		0.0088	0.1215	0.0022
L INT CON ELECT		0.0035	0.1398	0.0010
M INT CON ELECT		0.0011	0.1422	0.0003
K ALPHA-1 X-RAY		0.0441	0.0183	0.0017
K ALPHA-2 X-RAY		0.0221	0.0182	0.0008
K BETA-1 X-RAY		0.0105	0.0206	0.0004
KLL AUGER ELECT		0.0152	0.0154	0.0005
KLX AUGER ELECT		0.0055	0.0178	0.0002
LMM AUGER ELECT		0.1093	0.0019	0.0004
MXY AUGER ELECT		1.2359	0.0004	0.0011

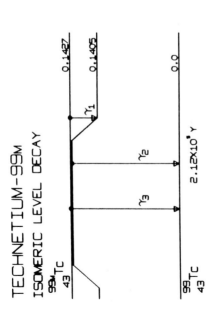

TECHNETIUM-99M
ISOMERIC LEVEL DECAY

$^{99m}_{43}$Tc

0.1427

0.1405

γ_1

γ_3 γ_2

$^{99}_{43}$Tc   2.12×10⁵ Y

0.0

INDIUM-111
ELECTRON CAPTURE DECAY

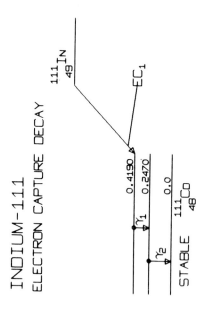

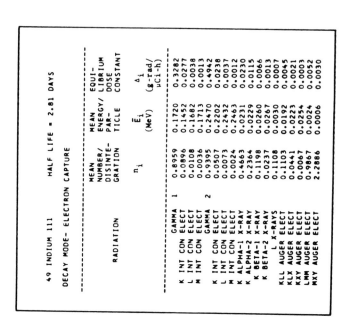

49 INDIUM 111   HALF LIFE = 2.81 DAYS

DECAY MODE- ELECTRON CAPTURE

RADIATION		MEAN NUMBER/ DISINTE- GRATION n_i	MEAN ENERGY/ PAR- TICLE $\bar{E}_i$ (MeV)	EQUI- LIBRIUM DOSE CONSTANT Δ_i (g-rad/ μCi-h)
GAMMA	1	0.8959	0.1720	0.3282
K INT CON ELECT		0.0896	0.1452	0.0277
L INT CON ELECT		0.0108	0.1682	0.0038
M INT CON ELECT		0.0036	0.1713	0.0013
GAMMA	2	0.9395	0.2470	0.4942
K INT CON ELECT		0.0507	0.2202	0.0238
L INT CON ELECT		0.0073	0.2432	0.0037
M INT CON ELECT		0.0024	0.2463	0.0012
K ALPHA-1 X-RAY		0.4663	0.0231	0.0230
K ALPHA-2 X-RAY		0.2364	0.0229	0.0115
K BETA-1 X-RAY		0.1198	0.0260	0.0066
K BETA-2 X-RAY		0.0237	0.0267	0.0013
L X-RAYS		0.1108	0.0030	0.0007
KLL AUGER ELECT		0.1103	0.0192	0.0045
KLX AUGER ELECT		0.0441	0.0223	0.0021
KXY AUGER ELECT		0.0067	0.0254	0.0003
LMM AUGER ELECT		0.9867	0.0024	0.0052
MXY AUGER ELECT		2.2886	0.0006	0.0030

IODINE-123
ELECTRON CAPTURE DECAY

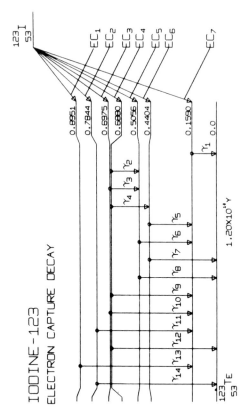

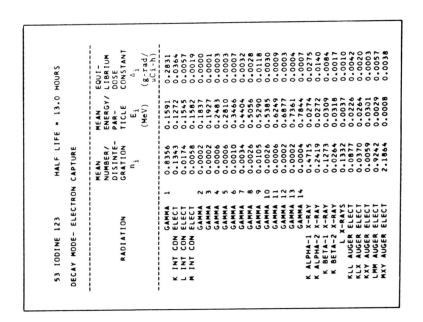

53 IODINE 123 HALF LIFE = 13.0 HOURS

DECAY MODE- ELECTRON CAPTURE

RADIATION		MEAN NUMBER/ DISINTE- GRATION n_i	MEAN ENERGY/ PAR- TICLE E_i (MeV)	EQUI- LIBRIUM DOSE CONSTANT Δ_i (g·rad/ μCi·h)
GAMMA	1	0.8356	0.1591	0.2831
K INT CON ELECT		0.1343	0.1272	0.0364
L INT CON ELECT		0.0174	0.1545	0.0057
M INT CON ELECT		0.0058	0.1582	0.0019
GAMMA	2	0.0002	0.1837	0.0000
GAMMA	3	0.0002	0.1927	0.0001
GAMMA	4	0.0006	0.2483	0.0003
GAMMA	5	0.0006	0.2810	0.0003
GAMMA	6	0.0010	0.3466	0.0007
GAMMA	7	0.0034	0.4404	0.0032
GAMMA	8	0.0026	0.5056	0.0028
GAMMA	9	0.0105	0.5290	0.0118
GAMMA	10	0.0026	0.5385	0.0030
GAMMA	11	0.0006	0.6249	0.0009
GAMMA	12	0.0002	0.6877	0.0003
GAMMA	13	0.0002	0.7361	0.0004
GAMMA	14	0.0004	0.7844	0.0007
K ALPHA-1 X-RAY		0.4715	0.0274	0.0275
K ALPHA-2 X-RAY		0.2419	0.0272	0.0140
K BETA-1 X-RAY		0.1273	0.0309	0.0084
K BETA-2 X-RAY		0.0264	0.0318	0.0017
L X-RAYS		0.1332	0.0037	0.0010
KLL AUGER ELECT		0.0877	0.0226	0.0042
KLX AUGER ELECT		0.0370	0.0264	0.0020
KXY AUGER ELECT		0.0059	0.0301	0.0003
LMM AUGER ELECT		0.9242	0.0029	0.0057
MXY AUGER ELECT		2.1864	0.0008	0.0038

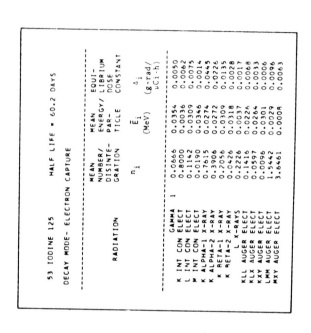

53 IODINE 125   HALF LIFE = 60.2 DAYS

DECAY MODE- ELECTRON CAPTURE

RADIATION	MEAN NUMBER/ DISINTE- GRATION n_i	MEAN ENERGY/ PAR- TICLE $\bar{E}_i$ (MeV)	EQUI- LIBRIUM DOSE CONSTANT Δ_i (g-rad/ μCi·h)
GAMMA 1	0.0666	0.0354	0.0050
K INT CON ELECT	0.8000	0.0036	0.0062
L INT CON ELECT	0.1142	0.0309	0.0075
M INT CON ELECT	0.0190	0.0346	0.0014
K ALPHA-1 X-RAY	0.7615	0.0274	0.0445
K ALPHA-2 X-RAY	0.3906	0.0272	0.0226
K BETA-1 X-RAY	0.2056	0.0309	0.0135
K BETA-2 X-RAY	0.0426	0.0318	0.0028
L X-RAYS	0.2226	0.0037	0.0017
KLL AUGER ELECT	0.1416	0.0226	0.0068
KLX AUGER ELECT	0.0597	0.0264	0.0033
KXY AUGER ELECT	0.0096	0.0301	0.0006
LMM AUGER ELECT	1.5442	0.0029	0.0096
MXY AUGER ELECT	3.6461	0.0008	0.0063

IODINE-125
ELECTRON CAPTURE DECAY

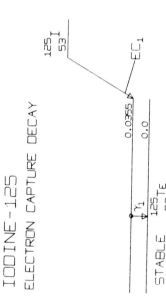

STABLE $^{125}_{52}$Te

IODINE-131
BETA-MINUS DECAY

53 IODINE 131   HALF LIFE = 8.06 DAYS

DECAY MODE- BETA MINUS

RADIATION	n_i MEAN NUMBER/ DISINTE- GRATION	$\bar{E}_i$ (MeV) MEAN ENERGY/ PAR- TICLE	Δ_i (g-rad/ μCi-h) EQUI- LIBRIUM DOSE CONSTANT
BETA MINUS 1	0.0200	0.0691	0.0029
BETA MINUS 2	0.0067	0.0867	0.0012
BETA MINUS 3	0.0664	0.0964	0.0136
BETA MINUS 5	0.8980	0.1916	0.3666
BETA MINUS 6	0.0080	0.2839	0.0048
GAMMA 1	0.0258	0.0801	0.0044
K INT CON ELECT	0.0343	0.0456	0.0033
L INT CON ELECT	0.0043	0.0751	0.0007
M INT CON ELECT	0.0014	0.0792	0.0002
GAMMA 2	0.0029	0.1772	0.0011
K INT CON ELECT	0.0004	0.1426	0.0002
GAMMA 3	0.0006	0.2723	0.0003
GAMMA 4	0.0004	0.2843	0.0002
K INT CON ELECT	0.0023	0.2497	0.0012
L INT CON ELECT	0.0004	0.2792	0.0002
GAMMA 6	0.0010	0.3180	0.0007
GAMMA 7	0.0036	0.3257	0.0025
GAMMA 8	0.0001	0.3585	0.0001
GAMMA 9	0.8201	0.3644	0.6366
K INT CON ELECT	0.0147	0.3299	0.0103
L INT CON ELECT	0.0023	0.3594	0.0017
M INT CON ELECT	0.0007	0.3635	0.0006
GAMMA 10	0.0006	0.4048	0.0005
GAMMA 11	0.0029	0.5029	0.0031
GAMMA 12	0.0653	0.6367	0.0886
K INT CON ELECT	0.0002	0.6021	0.0003
GAMMA 13	0.0014	0.6430	0.0020
GAMMA 14	0.0173	0.7228	0.0267
K ALPHA-1 X-RAY	0.0249	0.0297	0.0015
K ALPHA-2 X-RAY	0.0128	0.0294	0.0008
K BETA-1 X-RAY	0.0068	0.0336	0.0004
K BETA-2 X-RAY	0.0014	0.0345	0.0001
KLL AUGER ELECT	0.0041	0.0244	0.0002
KLX AUGER ELECT	0.0018	0.0285	0.0001
LMM AUGER ELECT	0.0477	0.0031	0.0001
MXY AUGER ELECT	0.1147	0.0009	0.0002

54 XENON 133   HALF LIFE = 5.31 DAYS

DECAY MODE- BETA MINUS

RADIATION		MEAN NUMBER/ DISINTE- GRATION n_i	MEAN ENERGY/ PAR- TICLE $\bar{E}_i$ (MeV)	EQUI- LIBRIUM DOSE CONSTANT Δ_i (g-rad/ μCi·h)
BETA MINUS	2	0.0163	0.0750	0.0026
BETA MINUS	3	0.9830	0.1006	0.2106
GAMMA	1	0.0061	0.0796	0.0010
K INT CON ELECT		0.0084	0.0436	0.0007
L INT CON ELECT		0.0012	0.0742	0.0001
GAMMA	2	0.3603	0.0809	0.0621
K INT CON ELECT		0.5261	0.0450	0.0504
L INT CON ELECT		0.0848	0.0756	0.0136
M INT CON ELECT		0.0282	0.0799	0.0048
GAMMA	3	0.0000	0.1606	0.0000
GAMMA	4	0.0000	0.2230	0.0000
GAMMA	5	0.0000	0.3028	0.0000
GAMMA	6	0.0002	0.3839	0.0001
K ALPHA-1 X-RAY		0.2552	0.0309	0.0168
K ALPHA-2 X-RAY		0.1321	0.0306	0.0086
K BETA-1 X-RAY		0.0712	0.0349	0.0053
K BETA-2 X-RAY		0.0150	0.0350	0.0011
L X-RAYS		0.0823	0.0043	0.0007
KLL AUGER ELECT		0.0402	0.0253	0.0021
KLX AUGER ELECT		0.0177	0.0296	0.0011
KXY AUGER ELECT		0.0029	0.0339	0.0002
LMM AUGER ELECT		0.4894	0.0033	0.0034
MXY AUGER ELECT		1.1867	0.0009	0.0025

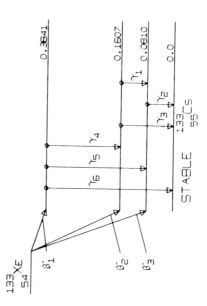

XENON-133
BETA-MINUS DECAY

CESIUM-137
BETA-MINUS DECAY

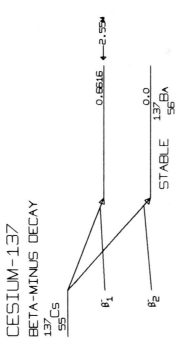

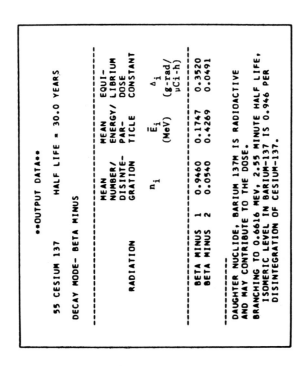

••OUTPUT DATA••

55 CESIUM 137   HALF LIFE = 30.0 YEARS

DECAY MODE- BETA MINUS

RADIATION	MEAN NUMBER/ DISINTE- GRATION n_i	MEAN ENERGY/ PAR- TICLE $\bar{E}_i$ (MeV)	EQUI- LIBRIUM DOSE CONSTANT Δ_i (g-rad/ μCi-h)
BETA MINUS 1	0.9460	0.1747	0.3520
BETA MINUS 2	0.0540	0.4269	0.0491

DAUGHTER NUCLIDE, BARIUM 137M IS RADIOACTIVE AND MAY CONTRIBUTE TO THE DOSE.
BRANCHING TO 0.6616 MEV, 2.55 MINUTE HALF LIFE, ISOMERIC LEVEL IN BARIUM-137 IS 0.946 PER DISINTEGRATION OF CESIUM-137.

TABLE 1. Tl-201 EC DECAY (3.044 D 9)*

Radiation type		Energy (keV)		Intensity (%)		Δ (gr-rad/μCi-h)
Ce-NOP-	1	0.78	4	38	22	0.0006
Auger-L		7.6		78	6	0.0123
Ce-L-	2	15.76	3	11.4	6	0.0038
Ce-L-	3	17.35	3	9.1	5	0.0033
Ce-MNO-	2	27.04	3	3.63	16	0.0021
Ce-MNO-	3	28.63	3	2.85	12	0.0017
Ce-K-	4	52.24	4	7.5	4	0.0083
Auger-K		53.8		3.3	20	0.0038
Ce-K-	5	82.78	7	0.29	4	0.0005
Ce-K-	6	84.33	7	15.5	4	0.0278
Ce-L-	4	120.50	4	1.27	6	0.0033
Ce-MNO-	4	131.78	4	0.397	15	0.0011
Ce-L-	6	152.59	7	2.62	7	0.0085
Ce-MNO-	6	163.87	7	0.810	14	0.0028
X-ray	L	10		47	6	0.0099
γ	2	30.60	3	0.310	13	0.0002
γ	3	32.19	3	0.285	12	0.0002
X-ray	Kα₂	68.8950	20	27.4	9	0.0402
X-ray	Kα₁	70.8190	20	46.6	14	0.0704
X-ray	Kβ	80.3		20.5	7	0.0351
γ	4	135.34	4	2.65	10	0.0076
γ	5	165.88	7	0.180	20	0.0006
γ	6	167.43	7	10.00	17	0.0357

* I (min) = 0.10%.
The intensity entry 10.00 17 is to be read as 10.00 ± .17; similarly, the energy entry 167.43 7 is to be read as 167.43 ± 0.07.

Reproduced, with permission, from: Nass HW: New Tl-201 nuclear decay data. J Nucl Med 18: 1047–1048, 1977.

Appendix C
Exponential Functions

x	e^{-x}	x	e^{-x}	x	e^{-x}
0.00	1.000	0.40	0.670	1.0	0.368
0.01	0.990	0.41	0.664	1.1	0.333
0.02	0.980	0.42	0.657	1.2	0.301
0.03	0.970	0.43	0.651	1.3	0.273
0.04	0.961	0.44	0.644	1.4	0.247
0.05	0.951	0.45	0.638	1.5	0.223
0.06	0.942	0.46	0.631	1.6	0.202
0.07	0.932	0.47	0.625	1.7	0.183
0.08	0.923	0.48	0.619	1.8	0.165
0.09	0.914	0.49	0.613	1.9	0.150
0.10	0.905	0.50	0.607	2.0	0.135
0.11	0.896	0.52	0.595	2.1	0.122
0.12	0.887	0.54	0.583	2.2	0.111
0.13	0.878	0.56	0.571	2.3	0.100
0.14	0.869	0.58	0.560	2.4	0.0907
0.15	0.861	0.60	0.549	2.5	0.0821
0.16	0.852	0.62	0.538	2.6	0.0743
0.17	0.844	0.64	0.527	2.7	0.0672
0.18	0.835	0.66	0.517	2.8	0.0608
0.19	0.827	0.68	0.507	2.9	0.0550
0.20	0.819	0.70	0.497	3.0	0.0498
0.21	0.811	0.72	0.487	3.2	0.0408
0.22	0.803	0.74	0.477	3.4	0.0334
0.23	0.795	0.76	0.468	3.6	0.0273
0.24	0.787	0.78	0.458	3.8	0.0224
0.25	0.779	0.80	0.449	4.0	0.0183
0.26	0.771	0.82	0.440	4.2	0.0150
0.27	0.763	0.84	0.432	4.4	0.0123
0.28	0.756	0.86	0.423	4.6	0.0101
0.29	0.748	0.88	0.415	4.8	0.0862
0.30	0.741	0.90	0.407	5.0	0.0067
0.31	0.733	0.92	0.399	5.5	0.0041
0.32	0.726	0.94	0.391	6.0	0.0025
0.33	0.719	0.96	0.383	6.5	0.0015
0.34	0.712	0.98	0.375	7.0	0.0009
0.35	0.705			7.5	0.0006
0.36	0.698			8.0	0.0003
0.37	0.691			8.5	0.0002
0.38	0.684			9.0	0.0001
0.39	0.677				

Properties of exponential functions: $e^1 = 2.71828\ldots$ $\quad e^x e^y = e^{x+y}$ $\quad \ln e^x = x$
$e^{-x} = 1/e^x$ $\quad e^{xy} = (e^x)^y$ $\quad e^{\ln x} = x$
$\exp x \equiv e^x$

559

Appendix D
Mass Attenuation Coefficients for Water, Sodium Iodide, and Lead

Photon Energy (MeV)	$\mu(cm^2/gm)$		
	H_2O $(\rho = 1.0 \ g/cm^3)$	$NaI(Tl)$ $(\rho = 3.67 \ g/cm^3)$	Pb $(\rho = 11.34 \ g/cm^3)$
0.010	4.99	136.	128.
0.015	1.48	45.9	112.
0.020	0.711	21.2	83.4
0.030	0.338	6.86	28.4
0.033†	—	5.19	—
0.033†	—	30.4	—
0.040	0.248	18.9	13.1
0.050	0.214	10.5	7.22
0.060	0.197	6.42	4.43
0.080	0.179	3.00	2.07
0.088†	—	—	1.62
0.088†	—	—	7.23
0.100	0.168	1.64	5.23
0.150	0.149	0.590	1.89
0.200	0.136	0.314	0.945
0.300	0.118	0.158	0.383
0.400	0.106	0.112	0.220
0.500	0.0967	0.0921	0.154
0.600	0.0895	0.0802	0.120
0.800	0.0786	0.0663	0.0856
1.000	0.0707	0.0580	0.0690
2.000	0.0494	0.0412	0.0450
4.000	0.0340	0.0350	0.0414
8.000	0.0277	0.0355	0.0459
10.000	0.0222	0.0368	0.0484

†K shell binding energies. L shell binding energies for lead omitted.

Values from Hubbell JH: Photon cross-sections, attenuation coefficients, and energy absorption coefficients from 10 keV to 100 GeV. Natl Bur Stand Ref Ser Natl Bur Stand 29, 1969, pp 62, 64, 66.

Appendix E
Radiation Absorbed Dose Estimates (mrad/μCi to Adult subjects) From Internally Administered Radionuclides

Radionuclide	Radiopharmaceutical	Route of Administration	Total Body	Red Bone Marrow	Gonads	Other	
^{32}P	Na phosphate	i.v.	7–10	20–40	20	Liver:	20–30
						Spleen:	20–30
^{67}Ga	Citrate	i.v.	0.2–0.4	0.6–0.8	0.02–0.04	Kidneys:	0.4–0.5
						Liver:	0.4–0.6
^{75}Se	Selenomethionine	i.v.	7–9	10^{+}	5–11	Kidneys:	18–26
						Liver:	21–29
						Pancreas:	10–14
^{99m}Tc	Pertechnetate	i.v.	0.01–0.02	0.022^{+}	0.01–0.02	Thyroid:	0.1‡–0.5
						Stomach:	0.1–0.3
	Sulfur colloid	i.v.	0.01–0.02	0.02–0.03	0.01–0.02	Liver:	0.2–0.4
						Spleen:	0.2–0.4
	MAA	i.v.	0.01–0.02		0.01–0.02	Lungs:	0.1–0.3
						Liver:	0.07–0.08
	Albumin	i.v.	0.01–0.02	0.02^{+}	0.02^{+}		
	Polyphosphate, methylene diphosphonate, pyrophosphate	i.v.	0.01	0.01	0.02	Bone:	0.05–0.07
						Kidneys:	0.09
						Bladder:	0.1–0.2

	Route				Organ	Dose
DTPA	i.v.	0.1–0.02	0.0095[†]	0.01–0.02	Kidneys: Bladder:	0.05–0.3 0.4–0.6
Microspheres	i.v.		0.015[†]	0.004–0.006[†]	Lungs:	0.21[†]
Glucoheptonate	i.v.		0.012[†]	0.004–0.007[†]	Kidneys:	0.30[†]
HIDA	i.v.		0.02[†]	0.003–0.05[†]	ULI:	0.55[†]
DMSA	i.v.		0.035[†]	0.01–0.02[†]	Kidneys:	0.75[†]
[111]In DTPA	Intrathecal (cistern.)	0.6[†]			Spinal cord:	12–20[†]
[123]I Na iodide	Oral		0.033[†]	0.015–0.021[†]	Thyroid:	20[†]
[131]I Na iodide	Oral	1–4	0.41[†]	0.18[†]	Thyroid:	1500–2000
Iodohippurate	i.v.	0.03–0.2		0.02–0.1	Kidneys: Bladder: Thyroid:	0.4–1.0 2–10 48[†]
[133]Xe Gas	Inhaled**		3.7[†]	3.7[†]	Lungs: Trachea:	39[†] 642[†]
[201]Tl Chloride	i.v.		0.25[†]	0.3[†]	Kidneys: Heart:	0.4[†] 0.2[†]

[†]Data reproduced with permission from Roedler HD, Kaul A, Hine GJ: Internal Radiation Dose in Diagnostic Nuclear Medicine. Berlin, Verlag H. Hoffman, 1978. All other data reproduced with permission from Hine GJ: A guide to the absorbed dose from internally administered radionuclides, in, Hine GJ, Sorenson JA (eds): Instrumentation in Nuclear Medicine (vol 2). New York, Academic Press, 1974, Appendix II.
[‡]Thyroid blocking agent used.
**Rebreathing 3 min of air containing 1 mCi/liter; doses in mrad.

Appendix F
**Nomograms for Converting Between
Conventional and SI Units**

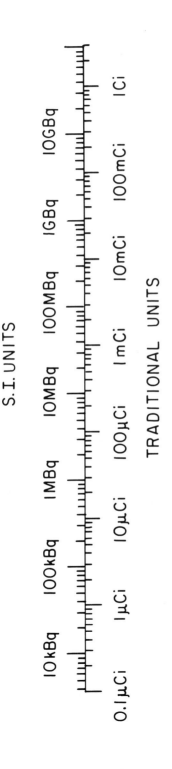

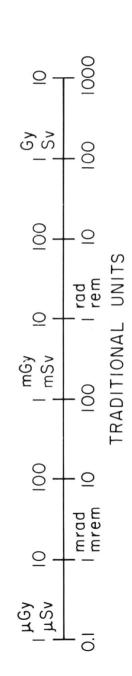

Appendix G

CONVOLUTION

The convolution of two functions $f(x)$ and $g(x)$ is given by:

$$h(x) = \int_{-\infty}^{+\infty} f(u)g(x - u)du \qquad \text{(G-1)}$$

Often this is denoted as:

$$h(x) = f(x) * g(x) \qquad \text{(G-2)}$$

Equation G-1 states that the convolution of two functions, $f(x)$ and $g(x)$, is obtained by changing the variables in the two functions, specifically, $h(x)$ is replaced by $h(u)$, and $g(x)$ by $g(x - u)$, and then integrating over the new variable, u. Note that Equation G-2 does not imply that the value of h is determined by the values of f and g at the same values of x. Rather, it indicates only that h, f, and g are functions of the same variable, e.g., time or distance.

Virtually all uses of convolution in nuclear medicine involve discrete, rather than continuous functions (e.g., a scan profile is a series of discrete numbers). Consider, two functions, each represented by a series of integers

$$f = a_1, a_2, a_3, \cdots a_m \qquad \text{(G-3)}$$

or

$$f(x) = a_x, x = 0,1,2, \cdots m \qquad \text{(G-4)}$$

and

$$g = b_1, b_2, b_3, \cdots b_n \qquad \text{(G-5)}$$

or

$$g(x) = b_x, x = 0,1,2, \cdots n \qquad \text{(G-6)}$$

The convolution of these two functions is given by:

$$h_i + 1 = \sum_{j=0}^{m} a_j b_{i-j} \qquad \text{(G-7)}$$

Where i and j range from 0 to n and m, respectively and $h_i + 1$ represents the numerical value of the convolution for a given value of i. Thus, the convolution of two discrete functions is a summation of the product of terms defined by equation G-7.

Among its properties, convolution is commutative (i.e., the order of operations can be reversed), distributive over addition, and associative, so that:

$$f(x) * g(x) = g(x) * f(x) \qquad \text{(G-8)}$$

$$f(x) * [g(x) + h(x)] = f(x) * g(x) + f(x) * h(x) \qquad \text{(G-9)}$$

$$f(x) * [g(x) * h(x)] = [f(x) * g(x)] * h(x) \qquad \text{(G-10)}$$

Analogous expressions exist for two-dimensional convolutions i.e., functions of two variables x and y rather than a single variable x. Two-dimensional convolutions frequently are used for image processing; however, the concept of convolution is most easily understood by considering a one-dimensional graphical example.

In Figure G-1A, the function $f(u)$ is plotted as a function of u. The convolving function, $g(u)$, is plotted in Figure G-2B. In Figure G-1C, $g(x - u)$ is reflected about the origin ($u = 0$), and in Figure G-2D it is shifted by a distance a, i.e., $x = a$ in Equation G-1. In Figure G-1E, the reflected and shifted function, $g(a - u)$, is superimposed on $f(u)$. From Equation G-1, the convolution, $h(x)$, at the value $x = a$, is the integral of the product of these two functions, which is shown in Figure G-1F. Whereas either f or g are zero, the product is zero. Therefore, the only values of $g(a - u)$ and $f(u)$ contributing to $h(a)$ are those where both functions are nonzero, the non-zero overlap of the two functions. Repeating this process (reflect and shift g, multiply by f, and integrate the product) for all values of x produces a complete set of values for $h(x)$. The convolving and stationary functions may be reversed in this process (Equation G-8).

Figure G-2 illustrates the convolution of two discrete functions $f(x) = [1,2,1]$ and $g(x) = [2,1]$. As in the example in Figure G-1, the convolving function $g(x)$ first is reflected, i.e., set equal to [1,2] and then shifted across the stationary function $f(x)$. The convolution $h(x)$ is the summation of the product of the values of these two functions. The resulting values for $h(x)$ are [2,5,4,1]. Note that the convolution $h(x)$ is non-zero over a wider range of values of x than either the stationary or convolving function. One of the effects of convolution is to create a new function that has a greater "spread" than the two original functions.

Figure G-3 illustrates the convolution of two Gaussian functions.

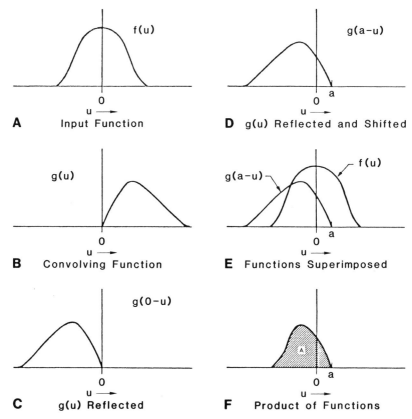

Fig. G-1. Illustration of the steps involved in determining the value of the convolution of two functions, $f(x)$ and $g(x)$, at $x = a$. (A) and (B): The variable x is replaced by u. (C): The convolving function is reflected about the origin, $u = 0$, (D) and then shifted a distance, $x = a$ to the right. (E): The overlapping functions are multiplied together. The area under the curve representing this product (F) is the value of the convolution at $x = a$. Reproduced, with permission, from Castleman KR, Digital Image Processing, Prentice Hall, 1979.

Gaussian functions are characterized by a mean value (μ) and variance (σ^2) and are of the form:

$$f(x) = (1/\sqrt{2\pi}\,\sigma)e^{-(x-\mu)^2/2\sigma^2} \qquad (G-11)$$

It can be shown that the convolution of two Gaussian functions with mean values μ_1 and μ_2 and variances σ_1^2 and σ_2^2 is another Gaussian function given by:

$$(1/\sqrt{2\pi}\,\sigma_3)\,e^{-(x-\mu_3)^2/2\sigma_3^2} \qquad (G-12)$$

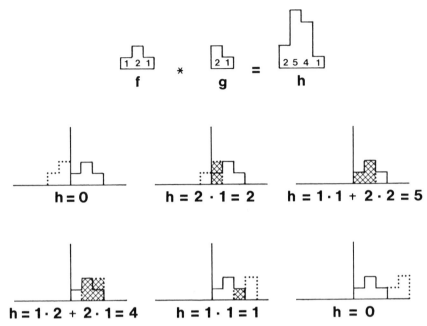

Fig. G-2. Convolution of two discrete functions, $f(x) = [1,2,1]$ and $g(x) = [2,1]$, is given by $h(x) = f(x) = [2,5,4,1]$. The convolving function, $g(x)$, is first reflected and shifted. Where this reflected and shifted function does not overlap with non-zero values of the stationary function ($x = 0$ and $x = 5$), $h(x) = 0$. Bottom two rows illustrate progressive, stepwise shifting of $g(x)$ across the stationary function, $f(x)$ to determine $h(x)$ for different values of x. In the regions of overlap, $h(x)$ is determined by summing the products of the two functions at each point of overlap.

where

$$\mu_3 = \mu_1 + \mu_2 \qquad \text{(G-13)}$$

and

$$\sigma_3^2 = \sigma_1^2 + \sigma_2^2 \qquad \text{(G-14)}$$

Therefore, the convolution of two Gaussian functions is another Gaussian with a mean value and variance equal to the sum of these values for the original two functions. This results in a function that is broader than the original functions, again demonstrating the "spreading" effect of convolution.

If two Gaussian functions f and g are characterized by full width half

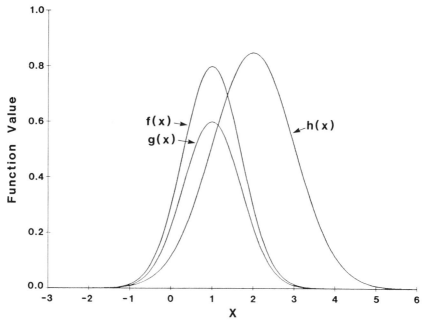

Fig. G-3.   The convolution of two Gaussian functions, $f(x)$ and $g(x)$, each having a mean value $\mu = 1.0$ and a variance $\sigma^2 = 0.5$, is a third Gaussian, $h(x)$, with $\mu = 2.0$ and $\sigma^2 = 1.0$.

maximum $FWHM(f)$ and $FWHM(g)$, then the full width half maximum of the convolution h of these two functions, $FWHM(h)$, is given by:

$$FWHM(h) = [FWHM(f)^2 + FWHM(g)^2]^{1/2} \qquad \text{(G-15)}$$

The process of convolution describes the effect of combining the spatial resolutions of two components in an imaging system. For example, if a scintillation camera has an intrinsic resolution of 4 mm $FWHM$, and a collimator resolution of 10 mm $FWHM$, and both are of Gaussian shape, then the convolution of these two functions would be a Gaussian function with a $FWHM$ of $(10^2 + 4^2)^{1/2} = 10.8$ mm. This would be the system resolution the detector/collimator combination (Chapter 16, Section B.3). Note also that the combined effect of the detector and collimator are not additive (i.e., $10 + 4 = 14$ mm).

An important property of convolution is given by the *convolution theorem*. If the Fourier transforms (Chapter 18, Section A.2) of two functions $f(x)$ and $g(x)$ are given by $F(v)$ and $G(v)$, where x is distance and v is spatial frequency, then:

$$\mathscr{F}\,[f(x) * g(x)] = F(v) \cdot G(v) \qquad \text{(G-16)}$$

and

$$\mathcal{F}^{-1}[F(v) \cdot G(v)] = f(x) * g(x) \qquad \text{(G-17)}$$

where $\mathcal{F}$ is the Fourier transform and $\mathcal{F}^{-1}$ is the inverse Fourier transform (see Equation 19-2). Therefore, convolution in the spatial domain corresponds to multiplication in the frequency domain. This is the basis for the property that the modulation transfer function (MTF) of a system is equal to the product of MTF's of the individual system components (Chapter 18, Section A.2). System resolution is described by the convolution of line- or point-spread functions in the spatial domain or, equivalently, by the product of their Fourier transforms in the frequency domain.

Index